Computers in Health Care

Kathryn J. Hannah   Marion J. Ball
Series Editors

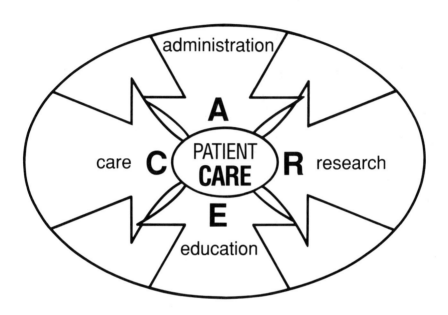

Computers in Health Care

Series Editors:
Kathryn J. Hannah   Marion J. Ball

Nursing Informatics
Where Caring and Technology Meet
M.J. Ball, K.J. Hannah, U. Gerdin, and H. Peterson (Eds.)

Healthcare Information Management Systems
A Practical Guide
M.J. Ball, J.V. Douglas, R.I. O'Desky, and J.W. Albright (Eds.)

Knowledge Coupling
New Premises and New Tools for Medical Care and Education
Lawrence L. Weed

Dental Informatics
Integrating Technology into the Dental Environment
Louis M. Abbey and John L. Zimmerman (Eds.)

Forthcoming Volume

Aspects of the Computer-Based Patient Record
Marion Ball and Morris Collen (Eds.)

Louis M. Abbey   John L. Zimmerman
Editors

Dental Informatics

Integrating Technology into the Dental Environment

With 63 Illustrations

Springer-Verlag
New York Berlin Heidelberg London Paris
Tokyo Hong Kong Barcelona Budapest

Louis M. Abbey, D.M.D., M.S.
Professor of Oral Pathology
School of Dentistry
Medical College of Virginia
Virginia Commonwealth University
Box 566 MCV Station
Richmond, VA 23298, USA

John L. Zimmerman, D.D.S.
Director
Academic Computing and Health Informatics
University of Maryland at Baltimore
610 West Lombard St.
Baltimore, MD 21201, USA

Cover Illustration: This is a crown restoration automatically generated from digitized data of the prepared tooth plus adjacent and occluding teeth. The crown is designed by an expert system, using an ideal morphology that is modified to fit the unique space and occlusion of each patient. Photo courtesy of DentiCAD, Inc. and the University of Maryland at Baltimore.

Library of Congress Cataloging-in-Publication Data
Dental informatics : integrating technology into the dental
    environment / [edited by] Louis M. Abbey, John Zimmerman.
        p.   cm.   (Computers in health care)
    includes bibliographical references and index.
    ISBN 0-387-97643-4. ISBN 3-540-97643-4
    1. Dentistry"Data processing. 2. Medical informatics.
I. Abbey, Louis M. II. Zimmerman, John L. III. Series: Computers
in health care (New York, N.Y.)
    [DNLM: 1. Dentistry. 2. Medical Informatics Applications. WU
26.5 D4135]
RK240.D45 1991
617.6'00285"dc20
DNLM/DLC   91-4931

Printed on acid-free paper.

Production managed by Christin R. Ciresi; Manufacturing supervised by Jacqui Ashri.
Typeset by Keefe and Associates, New York, NY.
Printed and bound by Edwards Brothers, Inc., Ann Arbor, MI.
Printed in the United States of America.

9 8 7 6 5 4 3 2 1

ISBN 0-387-97643-4 Springer-Verlag New York Berlin Heidelberg
ISBN 3-540-97643-4 Springer-Verlag Berlin Heidelberg New York

We dedicate this book,
with deep gratitude and affection, to our mentors,
Dr. Marion J. Ball and Dr. John J. Salley.

Acknowledgements

We are very grateful to a large number of people who were instrumental in bringing about this project. Our co-authors deserve a large thank you for their persistence, understanding and hard work in preparing what we consider to be a superior set of chapters. We wish to thank our department chairs, Dr. James C. Burns (L.M.A.) and Dr. James Craig (J.L.Z.) for understanding how much time it takes to put a work like this together. To our secretaries and all the secretaries, office personnel and artists who contributed to our chapters and those of our co-authors, we are extremely grateful. The editors at Springer-Verlag have been very understanding and helpful in instituting changes and adding chapters. Thank you very much. We will be eternally grateful to our mentors, Drs. Marion J. Ball and John J. Salley to whom we dedicate this book and without whom there would be no book. And finally, though certainly not least, we thank our families for their understanding and encouragement through our periods of anxiety with late nights and long days of writing and editing, when we could not be as present with them as we would have liked. To you all, thank you very much.

Contents

Section 3   Planning for the Future

Introduction

Recently, a bright, third year student knocked at my (L.M.A.) open, office door and asked if I knew the whereabouts of a fellow faculty member. I said the colleague had gone to lunch, but could I be of some help.

Well, the student said, perhaps I could ask you.

She showed me a good quality, panoramic radiograph and pointed to a radiolucency between the mandibular left first and second molars. The lesion was uniformly radiolucent, well-circumscribed and extended up into the alveolar bone between the two teeth and further into the interradicular bone between the roots of the first molar.

Is this a traumatic bone cyst? asked the student somewhat tentatively.

Well I don't know, I replied. Tell me, what makes you think it's a traumatic bone cyst?

Because it goes up between the roots, came the answer.

Is that all that tells you this is a traumatic bone cyst; just that it goes up between the roots? I asked, feeling my face beginning to flush. Can you tell me, what is a traumatic bone cyst? I continued, trying to think up openings I could give the student.

It's a radiolucency and goes up between the roots.

Is that all? I probed again. O.K. Step back for a moment, look at the radiograph and perhaps you can tell me what is going on in that area, in a pathophysiologic sense. I pointed to the radiolucency and felt myself gaining control of my initial emotional response.

You mean basic science? The student's voice began to fill with incredulity. I'm sorry, but I haven't reviewed that since first year, if you mean anatomy and physiology. Nobody ever asks us those questions in the clinic.

I reigned in my desire to explode and continued a bit further. But you passed those courses, did you not?

Yes I did, came the confident reply, bearing more than a hint of relief that the ordeal was in the past. Made Dean's list both first and second years.

Then the credentials with which you reported to the clinic say you should be able to answer my question. Tell me, I pursued, be perfectly honest, when you were confronted with this clinical problem, where you did not know what you were looking at, didn't your basic intellectual honesty tell you at least to look up the entity in a dictionary, or even possibly in a pathology book before you consulted with a faculty member?

Then came the incredible reply: I was unaware that I didn't know what I was looking at. I thought it was a traumatic bone cyst and all the instructor would do was confirm my suspicion.

How, then, did you know it was a traumatic bone cyst? I probed further.

I remembered it from Oral Pathology.

Then the predictable happened. The student paused, drawing a long breath, and said: I am so embarrassed, I feel so stupid.

No, I said, We, your teachers, should be embarrassed. You are the product of our educational system. You have succeeded, met our criteria, earned your credentials. All you have done is prove that a system based on memorized facts and testing on what you know is doomed to failure.

The point of failure in the system, as this example illustrates, is that if we require our students to use knowledge to help them care for people with dental problems, we need to give them the tools with which to make optimal use that knowledge, accurately and efficiently, to solve those problems. Further, if our aim is to provide the best possible care for our patients, then we should examine students on how well they use that knowledge in the care of patients. Thus we would increase the public's confidence in dentists and dentists' confidence in themselves.

This book is about knowledge. Knowledge is accumulated bits of information (facts) enhanced and made useful by understanding and arrangement in such a way that this information can be put to work.

We are fast approaching a time when dentists will need some memory aid to accumulate and process facts into knowledge to the degree necessary to provide exemplary patient care. This is not a recent or abrupt change. The increased incidence of malpractice litigation, creeping increases in liability insurance premiums and proliferation of dental specialities are all symptoms of this knowledge deficit. As the size of the knowledge base increases, those who use it need to specialize in progressively smaller portions of that knowledge base in order to feel in control of the problems with which they deal.

We now have a plethora of tools that can take over some of the fact accumulation, storage and arrangement functions. This leaves to dentists the task of putting knowledge to work, a function that humans always will do better than machines. Modern computers and other information management technologies will be at the heart of health care education, practice, research and administration paradigms for the foreseeable future.

In order to prepare for and participate productively in this evolution, the dental profession must begin to lay the groundwork and grease the skids for these changing paradigms. The change will be from a linear, hierarchical knowledge management paradigm to an integrated, three dimensional knowledge network based in electronic technology. What follows in this book are detailed discussions of a number of basic changes that will, to one degree or another, be critical in the transition.

We have attempted to deliver an even mix of conceptual changes and practical outcomes that have begun to emanate from some quarters where the paradigms have already begun to shift. It is our hope that readers will find this book useful in both helping decide what has to change in basic attitudes and philosophy as well as what can be put in place to fill some of the freshly opened ground created by philosophical and attitudinal change. We want this book to be a how to as well as a what's up resource.

One of the definitions associated with Advent is a coming or an arrival. We are privileged to bring you this volume in hopes that it represents an arrival of a new age upon the dental profession, the age of informatics.

L.M.A. and J.L.Z.

Section 1
Dental Informatics

1
Mastering Change

Louis M. Abbey

"The postindustrial society will be fueled not by oil but by a new commodity called artificial intelligence (AI). ...the knowledge imbedded in AI software and hardware architectures will become even more salient as a foundation of wealth than the raw materials that fueled the first Industrial Revolution. ...it has no material form. It can be a flow of information with no more physical reality than electrical vibrations in a wire."

Raymond Kurzweil

Virtually everything we do in dentistry that involves research, teaching, administration or patient care is based on generation, storage and manipulation of information (information management). The current paradigm for managing information in dentistry, as in most health care, is human memory backed by printed or written information stored in books or journals. We distribute and communicate information via printed or verbal channels.

There are numerous interfaces where technology has been added to this system to provide peripheral support and increased efficiency. Examples include various electronic storage media and film, electronic voice communication systems (telephones), electronic typewriters and word processors. In some sectors of society, computers have become the dominant mode for information storage, and in a more limited way, for information management and utilization. This trend has only begun to impact the dental profession.

Each one of the 140,000 practicing dentists in the United States makes an average of ten diagnostic and/or treatment decisions every day. These 1.4 million decisions are made using only human memory and an incomplete base of knowledge. Dentists gather and process information, make decisions about therapy and, through follow-up care, evaluate those decisions. Using the most up-to-date information, dentists educate patients, staff, colleagues and (as life-long learners) themselves. Consultations with colleagues are carried out by written or spoken communication from one site to another. This transfer must be accurate and rapid. Successful patient management requires that the dentist be a compassionate enabler, carefully guiding those who seek care through a complex maze of decisions about treatment, follow-up and prevention. A dental practice is both a care setting for people with health problems and a small business. Often dentists must choose what will benefit the patient over the business. This choice is frequently difficult and not clearly defined. To assure optimal, enduring patient care, dentists are skillful in technique and procedures. This requires vigorous pursuit of new techniques and materials. If a dentist is to contribute to the advancement of the profession and practice scientifically, a certain amount of research is necessary. All of these activities that weave together to form the dentist's practice involve information manipulation, and that information must be stored in such a way as to facilitate easy access. Paper records take up vast amounts of space, their access is cumbersome and there is growing concern for the impact on the forests from which the paper is made. Everything the dentist does requires access to several knowledge bases, data collection, recall at the time of action, and creative combining, reordering and integrating information from many sources. Dentists must do all this relying on memory, backed up only by written text. This system is taxed to the limit and hardly adequate for a growing profession looking toward the next century. Gathering, manipulating, communicating and storing information, inquiring, combining and synthesizing all should be done with the most up-to-date tools available. From now and into the foreseeable future, these tools are computers.

Change from a memory-based, paper-oriented paradigm to one grounded in technology will involve integration. Technology, being the "new kid on the block" will have to integrate into the environment of the establishment. We now have many technological capabilities but no environment that is hospitable for integrating a large variety of computer-based support tools. In dental education the classrooms and labs must be entirely refitted and rewired. Computers in the clinics are placed awkwardly in a corner, "out of the way." It is quite obvious that if computers are to be a cornerstone of function, they need to be within easy access where they will be highly useful. In private practices, there is never enough wiring or counter space. Most of the machines are too big to fit easily into the small amount of extra space in the office. We will know when integration is successful because computers will be as central to the office function as x-ray machines and far less noticeable.

Successful integration of electronic technology into dental health care practice, education and research will depend on several very important developments:

1) standards for communication, storage and processing information

2) effortless, accurate natural language communication

3) natural, familiar and invisible human-computer interfaces

4) large, accessible, centrally maintained databases

5) a fully supportive infrastructure within dental education that prepares people to practice within the new paradigms of electronic information management.

Let us now look at each one of these individually.

Standards Development

Development of standards in all aspects of computing is the foundation on which the rest of computer integration is built. It is arguable that natural, transparent interfaces are of equal importance; however, it seems that to encourage broad-based utilization and to provide a basis upon which to develop interfaces, standards must come first. Anyone who has contemplated purchasing a home computer has confronted the problem. Do you buy an Apple or an IBM? Is the clone 100% compatible or only 90%? Can I use this board in another type of computer? These are not new problems but have suddenly been brought home to the average user since the explosion in the micro-computer market. Everyone would like to use all the software on their one machine and have that machine be the lowest priced one as well. Standards need to be developed in hardware and software. A *de facto* standard was introduced when IBM adopted MS-DOS (a disk operating system written by Microsoft Corporation). This happened because IBM was the largest supplier of micro-computers in the industry and where they went, so went the industry. Now, however, with clones claiming an increasing percentage of the market, and with institutional computing operating on limited budgets, a new look must be taken at hardware compatibility standards. Hardware and software are not the only areas where standards should be adopted. Some would say that in the health care field, it is much more important to develop standard data elements and terminology. The problems posed by introduction of standards loom large and this is a simplified example, however, incompatibility in software and hardware has made the problem very real for the less-computer-sophisticated among us.

Standard means of communicating data over existing channels must be addressed. Whether data is sent by telephone line or satellite, what is sent out must arrive in flawless condition, and be available to multiple users. Standards relating to speed, packaging and routing of information must be developed in order for data to be transferred efficiently.

Storage and use of information also must be subjected to standards if computer technology is to achieve full effectiveness in dentistry. Standards must address what information is stored, how, and in what form it will be accessed. Who has access to what data (data security) is also critical. The first five chapters in this book will deal with aspects of standards and their impact on integrating aspects of information technology into the fiber of dental practice.

Effortless, Accurate Communication

Users must enter data into a computer in order for the machine to perform its functions. Today we transfer data in numerous ways including mouse, joy stick, keyboard, scanner and video camera among others. None of these data input methods is acceptable under all circumstances. All require some skill and familiarization. Most are limited to transmitting one kind of data better than others. Some work better with text and others are more suitable for graphics. For as long as dentistry has been around, dentists have been entering data into their records, mostly in the form of handwritten text, in their natural language. We use natural language without thinking and it allows the greatest flexibility and the largest number of options. Our skill in natural language transmission of data is perfected from childhood. Computer engineers are working to develop a smooth, accurate natural language means of entering patient data. This technology will be universally acceptable and will encourage the largest number of users.

Invisible Human-Computer Interfaces

Perhaps the best way to interact with a computer is not to realize you are interacting with one. This has been the objective in many commercial and industrial applications. We rarely are aware of the computer that is a vital part of directing and monitoring our fuel consumption, exhaust emissions, timing and carburetor control in most new automobiles; that is, until the computer fails, and our car will not run. Usually it is only at that time we realize how vital the computer is. We find we have been communicating very naturally, by starting the engine, pressing on the accelerator and using the normal controls with which we are familiar. Using the most widely used communications device of the 20th Century, the telephone, we are communicating almost entirely through a computer, yet few people are aware of this as they make their daily calls. McDonalds' Restaurant uses a very sophisticated, computer-linked ordering and inventory control system. All the communication is accomplished by very natural, cash register-like entries carried out by the clerk when you place your order.

Utilizing natural activities and long-familiar tasks, computer engineers have made modern human-computer interfaces effortless if not invisible. In dentistry we will see similar interface developments oriented around the standard data forms we use with patients, perhaps linked to some of the instruments we use every day. Already there are periodontal probes that read pocket depths directly into a computer, which in turn generates a graphic representation of the examination. There are instruments that can analyze occlusion using pressure sensitive media which interface directly with a computer. It is only a step to interface these readings with an expert system or artificial intellegence software that gathers all the data from the entire examination and renders a differential diagnosis and suggested treatment plan fully documented and up-to-date. Development of these interfaces is underway and available today on a small, experimental scale. This process should continue and eventually lead to full integration into practice.

Accessible Central Databases

With improved communications and invisible interfaces, there is no reason to saddle each user with the task of designing, maintaining and updating a separate database other than what might be absolutely necessary for local personal use. There are a number of databases that will be useful to dental practice in the age of

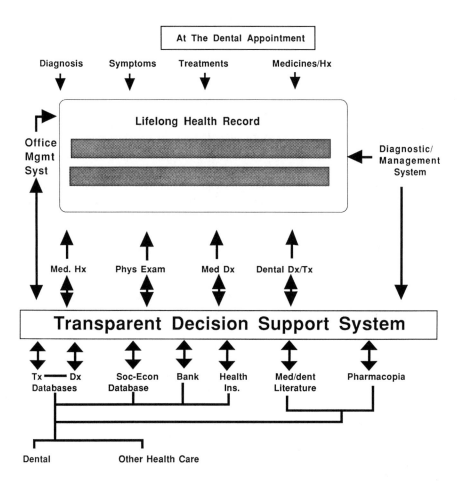

Figure 1.1. A diagram representing many elements that contribute to a patient health record and how, through a decision support system they can be related to shared databases through electronic bridges. Copyright 1991 American Association of Dental Schools, Office of Publications. Reprinted with permission from the *Journal of Dental Education*, April 1991.

information technology. It will not be long before a patient will possess a lifetime health record, of which the dental record will be a part. They will carry this record with them on some compact storage medium, perhaps no bigger than a credit card. In order to keep this record up-to-date, each health care station the patient visits will not only need to be equipped to enter all new data, but also access a number of national databases to keep the flow of information current and continuous. Figure 1.1 is a schematic representation of the pattern of information that may flow to and from this hub of the electronic, lifelong health record. Toward the bottom third of the diagram, some of the national databases are given that will be available in the future and that will make continuity possible in this web of health information. All of this information will be processed by invisible decision support systems through friendly, natural user interfaces.

Dental Education Infrastructure

Another critical hub will be the supportive infrastructure that must be built into dental education to accommodate and prepare students to practice in the information-intensive environment of the next century. In addition to the need to be technically skilled (which has always been necessary), the dentist of the future will need to be an expert in a number of arenas. For example, the Twenty-First Century dentist will need to be an expert at problem solving, identification and utilization of resources, interpersonal relations, counseling and decision making. The need to remember all the information necessary to practice will decline and be replaced by the need to access information and decision support systems through friendly, transparent computer systems. Dentists will need to be able to solve complex patient problems employing more data than is currently available. The choices will be more numerous and the dentist will have to guide patients through a very complex maze of information. So many resources will be at the dentist's disposal that it may be necessary to limit and choose carefully between resources according to the demands of the problem.

One of the major ways electronic technology will impact on dental education will be through integrating teaching, research, and patient care. Traditionally, teaching has taken place in the didactic mode through illustrated classroom lectures or small group activities. Clinical teaching is introduced in the pre-clinical laboratory with development of the instructor supervisor-demonstrator model. This is transported to the clinic by replacing the typodont with a live patient. The computer will change all that. Many laboratory exercises will be presented as computer simulations using three dimensional modeling. Automation of laboratory procedures will make it unnecessary for students to learn what will be completely automated in their clinical experience. Fully integrating patient care with research will be accomplished by developing automated patient treatment record systems that are linked to large, easily accessed smart databases. All treatments will be tracked, as will patient progress. The easy access to databases will allow cumulative records on all aspects of patient care, thus contributing to a fuller understanding of dental diseases, their epidemiology, treatment, and effectiveness of those treatments over the long term. With a few exceptions such as the National Library of Medicine's (NLM) Medline and Toxline, there are currently no easily accessible, large databases serving the general practicing dentist. This ubiquitous accumulation of usable patient care data will include insurance statistics and data from private practice and university data pools. This information reservoir will be stored and maintained by university-based dental schools and maintained by the institutional computer network. The major purpose will be to serve the local practicing community and augment national databanks. Figure 1.2 is a schematic representation of this relationship.

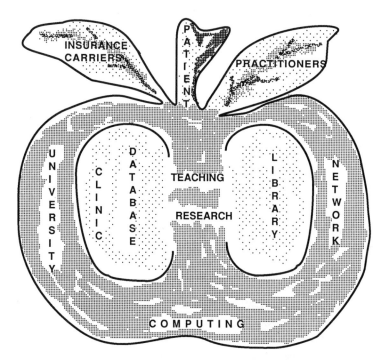

Figure 1.2. Schematic representation of the relationship between the four major components of dental health care: teaching, research, clinical practice and patients. There should be a continuous flow of information from one component to all the others through a conveniently accessed electronic network.

Not only is educational structure and the relationship between the school of dentistry and the practicing and researching communities going to change with the influx of modern information management tools, but the face of dental education itself will change. The single biggest failure in today's dental education is the way we teach. Curricula are still dependent on facts. Teachers are given factual topics on which to prepare lectures that consist of piles of facts expressed rapid-fire to bored passive students who sit in hot lecture halls in groups of one hundred or more. The knowledge base with which students must work is still fragmented into individual basic sciences, dental specialties and pre-clinical and clinical years. Examinations are administered in such a way that the students who succeed are those who have memorized most successfully and can choose between four or five alternatives on single answer, fact based, multiple choice examinations. What is worse, is that those who try to introduce any alternative learning strategies are either ignored or pressured by students and administrators to revert to the old ways because the new strategies are irrelevant to the methods of testing and of giving credentials.

If we can accept that the computer is with us to stay, then new paradigms associated with a technology-based education system will evolve. This list is not exhaustive. It is an interesting exercise to read the list and think of whether the paradigm is part of the dental education environment today.

Some Educational Paradigms that Will Emerge from an Informatics-Based Environment

- Students bear primary responsibility for their education
- Teachers can learn from students
- Students are colleagues
- Students will participate actively in their education
- Solving problems through consultation is standard procedure
- There may be more than one right answer to a problem
- Finding the answer with the help of a computer is standard procedure
- Teachers are resource managers and consultants and may not be the best resources
- The accumulation of facts is not knowledge
- Learning and play are not mutually exclusive
- Real play is not always easy
- Testing will emphasize how students use knowledge, information management tools and resources to solve real problems
- Computers are tools not human substitutes

The basic themes of the new educational paradigms will be sharing, cooperation, participation and building linkages. These are not necessarily meaningless in a technology-deficient education environment, but they have evolved to prominence as a result of computer-related technologies being used more frequently. Cooperative participants who consult, use resources and the most modern information-management tools will naturally emerge from a system based on integrated technologies.

Creative and courageous use of information technology in education will open the door for changes in the status quo. There are already movements in the early stages that aim to change the way dentists are tested and credentialed on an institutional and national basis. These changes will move dental schools to respond (a case of the tail wagging the dog) by altering the strategies and methods of dental education. The database that dentists must use in daily responsible practice is doubling every five years and some would say the speed will increase to every three years. Old knowledge is becoming obsolete. If the dentist's intellectual database remains primarily accumulated in texts, journals and clinical records and if it must be manipulated and stored for immediate use only in the human memory, then we are fast approaching the point where the information deficit may threaten responsible practice. If we believe that the dentist must be able to draw upon this knowledge base in patient care and that the time we need the knowledge is the time of application (i.e. when the patient is sitting in our chair) then we will soon be forced to employ modern knowledge management tools to store, manipulate, and make available the information we need to treat our patients.

An American Dental Association/American Heart Association poll[2] revealed that 71% of the dentists surveyed were not fully aware of the recommended penicillin regimen for prevention of secondary bacterial endocarditis in patients with rheumatic heart damage. The survey also revealed that approximately 1/3 of dentists interviewed did not know that patients with a history of congenital heart disease are at risk for bacterial endocarditis resulting from dental procedures. We can no longer expect human memory to function as the sole information manager for the entire database needed in clinical decision making. A computerized decision support system integrated with a problem-oriented record will give dentists the opportunity to overcome this inadequacy.

"The safest thing for a patient," Charles Mayo once said, "is to be in the hands of a man engaged in teaching medicine. In order to be a teacher of medicine the doctor must always be a student."[3] In the broadest sense, is this still the safest thing for a patient, and are we turning out dentists from our schools in whose hands patients are going to be safe? And further, are our graduates continuous students, and are we showing our students, by example, how to learn and keep learning for their entire lifetimes?

"Doctor" derives from the Latin word *docere* which means to teach. Not only are we charged with patient care, but we must teach as well, our patients, our communities, our colleagues and ourselves. If we are teaching and learning, then we must be open to examining the paradigms by which we carry out those activities, continuously asking how do we teach and how do we learn? These ongoing questions guarantee change to be a constant companion, thus binding us to the art of mastering change.

Dental practice in the 21st Century will be conducted using a fully integrated information management system based in the most current computer technology. This system will be a sophisticated merger of business applications and patient record keeping. An additional element and key to its smooth functioning will be a nearly invisible decision support system that will function a level below where the user and the computer interact.

A new patient in a dental practice will use a computer station in the reception area to enter all demographic data, medical and dental history and drug information by simply talking into a microphone, thereby creating or augmenting their permanent electronic health record. After this initial entry, only new information will be entered. The transparent decision support system will see to it that new data (entered only one time) goes to every place it is needed. On a yearly basis, possibly keyed to a clock, the patient's age will be updated. With a change in age or new medication entry, or if the patient is treated for a new disease or condition, the expert system will integrate the new data with all information in the patient's file and with all relevant disease and management databases. In updating the patient's health status, the computer will recognize diseases, conditions, medications and potential areas of drug interaction or disease history about which the dentist will need further information. The computer will offer to search the National Library of Medicine on-line databases for the most current articles on the topic. An updated report with references on the patient's health status will then be available for the dentist or other health professionals.

Such systems could function as teaching tools in dental schools. Students who learn using these information management systems would naturally use them in practice. Computerized decision support systems coupled with patient simulations create a natural vehicle for continuing professional education. Dentists and auxiliaries will enjoy continuing education programs in the familiar surroundings of the office, thus saving time and expense. This will also offer the opportunity to relate this education more directly to their personal experience. This form of continuing education will be equally as interactive and participatory as that which is attended in person.

Business management will take up less clerical time and more computer function in the dental practice of the next century. Correct billing information will be generated once standard terminology and procedure codes are adopted. Simply updating the treatment record will initiate payment to the dentist and debit the patient. This information will be transferred electronically directly to the insurance company. Coming decades will see more and more dental care paid for by sources other than the patient. Some practices already bill more than 80% of their accounts to third parties. In the case where patients pay their own bills, the dentist's computer will automatically transfer funds from the patient's bank account to the dentist's account, eliminating the need for checks, charge cards or direct billing. Electronic information transfer will be bi-directional, with the dentist's records updated when new information is entered into the patient's insurance records. Guided by invisibly-functioning expert systems, changes in patient data such as disease states, disabilities and classifications will flow freely from the central record storage facility to the patient chart, wherever that record may be. This will free office personnel from the tedious tasks of billing and filing claims.

One and one half million dentists world-wide, many practicing far from current sources of information, will benefit greatly from access to up-to-date knowledge bases to aid in daily decision making. With language translation and relatively minor modifications, these decision support systems and databases can be adapted to different styles of practice in other countries and cultures.

No one patient presents the dentist with an isolated problem. Dental practice is characterized by patients with multiple problems, some chronic, some acute, some within the therapeutic realm of the dentist and some not. Very few of these problems exist totally uninfluenced by the others. Regardless of their state upon presentation, every patient has the right to expect that their dentist is capable of bringing the most current knowledge to bear on any problem. Dentists and educators would do well to look at a study of the quality of American dental practice conducted by Morris and Bohannon in 1987.[4] They meticulously surveyed 300 United States dental practices representing all specialties, geographic and demographic areas and levels of income. They found, among other things, that 83%

of the records made provision for recording periodontal status, yet only 18% actually recorded the information. Sixty-one percent of the records provided space for occlusal analysis but only 7% contained record entries in this category. Only 53% of the records allowed for recording a treatment plan but only 24% actually recorded such a plan. In contrast, however, they found that nearly all of the records sampled from graduates since 1974 accurately recorded treatments and fees. Their study concluded: "...a wide gap exists between the way faculty believe dentistry should be practiced and the way it is practiced." Perhaps the underlying reason for this can be found in a dental curriculum preoccupied with providing answers and too little concerned with problem analysis.

No one would claim that dental practice is a simple-minded application of techniques or rote procedures to static, predictable deficiencies in tooth number and structure. But a look at dental curricula reveals that six times as many hours are devoted to technique laboratories in the first two years than is spent on behavioral science, patient management, special patient care and practice administration in the entire curriculum. Most would agree that the practice of dentistry is characterized by a careful integration of data gathering and interpretation for problem identification, problem sequencing and treatment. Most will go on to say that the responsible practitioner should have a built-in mechanism to evaluate the results of treatment and to continue education after leaving academia. No one would argue that a dentist does not have to be a very skilled operator to practice, but the Morris and Bohannon study and the dental school curriculum seem to indicate a minimal emphasis on diagnostics and a maximum emphasis on therapeutics (treatments). We are at a point in dental education where what we seem to be doing does not support what we should be doing.

Dentistry has a history of using technology to supplement human inadequacies as exemplified by the professions' dependence on radiography for diagnosis. We have known for years that human eyes were not adequate to spot early carious lesions. So we adopted radiography as a diagnostic tool and the relationship has been a productive one ever since. We now have another tool that will help us serve our patients more responsibly and efficiently. The computer is the perfect tool to help us solve our present and future expanding information management and integration problems.

The trend setters in current American Society have certainly indicated that the 21st Century U.S. Citizen will be the wealthiest, slimmest, most stylish, happiest, best smelling, most educated and most sought-after person our world has ever seen. These kinds of trends are precisely that, drifts and tendencies, subject to the whim and fancy of those (whomever they may be) who decide what will come into fashion next. These decisions are usually geared to what will be best for business. The age of information and communication, however, seems to have slipped from the realm of trend into a firmly established reality. During World War II, the United States began developing computers for military purposes. From these initial trials the general-purpose computer arrived in the marketplace in the early 1950s. Since this time, every advance having to do with information gathering, storage, processing and communication has involved computers. Information gathering has become easier, faster and more "friendly"; information storage devices have become infinitely smaller but have steadily increased in capacity, with faster access time and efficiency. Information processing has become magnitudes faster with no end in sight. The physical size of computers has decreased while capabilities have increased and data communication speed has begun to approach the speed of light with the introduction of fiber-optics. Increasing also is the range and distribution of communications. So it seems safe to say that henceforth, in one form or another, the computer will always be with us.

Health care, and dentistry in particular, stands to benefit enormously from this fact. Becoming a dentist, or any other health care professional, from this time forward promises to be an immense journey pregnant with challenge and opportunity. Computers are ready to serve us in every phase of dental research, education and practice. In many cases, computers are already playing a part in discovery of new knowledge, teaching that knowledge and putting that knowledge to work for the best interests of patients. This book will examine a number of the ways in which computers can serve and expand the horizons of the dental profession and the patients it serves.

Patients and their dental problems are the foundation upon which the existence of the dental profession depends. Without patients, there would be no need for dental schools, no practice of dentistry and no dentally-related research. So if we assume patients with dental problems, and resolve to provide the best care possible in cooperation with those patients, we must then look to the dental educational institutions as the fertile soil that nourishes and fuels the dental profession.

Preparing to Effect Change

Asked to comment on the preparedness of dental education for the 21st Century, Dr. Enid Neidel, Assistant Executive Director for Scientific Affairs of the American Dental Association, presented a vision of the future of dentistry as requiring four things from dental education:

1) Respect for science and research

2) A commitment to lifelong continuing education

3) An environment/curriculum that leads to a highly developed ethic that will welcome quality assurance and peer review

4) Superior dental students.[5]

These four expectations cut across all levels of the dental profession, and bear substantial implication for dental informatics.

First, what is *dental informatics*? To look for a formal source that provides a definition for *dental informatics* is fruitless; there is no such formally agreed-upon meaning. We must look to the field of Health Informatics and apply the obvious general principles surrounding the definition of informatics, adding specific qualifications for dentistry. It is useful to refer to Morris Collen, a pioneer in the field of informatics.[6] Collen defines *health informatics* as a new domain of knowledge combining computer and information sciences, engineering and technology in every field of health and medicine to include research, education and practice. If we go on to add that this definition can be applied to problem-solving and decision-making in dentistry, then we have *dental informatics*.

Obviously, Neidel's vision for the future of dentistry[4] includes investigation and research, a vision of an expanding basis for the care and treatment of patients. She also sees delivery of health care, specifically dental health care, and further involvement of third parties in this delivery as important. Another feature of her vision involves the profession's increasing involvement in ethical issues such as care of the aged with their multiplicity of problems, insuring quality of care and sharing review of records with peers. To carry out this vision, Dr. Neidel sees the need for a continuous supply of top quality, well-motivated younger generations who eagerly look forward to future challenges. There are several basic issues that will impact on the vision as a whole.

Sharing, Cooperation, and Connectivity

Sharing is an attitude that encompasses cooperative behavior and is enhanced by connectivity. This chain linkage is at the core of computer use, and is an essential paradigm for dental informatics. Dentistry is emerging from the shroud of the cottage industry shepherded by the "solo" practitioner with a covey of patients, tended with care and compassion over numerous years of service. This individual practitioner has been rewarded by loyalty and respect from patients, status in the community and prompt payment of most of the bills in cash. In retirement, this cottage industrialist reluctantly sold the practice to another person of like persuasion (often a junior partner taken on during the final years). The buyer always paid two fees for the practice, one for the land, building equipment and other tangible property and another fee for the "good will" and the patient pool generated over time. Sharing, cooperation and connectivity between professionals were not dominant characteristics of this model. In fact, dental practice of this ilk is still widely evident today. The relationships are linear, hierarchical and geared to self-preservation and isolation.

It is important to visualize this model because it then becomes easier to understand the changes that are being presented by computerization of dental practice and the difficulty that will be encountered in effecting those changes. The computer has changed modern society all around this solo practitioner and the dentist has not been oblivious to that change. In fact, independence-minded practicing dentists have been rapping the centralized government regulation or "publicization" of society and health care for years in the dental literature. Articles and letters on this theme are still fairly commonplace in the trade publications. Concepts of peer review and quality assurance have fired stiff resistance in the grass roots of dentistry, and dental insurance has only recently achieved unenthusiastic, begrudging acceptance among a large part of the practicing community.

The major reason for this acceptance, however, was more related to fee collection and economics than an endorsement of the third party payment concept. The sharing-cooperative-connected paradigm carries what many regard as a singular threat, relinquishing control. This runs somewhat counter to thousands of dentists who still, upon entering dental school, list independence and "being my own boss" high among their reasons for choosing dentistry as a profession. Computers will not force any dentist to relinquish their independence.

With wide-spread computerization and networking will come central databases, sharing information on patients and records and more opportunity for those outside the profession to gain access to a dentist's practice. Patients will store their own health records and will be better educated about their problems. Thus they will seek a larger say in what the dentists propose as treatment. This relatively mild concern will fuel more extreme views on ownership of records, data and the ability to sell a patient pool to an associate when there is a shared aspect to the data. Issues will arise that computerization of dental practice is just another means for government, insurance companies or both to regulate people's lives. "Big Brother" is a concept that is still alive and well in this society and particularly so among health care practitioners.

The point of this discussion is to say that with all the advantages electronic technology brings, mastering change to technologically-based practice will require a direct, sympathetic and humane confrontation of these issues. Some means must be devised, in anticipation of roadblocks, to construct detours in order to create the smoothest integration possible with an eye toward enlisting the highest level of cooperation. Fear, prejudice and suspicion will not evolve out of the society before the need to change the dental practice, and any plan to introduce the tools of electronic technology will necessitate acknowledgement that perhaps these emotional issues will present more of a barrier than technology and economics. Sharing, openness to cooperation and connectivity are attitudes absolutely essential to the success of integrating computer technology into dental education, practice and research.

Openness to Change and Taking Risks

It is not often that people get the opportunity in life to participate actively in something that is truly new, to break new ground. Involvement with integrating information management technology into dentistry is one of those rare occasions. The computer with its empowering capabilities offers us an unprecedented chance to change information gathering, storing and utilization. Billing, accounting and office management can be made simpler and more efficient, and patient records can be more comprehensive and informative.

The computer offers us a world of opportunity in undergraduate, graduate, and continuing dental education. No precedent has been set, and the possibilities are unlimited. The power of programming languages challenges us to analyze carefully what we are trying to do in an educational endeavor, to create a way to do it unhindered by the linearity of paper and pencil, and to evaluate its results. In the next century a great deal of emphasis will be placed on educational research, and the computer will be at its core.

No change is possible, however, without an attitude of openness, a posture that welcomes change and a willingness to take risk. Of course, where precedents are few or lacking altogether, there is always an increased possibility of failure. Those who are enamored of their power, their position or the security of doing the same thing over and over will have their foundations shaken. Probably it is not unreasonable to assume, if we choose our means carefully with an eye toward the whole picture, that more automation is better, even for dentistry. This requires a mindset that looks at all we do as an evolutionary process and seeks satisfaction in the feeling that things are always somewhat out of balance. This dynamic existence stimulates creativity. The computer is here to stay. It can be a pivotal tool to help us in continuing to offer patients the best care possible. To take advantage of this tool, we must change the way we do what we do. The challenge is how to master that change as smoothly as possible. The chapters that follow will deal specifically with various issues that will be important in the change to dental education, research, and practice based in informatics.

References

1. Kurzweil, R. The age of intelligent machines. Cambridge (MA), London (England), The MIT Press 1990; p.13.
2. Brooks, S.L. Survey of compliance with American Heart Association guidelines for prevention of bacterial endocarditis. JADA 1980;101:41-43.
3. Mayo, C.H. Quoted in: Proceedings of the Staff Meetings of the Mayo Clinic. 28 Sep 1927;2(39):233.
4. Morris, A.L., Bohannon, H.M. Assessment of private dental practice: implications for dental education. J Dent Educ 1987;51:661-667.
5. Neidel, E. On the brink — Will dental education be ready for the future? J Dent Educ 1990;54:564-566.
6. Collen, M. Dental informatics: What, why, who, where and when. In: Rienhoff, O and Lindberg, D. eds. Lecture Notes in Medical Informatics Vol 39: Salley, J., Zimmerman, J. and Ball, M. eds. Dental Informatics: Strategic Issues for the Dental Profession. Berlin Heidelberg: Springer-Verlag, 1990; p. 1.

2
Integrating Computing and Dentistry

Mark Diehl

After half a century of electronic automation, we should note that this is also the fifth decade of computer applications in dentistry. During this time dentistry has generally kept abreast of advances in automation theory and technology. Dental informatics has now matured to the point where these efforts can become self-sustaining and thus prepare dentistry for an even more extensively automated future. To do this we need a fundamental understanding of the processes of the profession, and only then may we plan how and where to have automation technology fit into the future of dentistry.

Throughout the past decade, dental automation was primarily task-oriented. As was the practice in other sectors of society, we computerized isolated managerial or clinical functions. We were reacting to our environment. Informatics theory has now evolved to a stage in which the future operation of an organization is anticipated, functional activities of the complete organization are evaluated and a coordinated, integrated automation solution is sought. In this approach we strategically plan the informatics future of our profession. We must determine where we are, where the profession will go through the next decade, and then create an informatics blueprint to help us get there.

We should view dental informatics as a means to determine how automation interacts and assists with the whole of patient health, wellness and total healthcare, in all aspects of organized dentistry. To accomplish this we must view dental informatics from the perspective of the whole of organized dentistry: clinical practice, academia, research, program management, our professional societies and supporting industries. As we prepare these models, we find that patient care is the common denominator, that is, the reason for which all facets of dentistry exist.

In dentistry as for our companion healthcare professions, the focus of patient care is the clinical process. The clinical process concentrates on the study of the patient with our particular attention directed toward the oral and maxillofacial environment. If we apply current informatics theory to the clinical process, its supporting functions and the ancillary services of dentistry, we may construct a strategy by which the whole of the profession may be optimally served by data automation.

An Informatics Model of the Clinical Process

As illustrated in Figure 2.1, the clinical process may be constructed as a waterfall model. The first step in the clinical process, data acquisition, involves developing an initial impression of the patient, obtaining historical data, conducting a physical examination and recording the data developed by these activities. The body of data thus produced must be organized into a systematic and often stylized database. It is essential that the manner of organizing this database does not overly influence the methods and procedures used for developing the data.

Data analysis is often termed the diagnostic process. It usually consists of both deductive and inductive activities whereby individual elements in the database are evaluated for significance and relevance, and then attempted to be fit into a pattern of knowledge. Analysis may occur as the practitioner conducts data acquisition, leading to a set of presumptive diagnoses. These are often used to exclude expanses of impossible or highly improbable relationships, thus guiding data acquisition more efficiently. Analysis frequently involves recursion, a return to the patient or other information resources for additional pieces of data. The product of data analysis is a differential diagnosis, being a set of possible conclusions each of which is associated with a probability of correct fit to the relevant data.

Frequently, each diagnosis is associated with one or more plans of actions. Likewise, each of these plans of action, or treatment plans, is associated with a prognosis. Each of the possible plans of action assumes one or more interventions may be undertaken. Ideally these choices include options to gather additional data and to perform no intervention.

Interventions are the technical and therapeutic measures undertaken by the practitioner or at the practitioner's direction for the benefit of the patient. Interventions are a complex interplay between dental arts and sciences. Interventions rely on finely-honed microsurgical skills, the employment of proven methods and techniques, and the availability of efficacious materials, devices and therapeutic agents. These interventions also have a foundation in the dental arts, as a human

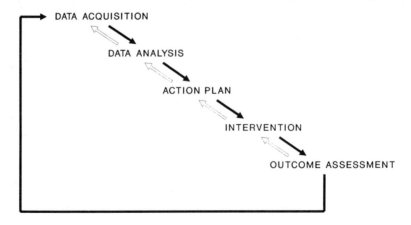

Figure 2.1. Waterfall model of the clinical process.

interaction between the needs of the patient and the perception and expertise of both the provider and the supporting staff.

Outcome assessment has evolved to viewing dentistry in terms of management models that measure the effectiveness and appropriateness of the services. It may indicate additional, unplanned services be provided. It may indicate a complete review of the case be undertaken either as a remedial step or as healthcare maintenance. This is a means to assure the quality of dental care and is undertaken by both the dental professional and regulatory entities.

How Computers Can Make the Dentist's Job Easier

Early in the computerization of dental private practice, there was a belief that merely automating specific tasks would provide efficiency and hence accrue economic benefits. Direct task replacement, such as automating insurance billing procedures, appeared deceptively successful. Automated insurance billing applications are characteristic of how not to automate dentistry. These applications have forced us to react to changing environments rather than creating a more ideal process and then making it work with information technology. Task replacement in this case has spawned additional labor intensive tasks such as redundant data entry where the clinician must make clinical data notes and then interpret clinical services in terms of coding conventions required by the various reimbursement mechanisms. The strategic, or proactive solution would have been to devise a common documentation method acceptable to both clinical practice and reimbursement mechanisms, and then apply automation technology. This approach translates to enhancement of the profession.

Ideally, applying informatics concepts to dentistry means blending information systems theory and technology, the dental arts and sciences, and the clinical process. The dental sciences deal with all factors supporting the physical practice of dentistry. The dental sciences include, among many other facets, the methods used to verify the presence or absence of disease, and the technical aspects of any intervention required to restore the patient to a condition of healthfulness. The dental arts are the humane component of dental healthcare. The dental arts concern how we manage the patient as a person and our contribution to maintaining health through the human dimension.

Within this model, dental informatics will make increasing contributions in areas ranging from applications in dental education, through computer assisted diagnosis and treatment planning, diagnostic systems and imaging, patient management, quality assurance and risk management, and the activities of the research and development community and the dental supporting industries. Following the experience of the PROMIS Laboratory, we can summarize the fundamental areas in which dentistry can best be automated as:

1. Information — Clinical information, and hence all information derived from it, is disorganized and incomplete because existing conventions for manually recording data are not widely adhered to. Automation technology can solve this problem

by gently compelling adherence to clinical documentation standards, using "legal" values in appropriate situations.

2. Memory — Most clinicians rely on their human initiative and memory to couple dental healthcare information to the case at hand. It is unrealistic to expect a clinician to retain complete details of potentially hundreds of active cases. Automated storage and retrieval, linked to computer-assisted clinical processing, can effectively improve practitioner case management.

3. Coordination — The need for extensive, coordinated care across healthcare disciplines continues to grow. For many patients, particularly in the outpatient setting of dental private practice, there is no rapid and effective means for the dental practitioner to interact with physicians, clinical laboratories or pharmacies. Automated data communications can provide the external linkages required to provide effective, coordinated, whole patient healthcare.

4. Feedback — Currently, it is difficult at best to gather evaluation data on specific cases or patient groups using manual techniques, even if partially automated. If clinical information is structured, electronically actuated, and maintained in an accessible database, automated systems could assist the practitioner to monitor case progress and realistically assess the long term outcome of services provided to both individuals and population groups.

As we expand the clinical process model, we find extensive interaction among informatics and the dental arts and sciences. The key aspect of the dental arts is the contribution made by professional and continuing dental education. The academic experience provides a wide range of interpersonal skills, the foundation of professional expertise, the analytical abilities needed for clinical judgement, and the survival skills required to maintain a professional business. In dental sciences, the academic experience also provides the technical skills required to perform the basic services demanded by the patient population. Here also the research establishment (academic, private and government supported) and the supporting dental industries provide the diagnostic devices and techniques, materials and methods required for proficient delivery of dental services. The key to fitting information technology to dentistry is determining what tasks are to be accomplished, which of these tasks are best handled by people, and which tasks are ideally suited to automation.

Dental Informatics as Combining People, Tasks, and Machines

Dental healthcare practices evolve regionally throughout the world. These conform to the cultural, social and political composition of nations, their geographic regions, the composition of their populations and the expectations of the people served by the profession. Great variance exists in the administration, regulation, delivery and support of dental healthcare. Those approaches which are optimally suited to one nation, region or state may not work as well in others. Methods which work well for one private practice, academic facility or research establishment may be a less optimal choice for another. Considering this range of diversity, a single automated solution for dentistry is neither likely nor desirable.

How then can this task be accomplished? By appropriately matching technology to the unique needs of the various users. Decades of experience in industry and commerce have shown that when computer programs or systems are developed, automation technologies must be tailored to specific organizational practices and organizations must adapt their operating methods to make best use of the technology. Applying this "systems approach" as an enterprise model to clinical dentistry, for example, requires that practitioners adapt the way in which they provide services to optimize the interaction between automation and clinical and practice-supporting activities. *Automation should be viewed as just another instrument in our armamentarium.*

Systems are composed of elements such as machines, programs, supporting equipment, human interaction, an operating environment, and supplies. In this system description, the key components are the human, the machine and its program elements. Automated systems do not replace personnel and human activities: they augment human capabilities and enhance their functions and operations. For the private practice or any other dental healthcare organization this should provide a substantial impact. For example, a good system that is judiciously employed will reduce the manual component of clerical workload. As a result it may permit retraining of an administrative staff person to take a more direct role in providing healthcare services. This means automation allows the conversion of a clerical or administrative cost center to a healthcare delivery revenue center. If it is appropriately used, automation will improve the economic profile of the organization. The organization will thus obtain a greater value from the automated system than its invests in acquisition, operation and maintenance costs.

Within the entire system, certain operations will be better performed primarily by human activity while others are best accomplished when left mostly to machines and programs. Emphasis on human capabilities is currently the best solution for tasks requiring creative, cogitive and judgmental activities. People perform these tasks far better than computers. They usually have a capacity to detect and solve inferential pattern recognition problems more rapidly and effectively than computer systems. Computers do not have a soul. They do not have emotions. They cannot feel. They cannot empathize with a patient as human practitioners do.

Humans live in the realm of *information*; machines operate in the realm of *data*. The data which our systems manipulate are symbolic surrogates which are generally agreed upon to represent items and concepts. Data are the raw facts. Information is data placed into a meaningful context for use by its human recipient. Humans handle information better than data and computers handle data better than information. Humans often make subjective observations, such as appraisal of the degree of inflammation of the gingiva or the vitality of a tooth. Computers make objective assessments of these events, which when coupled with precisely designed diagnostic systems accurately record the extent of gingival inflammation or the degree of pulp vitality. There are eleven fundamental data operations which, as logical processing steps, a computer uses to prepare data for human use as information. These are given with examples appropriate to dental informatics:

1. *Data Capture* obtains or records the data from an event or observation, as in an automated recording of examination observations.

2. *Data Verification* checks or validates the data to ensure that it is a true representation of the event or observation, such as a feedback step in an automated dental examination which confirms that a recording occurred and that the stated event was in fact recorded.

3. *Classification* places data elements into specific categories which have meaning to a user, such as demographic categories in a patient database.

4. *Arrangement* places data elements in a predetermined sequence as deemed desirable by a user, as in sorting patient addresses by Zip Code.

5. *Aggregation* combines or summarizes data either as a mathematical accumulation or a logical compilation, such as in totalling the prosthodontic caseload in a graduate school clinic.

6. *Decomposition* breaks grouped data into smaller components, such as in an epidemiology study of the prevalence of dental restorations.

7. *Calculation* entails the arithmetic or logical manipulation of data, as would be performed in an automated orthognathic analysis.

8. *Storing* places data in a temporary or permanent holding condition, readily available for further manipulation, typically using some form of automated storage media.

9. *Retrieval* searches out and accesses specific data elements from their storage condition, usually by some electronic device which performs the inverse of storage functions.

10. *Reproduction* duplicates data from one form or medium to another within user-specified limits, as in printing patient billing forms.

11. *Communication* disseminates or transfers data from one place to another, ultimately arriving at the final user. An example of such communication is displaying the results of an analysis of a research database on the video monitor.

Computers perform best as function multipliers. They accomplish mundane, iterative, and repetitive tasks consistently well where human performance would likely decline over time. They can perform routine communications with greater speed and accuracy than humanly possible. They are able to accomplish massive computation activities, including calculations used in image processing more rapidly than humans can. They have a greater capability for accuracy and rapidity as used in instrument sensing and control operations. Their processing forte is management of large amounts of disconnected pieces of data, with retrieval,

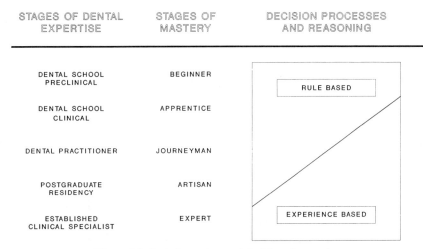

STAGES OF DENTAL EXPERTISE	STAGES OF MASTERY	DECISION PROCESSES AND REASONING
DENTAL SCHOOL PRECLINICAL	BEGINNER	RULE BASED
DENTAL SCHOOL CLINICAL	APPRENTICE	
DENTAL PRACTITIONER	JOURNEYMAN	
POSTGRADUATE RESIDENCY	ARTISAN	
ESTABLISHED CLINICAL SPECIALIST	EXPERT	EXPERIENCE BASED

Figure 2.2. An informatics model of dental expertise

rearrangement, and relocation in storage areas. They consistently interpret rule patterns and as such can emulate basic deductive thought processes.

Most currently used computer systems are based on the Von Neumann architecture. They accomplish their tasks as small, discrete elements. This frequently involves sequential processes and conditional program direction steps for operation and control. This is the reason computers are best suited for repetitious, iterative tasks, such as ALWAYS printing the dental practice address in exactly the same place on the insurance claim form.

Those computer architectures which do not follow the Von Neumann architecture, such as parallel processing computers, are not commonly used in dentistry. We can, however, expect that application of these systems will grow in specific applications like pattern recognition (as in speech recognition) where the performance of Von Neumann technology degrades. Technologists throughout the industry expect that computers based on alternatives to the Von Neumann design, such as those employing neural network, optical and photochemical technologies, will eventually evolve to more closely emulate and even exceed certain human information processing capabilities.

To better understand the relationship between human and computer capabilities, let us examine one approach to computer assisted dental diagnosis. This is the dental informatics realm of artificial intelligence or *expert systems* where automation is used to enhance diagnostic performance of a practitioner. The "apprentice-journeyman" model of dental diagnostic expertise, Figure 2.2, illustrates the environment in which a desired dental expert system is to perform. The apprentice by analogy would be the neophyte dental student who when confronted by a first case in the oral medicine clinic would rely on sets of precise rules to accomplish a diagnostic task. This student is performing a *rule-based* diagnostic task. As the level of formal knowledge and experience, collectively *expertise*, grows through the apprenticeship of dental school, the student begins to rely less on rules and more on *experience-based* decision making. Upon post-graduate education and residency training the dentist is on the artisan plane where most such decisions are experiential.

It is very easy for computers to make decisions based upon precise rules. Computers therefore have proven highly competent within the limits of *rule-based* diagnostic systems. Von Neumann technologies have a far more difficult time, both in processing speed and accuracy, when emulating *experience-based* decision processes. Their performance fails on comparison to the expert human practitioner.

If the strengths of both the computer and the human practitioner were collectively exploited, a true *expert system* would result. Herein the computer performs those tasks for which it is best suited, such as data storage, retrieval and manipulation. Likewise the human would perform those tasks involving observational, induction, interpretation, and similar processes. The computer would not permit the practitioner to make errors of omission and perhaps caution when mutually exclusive observations are considered. Hence arises the phrase *computer assisted diagnosis* where the computer *augments* the practitioner's diagnostic capabilities, and a man-machine system is created.

How well this man-machine system works is a function of how closely the machine interacts with its human master. The Turing Test is a generally accepted criterion which may be applied to determine an optimal man-machine interaction. In this test, an operator placed at a system interface would be unable to distinguish between interactions with another human or with a machine. How well system designers approach this criterion is one of many predictors for human acceptance of an intelligent or expert system. This gives rise to plain English (actually, native language) dialogue with the system and a requirement for the system to perform mental functions as a human. Whether a true Turing system is achievable is a matter of philosophical debate, yet it gives system designers a goal to strive for.

The Movement Toward Standards

All components of dentistry have unique information requirements. There are fundamental differences in the functional requirements to support clinical practice in the private sector, in governmental programs and in research and academia. Likewise, there are many social and geopolitical variations in the international dental healthcare environment. To fill this diverse demand, there are approximately 20 trained dental informaticians and individuals with dual dental and advanced computer degrees. Many more enthusiasts are active in the field of dental informatics research, education and the development of a wide range of systems and applications. In addition, there are tens of thousands of dental practitioners with varying degrees of computer literacy who use automated systems throughout the world. Each of these individuals have unique needs for automation and many employ a distinctive creative style and a technologic orientation to meet their needs.

Such diversity predicts a rapid and successful growth of dental informatics as a discipline. Yet without *discipline* such diversity also predicts chaos. Without some form of direction and oversight control there will be (and has been) considerable redundancy in research and development, waste of precious resources, and a need to resolve numerous conflicting opinions.

Standards provide a convenient and efficient mechanism to achieve progress in the various endeavors of dental informatics while providing wide-ranging freedom for both creators and users. Standards boost user confidence, facilitate versatility in system design, foster competition in the marketplace and provide a yardstick against which system designers may develop products. For dental informatics to remain a vital entity, these standards must not constrain development nor stifle innovation. Standards must, however, provide a common avenue upon which to pass along their creations. On the pragmatic side, for dental informatics to benefit the primary user, the clinical practitioner, standards must provide the common measure for the countless automated products and services found in the marketplace.

How Standards are Developed

Numerous routes to achieving standardization exist. These include the government and its regulatory agencies, the courts, public and private standards organizations and the commercial marketplace. Each route has a target segment of technology and users, and each has specific advantages and disadvantages.

First and foremost is the power of the government to regulate the practice of dentistry and hence all its component practices. This may be accomplished by law, as through the state dental practice acts, or by a regulatory agency of the government. For example, the United States Food and Drug Administration in the 1980s began regulation of automated patient care equipment. Dental informatics might be affected by this form of regulation. For example, there may be a constraint on the use of digital panoramic radiograph devices using AI technology to assess X-Ray dosage level. Additionally, the government may contribute to standards development through the courts, as indicated by the growing list of judicial opinions regarding automated clinical records.

In the courts, dental informatics standards may become linked with accepted standards of care. For example, a dentist who fails to use an accepted, proven, and available automated technique or device, to the detriment of a patient, might be held liable under the Hooper Doctrine. The Hooper Doctrine stems from a maritime incident of the late 1920s: the owner-captain of a ship was held liable for the loss of cargo because he did not employ a radio to learn about the approach of a storm. This principle is not limited to automation. It may include the failure to use any proven, readily available and generally accepted technology. The Hooper Doctrine could have applied in the past to those practitioners whose failure to use dental radiography resulted in an avoidable diagnostic omission. For the future practitioner it might apply to the failure to employ those biochemical tests or diagnostic devices that the majority of the profession will use for the detection and diagnosis of periodontal disease. As automated systems become increasingly commercially available and widely used in routine patient care, dental informatics standards will become a central issue in professional standards through application of the Hooper Doctrine.

Market-driven, "de facto" or "industry" standards respond to current marketplace conditions which for dental automation are exceptionally volatile. These are REACTIVE measures and manifest conflict among proponents of competing technologies which meet similar needs. De facto standards are efficient, but tend to define "validity" in terms of the products or services of major industrial or institutional organizations. These standards only measure success in the marketplace.

Consensus standards, conversely, are PROACTIVE. These bear a substantial resemblance to strategic planning. The consensus standards *process* derives its authority from the philosophical premises concerning the rights of the governed, or the right of those regulated to determine the means and method of regulation. Consensus standards provide a process whereby users, industry and academia collaborate to develop a standard that carries the weight of voluntary, majority acceptance. In systems design there is a premise that a dissatisfied user will not accept a system. Likewise, a dissatisfied user will dismiss an unacceptable standard and its effect will be meaningless.

Today there are countless standards organizations. Major organizations in the United States include the American National Standards Institute (ANSI), which is the official organization that represents the United States in the International Standards Organization (ISO). Professional, technical and trade organizations often participate in some form of standardization. Technical societies contribute specific standards such as a standard for data communications among automated medical devices. The American Dental Association represents the profession in the United States for the development of American standards and adoption of world-wide ISO standards. Professional organizations may also participate in the standards process by developing specific, focused standards, such as a standard terminology for periodontics or prosthodontics and also standards of care and ethical conduct. Several national standards organizations such as the American Society for Testing and Materials (ASTM) prepare and publish *voluntary consensus standards*. Consensus standards organizations tend to use the word standard as an adjective, as in a standard algorithm, a standard interface protocol, and a standard file structure.

There are numerous smaller standards organizations, industry associations and user groups. These generally have a narrow focus, such as the technical specifications of optical media for patient record cards. An individual with sufficient investment or influence might be able to "buy into" these standards-making activities. This standardization process thus risks promoting specific interests to the exclusion of the typical user. The resulting standards are "skewed" toward this specific interest and are more likely to be unacceptable to the affected population in general. When such standards are not widely accepted, they have little force of merit. Beyond being hollow, meaningless standards, these may risk "poisoning" the area for those future activities that intend to devise more acceptable standards.

The standardization process will affect all aspects of the medical and dental professions. Data communication standards in electronic pharmacy, clinical laboratory, and professional consultation will impact on how the practitioner interacts with healthcare systems outside his practice environment. Standards for electronic eligibility and preauthorization, claims submission and funds transfer will affect practice management. Standards for clinical and practice management automation will provide the yardstick against which vendors will develop future systems. A common data standard for the import and export of records will enable practitioners to avoid costly re-entry of data when they convert to a new practice management system.

Impediments to and the Potential for Standards

Historically, a fear of unconstrained control is the single greatest obstacle to an effective standardization program. Designers and researchers fear their creative activities will be stifled. Developers and manufacturers fear that a loss caused by not having invested in a specific technology or product inventory following the accepted standard will place them in an inferior competitive position. The entrepreneurial private practitioners fear the loss of both personal freedom and independence to conduct their practice according to their own personal desires.

Despite these fears, many dental informaticians believe in the necessity of standardization. Seven general concepts, as outlined in Table 2.1, form the foundation for a standardization process. Recently, preliminary activities have suggested standards are indicated for specific technological areas. Interest has been shown in academia and research, hospital and teaching clinic systems, automated records and clinical systems, private practice systems, and diagnostic technology. Table 2.2 illustrates some of the suggested standards from these interest areas.

The concept of standardized databases and a nosology for dentistry is appealing to academicians. However, the majority of dentists (the private practitioners) and

Table 2.1. The seven Golden Rules for dental informatics standardization.

1. Dental informatics standards do not dictate standards of professional care.
2. Standards must not constrain research, impede creativity or obstruct intellectual activity.
3. Standards are an inappropriate vehicle for promotion of personal viewpoints, techniques, methodologies, technologies or systems.
4. Standards should provide a common avenue for innovators and developers to pass information to unlimited users.
5. Standards should be developed as a consensus among all interested parties.
6. The protocols and accepted processes of consensus standards organizations should provide a framework for standards development.
7. Standards are dynamic, requiring continuous revision to retain validity and avoid stagnation.

Table 2.2. Possible standards for dental informatics.

---

1. A standard informatics curricula for professional education and graduate dental informatics education.
2. A standard configuration for dental school automated clinical systems.
3. A standard representation and format for symbolic and graphic clinical documentation.
4. A standard nosology to structure knowledge in dental informatics.
5. Standard diagnostic device parameters such as probing force for automated periodontal probes, wavelengths for optical pulp testing, and image densities for digital dental radiography.
6. A safety standard for X-Ray exposure limit in digital radiography.
7. A standard file structure for data import and export among private practice dental systems.
8. A standard data communications protocol for text and image data between a practitioner system and external systems such as third-party reimbursement programs.

---

the insurance industry are interested in effective standards for practice management systems. Private practitioners appear to desire established standards for system performance and for the support and maintenance functions expected of vendors. Furthermore, private practitioners desire a system-to-system data import/export protocol to permit easy conversion among practice management systems. Vendors desire design yardsticks against which they can develop commercial dental systems. The insurance industry desires standard protocols for electronic claims submission, treatment plan preauthorization and claim payment.

A distinct trend which has been evolving for the past several years is toward compartmentalized healthcare systems. These *niche* systems permit development to meet specific local needs, while retaining a high degree of communication capability for data transfer to companion and external systems. Dentistry would do well to adopt this approach rather than focus on a single "universal" automated system. Standards are crucial for niche systems to succeed. While a standard *internal* dataset is not required (and would impede user creativity), a set of standards for communications interfaces and protocols is essential. Such standard interfaces and protocols would readily carry over as a file transfer specification for commercial dental practice systems.

Summary

Dental informatics has become self-sustaining and capable of supporting the unique needs of the dental profession. All activities in dentistry, and hence dental informatics, ultimately affect or are affected by patient care. The focal point in dental informatics thus becomes the clinical process and all other areas ultimately support or are driven by these aspects of patient care. Informatics is important to all personnel in organized dentistry through the enhancement and augmentation of human activities rather than by replacing the human component in specific areas of the profession. Automation improves the economic position of an organization by allowing the conversion of human activity cost centers in an organization to human-oriented revenue centers. For example, if automating the clerical processes in a practice allowed a data entry employee to be retrained to provide income-generating preventive dental services, the practice would have a greater earning potential.

In dental informatics the *system* consists of data processing hardware and software, personnel, material and information resources and products, and the processes of the organization. Humans perform certain tasks in this system better than computers and computers handle specific tasks better than people. Automated technologies should thus be part of the instrumentation available in our armamentarium. Specific technologies must be appropriately selected from this armamentarium to satisfy specific user needs. Likewise, users must change their activities to best employ these technologies. The resultant fit of technology to user operations must be a dynamic and proactive process.

Incorporating informatics technology into all aspects of dentistry will be facilitated by standardization activities. Of all means available for creating standards, the most likely to affect dental informatics are governmental activities (being administrative, regulatory, legislative and judicial actions) and the development of voluntary consensus standards from within the profession. Dental informatics standards will impact heavily on future standards of care. Practitioners who fail to employ standardized and accepted dental informatics technologies may risk liability under the Hooper Doctrine. Areas in which standards are imperative are for data communication both within and outside of the practitioner systems. These include file and image transfer to third party reimbursement agents, other medical and dental practitioner systems, and to pharmacies, clinical laboratories and dental prosthetic laboratories. Standards for interactive communications with academic, research, and bibliographic databases, when coupled with computer assisted diagnostic capabilities in a practitioner system, will facilitate enhanced quality of care through access to a wide range of human and machine information resources.

3
Dental Informatics: The Corporate Perspective

Leslie A. Jones

"Time is like a river made up of the events that happen and its current is strong; no sooner does anything appear than it is swept away, and another comes in its place, and will be swept away too."

Marcus Aurelius Antoninus, *Meditations*

Computers in Business

The once rare computer is now the most ubiquitous tool in the American office—second only to the telephone.

Computers have become prime tools for every aspect of business control, in particular for the counting, receiving, comparing, recording and banking of money. Computers allow today's busy managers to monitor activity the *very* second it is happening. For the first time in history managers can make decisions *during* the event. Elsewhere in business, researchers, designers, draftsmen and engineers use computers to develop and modify products, testing their ideas on cathode ray tube (CRT) screens at a fraction of the former design cost. In production plants computers control machines, measure output, order materials and parts, and control inventory.

As the cost of computing power has declined during the last decade the cost/benefit ratio of computers has changed so beneficially that most businesses in the United States can now ill afford to be without some computing power. Today's business managers receive copious quantities of fast, accurate data of a quality their predecessors only dreamed about. Through computers they control encyclopaedic volumes of historical data, accessible in fractions of a second. They manage and manipulate images and ideas, reducing even the most complex business problem down to a few simple keystrokes.

As recently as 1968 businessmen were still waiting for the computer revolution to occur. They knew that this powerful new resource was coming but only a few visionaries foresaw how business would be transformed by the ability to digitally control and communicate huge volumes of information.

Today no business can effectively compete without computer power because computers supplement and multiply human output many times. For example, computers allow instant access to vital customer information about credit, client preferences, and shipping information, thus resulting in massive efficiency improvements in customer service.

It has become routine in most businesses to enter customer orders into a computer programmed to use the information in diverse ways. While the computer signals the plant to ship the product, it also updates accounting records for the value of the goods invoiced, calculates the weight and cost of shipping, prints a label and tells a postage meter to debit itself for the mailing expense. All this happens with one data entry. Elsewhere in the organization computers are updating marketing and sales statistics to record the sale. The computer calculates the business's profit on the transaction, and this data is added to all the other orders it processes to tabulate the company's overall results. This whole process, which once took hours, even days to complete, is now over in a matter of seconds using a computer.

Before computers, managers could only react *after* the event had happened and were forced to wait until data had been reported and analyzed. Today computers are programmed to "flag" key events, calling attention the moment something occurs, offering the opportunity for immediate action. This "hands on" management style is not the exclusive realm of high-tech Wall Street offices. It is becoming more and more usual to see computers on executive's desks monitoring what is happening in the business.

Many businesses operate through "decision trees" passing control from one management level to the next as the dimensions of the opportunity or problem become larger and more risky. For example, routine orders from existing customers with good credit are accepted by customer service department operators without reference to management. Once the size of the order exceeds a pre-arranged ceiling or a new customer places an order, typically a supervisor determines the business risk of the new event and "signs off" on the decision. As the stakes get higher so does the level of approval, but instead of taking weeks for paperwork to pass through "channels", businesses using computers can request and receive decisions immediately between one executive level and another in the company.

This revolution in business operations is seldom credited as one of the reasons for the dynamic growth the US has experienced since the early 1970s, but there is no doubt that new computer-aided business management techniques have greatly improved individual productivity in all sectors of the marketplace. Businesses who have computerized their operations have seen their investment paid back many times by improvements in customer relations, and availability of faster and more accurate information which has produced faster decision-making. Perhaps in the future it will become more apparent that the last few decades have been a great time of transition in business, from paper and verbal communication methods to the beginning of digital control. In 1991 we are only at the beginning of that transition.

Computers in Use

As personal computers (PCs) have proliferated in industry many managers have learned to use keyboards themselves, becoming in the process less dependent on secretarial aid. This has spurred a quantum increase in individual output because documents can now be retrieved from storage, amended and dispatched with just a few keystrokes. Memoranda can be exchanged between executives through computer to computer "networks" which sometimes link hundreds of machines, often many thousands of miles apart.

PCs are not confined to working only with words or numbers. In advertising agencies, graphic design houses and architects' offices around the US, computers have replaced pencils and paintbrushes as the creative medium of choice. Frequently used images can be stored and retrieved as needed. A huge library of "scanned" digital images exists suitable to illustrate publications of any type, from religious mailings to financial newsletters. Special software allows graphic designers to create high-quality images with color separations produced by the computer ready for printing. Designers can mix type with colored photographs and other graphics and send these images to their printer by modem/telephone connection where, with no further human aid, the document can be produced. This technology has spawned both a new type of printing house and multifarious newsletters. Almost every organization now has the ability to create a newsletter and most of them do!

Engineers also use the computer's marvelous graphic capability to design. Using software called CAD/CAM for "computer aided design/computer aided manufacturing", engineers can create three-dimensional images detailed to the last screw and rivet. They can even simulate operation using a computer technique called "precision animation" which appears to make the all the devices's components work together. CAD/CAM saves industry millions of dollars of model making and hardware design costs. Electronics engineers use computers to simulate various electronic components working together on a screen before they assemble them in real life. The computer calculates how diodes, transistors and other components will function in a circuit and even suggests modifications. Once the engineer accepts the design the computer will produce detailed drawings of the individual parts, suggest sources for standard hardware, list components of each sub-assembly and the sequence of manufacturing and produce cost estimates for the work.

New applications for this technology are being applied to home construction and in the future will enable the buyer to chose the house design, even testing the selection by viewing each room from inside the room on a computer screen. This technique employs new technology called "virtual reality" which produces an apparent 3-D image. When coupled with CAD/CAM, "virtual reality" is a powerful tool for exploring design concepts and is certain to become more and more popular as computer power continues to decline in cost. Virtual reality requires large amounts of memory for each image.

It is in the crucial area of financial management that computers are still most widely used in business and have proven themselves completely indispensable. It would be inconceivable today for a bank to operate without a computer, for example. Financial control of a business is impossible without some level of computer power; even the smallest concern needs computers to generate invoices, customer statements, reports, balance sheets and to coordinate all the essential financial information it needs. Computers also enable comparison spreadsheet techniques and the graphic presentation of data which so simplifies its interpretation. Computers save their users hours of tedious compilation and calculation every day; time which can be used for more creative and intuitive activity.

Data Entry Methods

There are many ways of entering information into a computer. In fact, input/output (I/O) science is a whole new computer sub-industry diversified into various different technologies.

For example:

- Laser devices can interpret numbers from printed "bar codes" — these appear on all product packages today and supermarkets use them in new faster check-out counters.
- Optical scanners which digitize images can read and reproduce both graphics and the printed word. "Optical Character Reader" software can be "taught" to recognize and interpret many different scanned typefaces.
- Data can be entered using voice input, and computers can be designed to accept and digitally store both frozen and animated television images.

These are just the samples of I/O technology. Computers also accept digitized information from discs, VCR and audio tapes, telephone and a variety of other sources. In the future new I/O methodologies can be expected, including fibre optic laser sources.

Once data is entered into the computer, the user can modify it using graphic or word processing software, and can change shapes, sounds, colors, words and any part of the stored information in any almost imaginable fashion.

PCs can multiply their usefulness by linking them together in local area networks (LAN). In a typical system specially designed software stores and holds data and messages sent between devices using one of the computers as a "host" machine for the others. Through this innovation different users can share the same information. For example, an accountant could create and share a report of sales results with others in the same network. Someone on the network may decide to print the information (there is usually at least one printer in every LAN) or may send it by telephone via a "modem" or "computerfax" to a distant location. The possible permutations of these systems are only just beginning to be explored. What is already clear to businessmen is that LANs are a proven productivity tool.

Computers in the Dental Industry

Dental Dealers

In the dental industry computers have been proliferating in offices, warehouses and factories during the last decade.

Almost all dental dealers use mini-computers to control their buying and invoicing systems and many have graduated to very large scale systems to which their customers can gain direct access. In addition PCs are being used for letter writing and to create price lists and catalogs. Many managers use computers to measure hourly business activity, to monitor price changes and to control purchasing and inventory.

When you call your local dental dealer there is a high chance that whoever answers the telephone is looking at your account details on a CRT as you speak to them. The screen will tell them who you are, what you buy and how much, what you owe and what you have paid and may even offer suggestions about what the customer service clerk should talk to you about.

You may already know that the local order number you called may not be answered locally. The person you are speaking to may even be in another state, maybe even across the country. Many dealers have centralized customer records and can access your account details no matter who answers the call or where. When you place your order the clerk will be able to tell you if the item is in inventory, since most dealers have their inventory list on computer and can tell you the up-to-the-minute price for that item. It is vital for the dealer to stay up-to-date on pricing. If the selling price is too low, not taking account of the latest buying price, the dealer could lose money, but he can not overprice either. Adjusting and balancing product prices is an important task for the dealer's computer and this feature has handsomely rewarded those dealers who invested in enough computer power for this function.

Bar-Coding

You may have begun to notice that many dental packages now have the familiar black and white, variable width bar-code marks you see on other packaged goods (see Figure 3.1). An agreement within the American Dental Trade led to the nationwide acceptance of a bar code standard. Ultimately bar-coding will be used by the dental industry for the same reason as your local supermarket, for digitally recording credits and debits to inventory. Computers and bar code readers can do this much more accurately than people. Presently, on receipt of stock the dealer enters the information in the computer through the computer keyboard. As each item is sold it is recorded as a debit from the inventory by an operator who enters the information with a keyboard. In contrast, a bar code laser "wand" will recognize the package. It will also read the bar code attached to a manufacturer's label or invoice indicating quantities and prices and will store the digital information in the dealer's computer. As each item is sold, another bar code reader checks the item

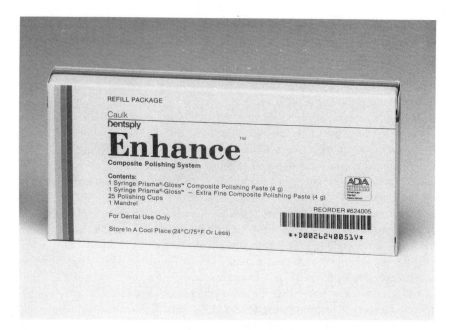

Figure 3.1. A typical bar code symbol used on dental packaging—in this case a box of L.D. Caulk's "Enhance". Manufacturers and dental dealers use these symbols and a laser "wand" to identify the product.

out of inventory, accesses the pricing information record and produces packing slips and invoices. It will also generate an automatic re-order to the manufacturer once the inventory is depleted.

Remote Order Entry

During the last few years some dealers have begun to offer dentists and laboratories direct access to their mainframe computers. Typical of these programs is Patterson Dental Company's REMO Remote Order Entry System (see Figure 3.2). Instead of calling your local Patterson store to place an order, REMO allows you to order directly through your computer and if you don't already have one, Patterson will provide the computer too! REMO allows you to search Patterson's inventory of 32,000 items for the product you want. A clever cross-reference system helps you find what you are looking for even if you do not know the brand name. You can place orders or check the status of your orders at any time of the day or night, seven days a week and receive a report each month which tells you if you are buying enough to qualify for the best prices.

This kind of direct link system is a major trend in computer use and you should expect dental dealers and manufacturers to take full advantage of it. Obvious expansions to these data bases in the future include "on-line" technical and clinical

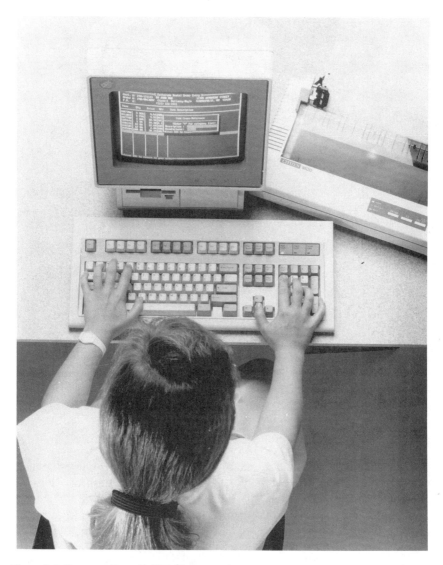

Figure 3.2. Patterson Dental's REMO is one of several dealer "direct entry" hardware and software systems for dental office use. Subscribers can check delivery and prices and place an order from a computer screen in their office for anything from Patterson Dental's 32,000 product inventory.

performance data for dental products, "expert" advice concerning clinical techniques, diagnosis and aid with treatment planning, as well as financial and tax planning.

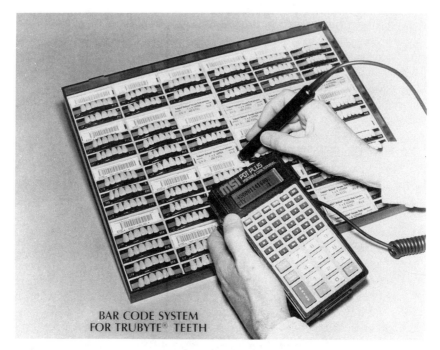

Figure 3.3. Dentsply's Trubyte automated tooth ordering system allows dental dealers to check their tooth inventory with a special bar code wand and place replacement orders through a dedicated telephone computer system.

Dental Manufacturers

Manufacturers have been quick to adopt computers. Beginning first in the financial departments, both mainframes and PCs have spread into every aspect of business management in dental manufacturing .

For example, a leading prosthetic tooth manufacturer has replaced an old ordering system with bar-coded re-order cards in dealer tooth inventories and has provided a bar code reader linked to a hand-held computer (see Figure 3.3). The dealer merely records items "missing" from inventory by passing a bar code "wand" over the visible record cards. When the task is complete a telephone line is plugged into the hand-held computer and the stored bar code information is downloaded to a dedicated computer at the manufacturing plant. The manufacturer's computer recognizes the caller, the digital information is passed between computers usually in less than a minute and becomes the dealer's order ready for overnight processing and next day shipment. This system replaces an error-prone and tedious daily re-ordering process, saving dealers valuable time and money as well as greatly improving the accuracy of in-coming orders.

Widely used by dental manufacturers are computer systems for controlling production and for managing in-coming raw and processed materials. Such programs as IBM's Materials Processing Inventory Control System (MAPICS) have become standards in the dental industry. Using linked modules these programs can systematize almost every aspect of production, coupling actual output to demand as orders are received and processed by the computer. This in-coming order data begins the chain of information processing, and everything else is cross-referenced back to that original entry. These highly sophisticated programs produce detailed reports, prompting managers to make key decisions concerning inventory investment, purchasing, production choices between different products, and many other vital elements of manufacturing control.

The MAPICS program was originally developed for use on IBM's System 34 family of "micro" mainframe computers but has been gradually transformed to work on the latest, much larger and much faster devices IBM is now selling. Thus information can be transferred between each generation of computer without the need to re-enter all the important historical records which have been developed during the use of the program.

Dental manufacturers often use CAD/CAM systems, at least in the "CAD" mode. In less than a generation hand drafting skills have begun to disappear as engineers turn more and more to computers to help develop designs and to produce drawings from which machine shops can turn out the finished products. Many of the machining devices themselves are also computer driven. These Computer/Numerical Control (CNC) devices use digitally stored information to control tool and raw material choice and then to guide fine cutting tools to produce the finished product. Their big advantage is that they can be set to work without human intervention until they run out of material and will repeatedly and accurately keep producing the same part. These machines can also be more easily reprogrammed than earlier machinery so even short "runs" can be economical. In fact they allow manufacturers to begin to make components as they are needed instead of producing large quantities each time the machinery is reset. You may hear this termed "Just In Time" manufacturing because the components are made available just when they are needed, not before and not after.

In the more advanced manufacturing plants, especially those repetitively making complex components, digitally controlled robots can be seen loading and unloading machines, twisting and turning components for machining and cross-checking that the machined output conforms to the required quality standards. Far from eliminating jobs in manufacturing plants, CAD/CAM, CNC devices and robots have generated a need for new, highly trained workers whose jobs are more challenging and rewarding.

Computers for the Dental Office

System Choices

In search of competitive advantages, the giant corporations at the center of the evolving computer industry have developed unique, sometimes copyrighted "operating systems". Because products designed for one operating system will not work on another, hardware and software designers, as well as computer buyers must choose which system they prefer.

Although there are as many systems as there are computer manufacturers, there are really only two system choices from which to select for dental office applications.

The most widely used is MS/DOS (Microsoft Disc Operating System) sometimes wrongly referred to as the "IBM System" and more frequently advertised as "IBM compatible". This operating system was adopted by IBM for its first generation of computers and retained for the "XT" and "AT" model series. Other computer manufacturers including Tandy, NEC and Compaq have been able to produce IBM style computers, called "clones", sometimes at much lower cost than IBM. Recently IBM began marketing new, proprietary operating systems labelled "PS/1" and "PS/2". No widely used dental office products have appeared using these new systems yet.

The other operating system used in dentistry is Apple's Macintosh system. This system was developed by the company for its Macintosh computer products and is Apple's exclusive property, so no Macintosh clones have been produced. This means that only Apple Macintosh computers can be used but it offers good compensation for this restricted access. The Macintosh operating system enforces strict rules for software designers. The result is that all Macintosh software works in precisely the same way, using "pull down" menus operated by the Macintosh "mouse" to display the program's various options. For example, to print a document the Macintosh user clicks the moveable cursor over the word "File" which appears in every program. This displays a list of options including "Print". Clicking on "Print" causes the computer to print a copy of the document on the computer screen.

Because software designers for MS/DOS products are not restricted in the way they make their programs work, every MS/DOS program is different and must be individually learned.

Before choosing between operating systems the computer buyer must first decide what the computer is intended to do. This will lead to decisions about software and that choice will determine which computer to buy and how powerful it needs to be.

It is unlikely that the dental office computer will be used for only one "dedicated" application such as bookkeeping or patient records. Computers are such versatile business tools that letter writing ("word processing") or other accounting tasks ("spreadsheets"), are certain to be future applications. Choosing a computer which can function equally well for all present and future needs is difficult.

The decision comes down to this:

There are more MS/DOS programs available than Macintosh programs and many more MS/DOS users so you can usually get help if you need it. The disadvantage is that it will take twice as long to learn how to use MS/DOS programs compared to Macintosh. Few people have the time or patience to learn how to use more than one MS/DOS program thoroughly. Aware of this deficiency, Apple advertises that the average Macintosh user routinely uses three or four different programs because they are so much easier to learn.

In an effort to overcome the MS/DOS system's long learning curve, the Microsoft Corporation has recently launched Windows for MS/DOS which simulates some of the Macintosh user benefits. Most reviewers are giving the company an "A" for effort but comment that it falls short of the Macintosh product in many important ways.

Other operating systems of importance in the dental market are UNIX and Xenix.

Dental Office Software

Programs for dental office management are available for IBM and Macintosh as well as other computers. Developers of dental office software have shown the same ingenuity as others in this dynamic new industry and offer dozens of features in their dedicated dental office programs. Software developers spend thousands of hours scrutinizing dental offices to determine how they operate and discuss their needs with hundreds of dentists. This ensures that the program simulates the regular office routines and includes the key features dentists want.

Many different programs are available, each taking a slightly different point of view and each operating on different computers or using different operating systems. Many providers do "Turnkey" operations, supplying the hardware and software, keying in the dental office's records and teaching the office staff how to use the equipment. This can save hundreds of learning hours and lots of frustration for the first time computer buyer, but it is expensive. Other vendors supply only the software and telephone support and the buyer must do the rest.

Today there are many programs with many features to select from. A good rule of thumb is to pick a system which does what is needed today but has the capability for further expansion. Some vendors offer their products in "modules", allowing future expansion of the system. For example the dentist may wish to begin with an appointment scheduling, recall, and insurance system first. Once these features are integrated into the office routine, modules for financial management of the business, payables, receivables, payroll and even materials inventory management can be added.

Updating software is important because change is a constant in computers and it is vital that software and hardware stay up to date. Having the current version of software facilitates faster help if something goes wrong. One of the major reasons for updating is to fix the "glitches" which are a regrettable part of most programs. Purchasing a system from a vendor who offers a guaranteed update service is prudent, and it is good advice to buy and use the updates when they are issued. Some software vendors insist that their customers subscribe to an updating service and pay for telephone help. The cost for updating and future access to technical help must be taken into account when determining the true expense of a dental office system.

Table 3.1. Dental software products.

Product	Source	Finance Module	Payroll	General Ledger	Accounts Payable	Accounts Receivable with aging	Treatment Planning	Claim Forms Generation	On-line Claims Processing	Ins Benefits Co-pay Estimator	Patient Budget Planning	Appointment	Recall Management
DDX®	Calyx Corp 150 N. Sunnyslope Rd Suite 375 Brookfield WI 53005 (800) 558 2208 (414) 782 0300	Yes	Option	Option	Yes	Yes	Yes	Yes	Option	Yes	Option	Option	Option
Easy Dental®	Dental Plan Inc 3633 Broadway, Suite B, Garland, TX 75043 (800) 824 6375 (214) 271 0457	No	No	Yes	No	Yes	Yes	Yes	Yes	Yes	Yes	Yes	Yes
QSI®	Quality Systems Inc 17822 E 17th St Tustin, CA 92680 (800) 327 2299 (800) 631 1751 In CA	No	Option	Option	Option	Yes	Yes	Yes	Yes	Yes	No	Yes	Yes
Softdent®	Professional Software Solutions Inc 2113 Emmorton Park Road Suite 104 Edgewood MD 21040 (800) 433 2409 (301) 679 3835	No	No	No	No	Yes	Yes	Yes	No	No	No	Yes	Yes
Three Star®	Three Star Dental Systems 26851 Oak Hollow Road Laguna Hills, CA 92653 (714) 582 5011	No	No	No	No	Yes	Yes	Yes	No	No	No	No	Yes
Triad®	Triad Systems Corporation 3055 Triad Drive Livermore, CA 94550 (800) 338 7423	Option	Option	Option	Yes	Yes	Yes	Yes	No	Yes	Yes	Yes	Yes
DentalMac®	Healthcare Communications Inc 301 S 68th St Ste 500 Lincoln, NE 68510 (402) 489 0391 (800) 888 4344	Option	Option	Option	Option	Yes	Yes	Yes	No	Yes	Yes	Yes	Yes

Table 3.1. (continued)

Product	Patient Clinical Records	Inventory Management	Word Processing	Specialist Programming Option	Training On-Site	Off-Site	Computer Assisted Help	Telephone Support	Automatic Software Updating	Software Leasing	Turnkey Package	Operating System	Computer	Misc Features
DDX®	Option	No	Option Letter Module	Yes	Yes	Yes	Yes Full Manual on system Prompt	Yes	Yes Yearly Maint & Enhance Fee	Yes	Yes through Local Reseller	UNIX/ XENIX	IBM Compatible	
Easy Dental®	Yes	Avail in the near future	Dedicated Will merge with other WP programs	No	Yes	Yes	Yes	Yes	Optional $50 - $150 each 6-8 months	No	No	MS/DOS	IBM Compatible	On-Line Support & Upgrades
QSI®	Yes	Option	Yes	Option Custom design feature	Yes	Yes	Yes	Yes	Yes Included in monthly fee	No	Yes	AIX/UNIX	IBM RS® or Macintosh	Streaming Tape back-up
Softdent®	No	No	Not Included	No	No	No	Yes	Yes	For One Year	No	No	MS/DOS	IBM AT®	
Three Star®	No	No	Not Included	No	No	No	Yes Built-in Tutorial	Free first Year then $95 p.a.	"Non-Profit" Policy	No	No	MS/DOS	IBM Compatible	
Triad®	Yes	Yes	Dedicated	Option Custom design feature	Yes	Option	Yes	Yes	Included in Service Plan	Yes	Yes	Theos	Altos-Dedicated system	Streaming Tape back-up Custom reports option
DentalMac®	No	No	Yes	No	Yes	Yes	Yes	Free first 90 days then by contract Healthtalk® Optional 24hr access	Yes	Yes	Yes	Apple Macintosh	Macintosh SE/30 or larger 2 Meg RAM min	Graphic Interface Easy merging with other software

Buying from a local "reseller" has merit because that person is usually available when needed. But people move about a lot in the growing computer business, so be sure that your faithful computer expert is not planning to quit his job the day after your system is ordered!

The following is a brief outline of some of the most popular dental software products currently available. Buyers are recommended to scrutinize the dental press closely for currently available products before making their own choice. (See Table 3.1)

Dramatic efficiency improvements have been brought about in the relatively low volume dental office environment, which for years has been resistant to many of the changes. The arrival of the personal computer and the proliferation of dental office management software has begun a process of change which will have far reaching benefits in costs and efficiency. Already the unit cost of patient administration has shown considerable improvement (with much more to come) as computers continue to grow in power and reduce in cost. Despite the easy to calculate benefits of computerizing the dental office, many dentists have stuck to the old paper-pushing techniques. Research into the dental program alternatives commercially available can be done from the office desk just by calling telephone numbers widely advertised in dental publications. The reputable vendors are very helpful about mailing out printed information and answering questions about their systems. A dentist who may be considering the purchase of an office computer system should include conversations with some of the many knowledgeable vendor telephone marketing people before making a decision.

Plugging your Computer into the World

Both Macintosh and IBM computers can be made to communicate with the outside world—to dental dealers or to information data bases. Predictions are that in the future being able to communicate with other computers will have increasing importance to the dental office user. Of immediate use is the ability to electronically send dental insurance information from the office computer directly to the third party payment insurance source. This ensures faster payment than mailing insurance forms and enables billings and receipts to be monitored directly by the computer so payments can be tracked until completely paid. Many dental software packages offer this useful add-on feature which quickly pays for itself.

New information sources of interest to the dentist will become available in the future. Already available are public data bases of many kinds with encyclopaedic memory banks on subjects as diverse as engineering, the stock market and law. In preparation are dental clinical and statistical data sources which dentists can use to stay up-to-date on research and even to compare a diagnosis with that of an expert or to seek expert help for difficult clinical situations.

German dentists can already access a trial program of scientific and commercial product information organized by the German Post Office. Data is supplied by manufacturers and can be brought to a dedicated computer screen through a series of easy "menus". This data base also enables pharmacists to shop among different sources for the best price or fastest delivery. The system will find the cheapest source for the drugstore product and prompts the pharmacist for a buying decision.

Oral Imaging Systems

New to dentistry but widely used in medicine are computer-driven digitized imaging devices which produce magnified images of the oral environment both dentist and patient can see. Using very small Charge Couple Device (CCD) cameras which can reach into every area of the mouth, these devices convert images into a television-like full color picture. They are most useful for demonstrating clinical procedures to an apprehensive patient or as part of a treatment planning discussion. Their major benefit though may be in capturing "before and after" images on discs or videotape for patient files, thus permitting the dentist to review the patient's oral situation before an appointment. Stored images provide highly detailed clinical records for a variety of possible purposes, including evidence for the increasing possibility of malpractice suits.

Oral imaging devices were first launched in 1987 and despite a high initial price many dentists found the technology appealing. In concert with other integrated circuit driven products, the cost of oral imaging has declined rapidly so that today it is well within the budget of every dentist.

One application for which digitized images have been used is to record the pre-operative oral condition of a patient for use in constructing prosthetic work. These images are stored on a regular video cassette and sent along with other instructions to the dental laboratory. This is particularly valuable when the laboratory is out of town.

Digitized images can be manipulated in a number of useful ways. Merging oral image technology with computer imaging systems allows the dentist to change captured images to predict, for example, the outcome of a restorative procedure. A common use for this technology, which is already on the market, is to demonstrate the after-effect of veneering or bonding to the diastema patient. Experimentation with various aesthetic alternatives is also possible using captured images of the patient's dentition or whole face. These are very useful devices for treatment planning and have the potential to benefit dentists' productivity greatly.

X-Ray Image Enhancement

Imaging products that will scan X-rays to produce digital images are currently being researched. Using image enhancement algorithms developed by NASA for astronomical and satellite photographic enhancement, the processing of the digitized X-ray image highlights or eliminates unusual features. These can be enlarged and even colored for clarification. A big advantage of these devices is that images can be electronically stored along with other patient clinical information, including full color oral images as discussed above.

Further into the future it is possible to anticipate coupling X-ray machines directly to imaging computers, eliminating the photographic stage entirely. It is calculated that digital images can be produced with much less exposure of the patient to X-ray radiation than at present. Imaging techniques will allow the resulting picture to be manipulated in many ways, perhaps using colors to represent variations in tissue density. Merging three-dimensional computer programs with digital X-ray technology offers the possibility of rotating images on the screen. The image could then be viewed from different angles. Precise measuring techniques are also possible. Researchers are already using X-ray subtraction techniques to measure changes in tissue and it is certain that this will soon become available for everyday office use.

The dentist of the future will be able to capture images of soft and hard tissue by a variety of digital collection techniques. Computer programs will process the images for immediate viewing at chairside. Digitized images of the same site or the same oral view will be retrieved and visual and electronic comparisons made of the various features. It will be possible to establish precise depths of periodontal pockets and their shape and to accurately monitor any changes. Camera miniaturization will allow exploration of subgingival areas and root canals. Images of the patient's soft tissue will be electronically compared with stored images of soft tissue disease pathology, alerting the dentist to possible problems.

Image enhancement techniques also offer the prospect of identifying and treating dental conditions at an earlier stage than is presently possible. For example, a semi-automatic technique locating and completely cataloging a patient's white spot lesions is feasible. New micro-restorative methods and materials need to be developed to keep up with image enhancement technology, providing the opportunity for much earlier and less radical hard tissue treatment.

Very little research has yet been done using image enhancement in the field of oral bacteriology. It is already practically possible selectively to stain and digitally identify pathological microorganisms in situ. Using this methodology in the dental office, stained anaerobic bacteria associated with periodontal disease could be detected and monitored, before and after prophylaxis, by a subgingival digital camera with the image magnified, displayed and stored for future use. Similar techniques could quickly establish the sterility of root canals prior to obturation.

The visually dependent nature of clinical dentistry suggests that many exciting uses can be found for digital imaging techniques. More research work in this field by dental schools and dental manufacturers should be encouraged.

New Input/Output (I/0) Devices

As the cost/density ratio of integrated circuitry devices continues its decline the increasing power and speed of computers has opened doors to technology which has long been contemplated but never previously affordable. One such technology is the interpretation of scanned script or typewritten documents into the computer's memory where it can be edited like a regular word processing document. There have recently been big improvements in the quality of scanned computer images, up from just a few hundred dots or "pixels" of information per inch of image to many thousand. As the quality of the scanned image improves it becomes increasingly possible to interpret the information. One interpretation program is called an "Optical Character Reader" (OCR). This clever program compares scanned digital images of letters and numbers with images stored in its memory, in effect "reading" the scanned document. The usefulness of this program is readily apparent. As well as storing the information in accessible, editable computer form it offers the possibility of using the stored data in other computer programs.

A practical use for this program is to scan and store patient clinical histories. As well as entering the data many times faster than a typist can hit keys and thus saving much expense, the document is available for review, amendment and for future additions that may be offered to the computer by other I/O means. Additionally, scanning can produce images of dental charts which can be recalled for future use.

Already available to dentists is a patient charting computer program which uses only the dentist's voice to input information. This or "Voice Activated" (VA) input scheme offers many future possibilities for quick and easy, hands off, data input applications in the dental office. To use the product the dentist accesses the patient's records on the computer and makes changes and additions by speaking into a microphone which digitizes the audio signal, compares it to stored signals and triggers a program function. For example, the dentist says "Distal surface on tooth number four is restored" and the computer analyses the digitized signal made by each separate word, sorts the information, and creates a record on the stored patient chart that tooth number four has a distal restoration.

Updating patient clinical and financial records which have been entered by OCR is one possible application for VA that would benefit the unit cost and possibly improve the quality of patient record-keeping.

Miniature Circuitry Applications

Other computer input/output schemes with future dental applications include miniature circuitry that can be implanted in teeth (or elsewhere in the mouth) recording and storing important physiological data ready for downloading to a computer. Manufacturers build sensors and computers into modern automobiles so that auto mechanics can analyze the vehicle for problems; it is speculated that orally implanted circuits (IC) could also diagnose and alert patients and dentists to potentially hazardous oral or general physiological conditions.

For example, using a telemetric signal to trigger an audible reaction in an interpreter device carried elsewhere on the body, constant saliva analysis could alert the user to elevated blood sugar or to undesirable physical, bacterial or chemical developments.

In a very simple dental application of this idea an IC could be fitted to a miniature strain gauge attached to delicate prosthetic work. If the bridge is subjected to undue masticatory stress the device would trigger a telemetric signal warning the patient to relax the jaw pressure or to move the food bolus away from the site.

Another application would be as an aid in birth control. Storing patient temperature patterns in an IC and coupling this to an oral temperature sensor would allow comparison with real time temperature patterns and could signal the patient's optimum conditions to facilitate or avoid conception.

It seems likely that the dentist of the future will play an important role in general medicine by implanting and servicing IC devices placed in the oral environment for data collection about the whole body.

A Walk through a Dental Office in the Year 2005

Computers have already had a profound effect on the practice of dentistry and it seems certain that they will revolutionize future dental practise. It is interesting to speculate what a dental office will look like 15 years from now.

There is no receptionist in this office. The dentist's image appears on a television screen as the patient enters the waiting room and greets the patient directly from the chairside. The patient relaxes into a Transcutaneous Electroneural Stimulator (TENS) chair, swinging the electrodes attached to the chair headrest until they touch his forehead. Back in his office the dentist notes that the TENS chair is in use by the new patient and waits for a signal that low level sedation has been achieved.

While the patient relaxes the dentist calls up the patient's clinical records by pronouncing his surname, apparently into the air. A screen on his desk displays the patient's full face picture and runs an accelerated video of the last treatment visit. Other parts of the screen show graphics of the patient's upper and lower arches and review multicolored X-rays. The dentist's notes occupy the final section of the screen, highlighting important physiological issues, then suggesting a series of treatment options for the present visit and noting that payment for past treatment is up-to-date.

A signal alerts the dentist that his patient has achieved TENS sedation and displays pulse and blood pressure data collected by the TENS chair. No action is required except to invite the patient into the clinical area.

The route to the clinical area of the office includes a pause for the patient to don disposable head, shoes, and clothing covers. The dental office of 2005 is very conscious of patient cross-contamination risk and attempts to keep the operating environment as sterile as possible. Office air is circulated through scrubbers and the very few operating surfaces in the room are draped with disposable film which sterilizes surfaces on contact. Despite this the area is bright and humanly cheerful.

The patient enters the operating area and is greeted by the dentist without a handshake. Hands have already been scrubbed, sterilized and barrier coated. Uncomfortable, non-tactile operating gloves have been obsoleted.

The patient reclines on the operating chair in front of the dentist. Because the patient has already been recognized by the office computer the chair and dentist's stool move to the operating position stored in memory. The first action is to check the implanted monitor. An electronic "reader" is touched to the surface of a crown, downloading stored data which is immediately analyzed and displayed graphically. A graph of fluoride ion concentration in the patient's saliva since the last visit reveals that a fluoride releasing implant needs servicing and the dentist notes an unusual decrease in pH for various periods, hovering at enamel erosion levels for some time. Enquiry reveals that this patient enjoys fresh oranges and indulged himself liberally on a recent trip to Florida. The dentist explains the risk. Elevated enzyme concentrations suggest a possible recurrence of a periodontal condition which will require further examination.

As they talk a video camera attached to the dentist's spectacles records the oral condition. The dentist fits a customized device to the patient's upper anterior teeth. Attached to this is a camera which begins to scan the mouth, extending and retracting so that images of all the teeth and soft tissue surfaces can be recorded. The dentist aids the process by retracting buccal and lingual tissue for the camera to capture. As it works, the new images are compared to stored information and a series of questions and suggestions for further examination and treatment appear on a screen opposite the dental chair.

Other sensors confirm the dentist's visual observation that the soft tissue is in good condition. A miniature camera makes an excursion into a pocket to reveal that surgical reattachment of connective tissue performed at an earlier visit is progressing well. The camera's scan of hard tissue surfaces discloses hardened plaque in the lower lingual area which must be removed and the dentist dispenses a gel solution to soften this before blasting the area with an air/water/abrasive concentration delivered by a miniature, disposable air jet device. No other major hard or soft tissue problems are noted by the camera scan or by the dentist's confirming examination.

After replenishing the aging fluoride implant, reprogramming the monitoring implant and suggesting the patient go easy on the oranges, the visit is over. They agree on a future appointment and the patient leaves the operatory.

As the patient heads towards the waiting room, disposing the cap and gown in a waiting receptacle, the dentist is preparing the office for the next patient. All the operating surfaces receive a new sterile film, instruments and other materials used on the patient are placed in the office medical waste incinerator which automatically sorts, cleans, crushes, and forms them into a reusable plastic mass. As the dentist works he dictates his notes to the ubiquitous computer which immediately transcribes them, creates a billing for his services and stores all the data together with the video images and other information for this patient.

Before the patient leaves the waiting room a "hard" copy of the charges, which have already been electronically sent to the third party payment source, is printed and the patient tears it off, reads it, noting the time and date of the next appointment and exits the office.[*]

---

[*]Who can doubt that computers will play an increasingly important role in dentistry?

In the early 1990s we have only begun to see the possibilities for the integrated circuit in the dental environment. The continuing application of human ingenuity welded to practical interpretation of real needs will produce uses for computer technology which this writer cannot begin to conceive, but none of the devices described in this chapter are "science fiction". They are based on ideas already conceived and in many cases, already in research for dentistry or in use in related sciences. Devices which electronically measure molecular level chemical changes and can interpret and store the data already exist. Fluoride-releasing oral implants have been the elusive "chalice" of many a researcher and are just a small research and development investment away from fruition. The digital collection, enhancement, and storage of visual, X-ray, and document images has already arrived and is in use in other fields. Dentistry will certainly be next.

What is sadly missing are enough champions of the computer in dentistry. Far too many graduating students know little more about computers than how to make a word processor work and too many practising dentists tell themselves they are too busy to learn more. What the profession needs are practical computer gurus to do the "imagineering" which will integrate dentistry into the computer age.

4
Dental Informatics and the Evolution of Computers—the Roles of Organized Dentistry

Anthony L. Kiser

Prior to 1980 computers were used sparingly in private dental practices. When I was collecting information for my master's thesis on computers in dentistry in 1978 (Kiser, A. Computer Applications for Dental Practice and Program Management, University of North Carolina Health Sciences Library, Chapel Hill) a practice management consulting firm with hundreds of clients in the southeastern United States could identify just one computerized dental practice for me to visit. That dentist had invested over $100,000 to build a customized system that performed only very basic office management functions. During the 1970s computers were not practical for most dental practices because home computers were too slow and minicomputers and mainframes were too expensive. The first offices to computerize tended to be group practices where the volume of administrative work was greater and the computer costs could be shared among several dentists.

That scenario changed dramatically during the 1980s due to improved technology and lower prices. In the decade following 1980 computer use in dental practices grew steadily. In 1984, the first year when information was collected about computer usage through the American Dental Association's Survey of Dental Practice, approximately 11.1% of all practicing dentists utilized in-house computers and another 9.6% used computer services housed outside the office. By 1990 the percentage of practices using inside or outside computers had grown to 43.2%.

Figure 4.1 vividly illustrates the steady growth in dental practices using computers and particularly the growth in the use of in-house computers.

A look at which practices are purchasing computers is revealing. In 1987, 26.1% of all solo dental practices and 44.5% of all group practices used computers. The dental practices with the higher gross billings are also more likely to use computers as illustrated by the Figure 4.2.

The use of computers also varies by geographic region as illustrated in Table 4.1. Dentists in the western United States are almost twice as likely to own a computer than dentists in other regions. Looking at the characteristics of geographic location and gross income simultaneously, one finds that only 4.7% of the small practices in the southern region of the United States use computers, in marked contrast to large practices in the western region where 88.3% are computerized.[3]

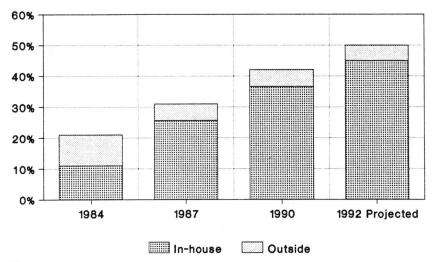

Figure 4.1. Percentage of dentists using in-house and outside Computers by Year. ©1990 RRC, Inc. Reprinted with permission from Dental Outlook, Vol. III, No. 10.

Younger dentists may be the more computer literate segment of the profession, but computer utilization in practice does not reach its peak among that group. Almost 50% of the practicing dentists between the age of 45 and 54 utilized computers, but only 42.5% of dentists under the age of 35 use computers. Above the age of 54 computer utilization falls off rapidly.[5]

The use of dental computers has changed since 1984. Patient accounting has been the most popular use of computers for all years. Preparation of insurance forms has grown steadily, while office newsletters seem to be falling from favor. Table 4.2 illustrates the trends for dentists utilizing computers for selected tasks since 1984.

Gross Billings

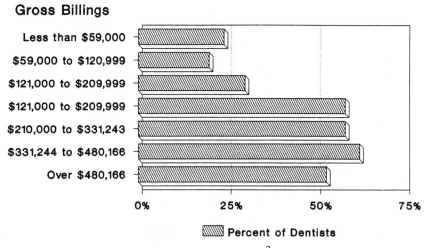

Figure 4.2. Computer utilization by annual gross billings.[2] ©1990 RRC, Inc. Reprinted with permission from Dental Practice Outlook, Vol. III, No. 10.

Table 4.1. Percentage of dentists using in-house computer by region[4].

Region	Percentage
Northeast	16.5%
Midwest	19.4%
South	20.7%
West	35.8%

Source: ©1990 RRC, Inc. Reprinted with permission from Dental Practice Outlook, Vol. III, No. 10.

Price is dissolving as a barrier to the use of dental office management systems, but a level of resistance to computerizing remains. Over 250 different vendors sell medical and dental office management systems, making the time and learning curve required just to assess a practice's needs, research the market, and select a system substantial. With the additional investment of time for system installation and staff training, significant barriers to computerization remain. Before dentists will make the decision to computerize, they must be convinced that there will be benefits—increased production, improved marketing or administrative cost savings—to justify the time, money and effort required to select and install a system. Other intangible barriers such as discomfort with or mistrust of computers represent special challenges for the computer industry to overcome.

Future Trends in Dental Office Computing

The information presented above is intended to illustrate the past and present trends in the use of computers in dental offices. The current growth rate of first-time dental office computer purchasers is 11 percentage points every three years.[7] At this rate a majority of the dental offices in the United States will have a dental office management computer system by 1992.

Table 4.2. Percentage of dentists utilizing computers for selected tasks by year[6].

Tasks in the Dental Office	1984	1987	1990
Patient Accounting	84.8	89.6	91.9
Maintain Expense Records	49.2	43.1	47.6
Process Insurance Forms	46.8	64.0	73.5
Maintain Treatment Records	22.9	34.0	32.9
Diagnosis and Monitoring Treatment	8.4	18.3	17.9
Scheduling Patients	11.2	20.7	16.7
Office Newsletters		24.7	13.7
Form Letters		49.6	60.1

Source: ©1990 RRC, Inc. Reprinted with permission from Dental Practice Outlook, Vol. III, No. 10.

Although no perfect crystal ball for forecasting the future exists, the experiences of hospitals and medical practices using computers give some indication of how dental office computing may grow and change. Medical computing has evolved ahead of dental computing due to the greater ability of hospitals to afford first-generation computer systems. Those computer capabilities later become affordable for private dental offices. The following five general trends are likely to characterize the future evolution of dental office computing.

Free-Standing to Networked Systems

Hospitals are moving away from the mainframe computer to a system called a local area network or LAN. One LAN may connect dozens of personal computers cabled to a file server, which directs data traffic on the lines. Although the evolution from mainframes to LANs will not be part of dental computing's history (since mainframes were never affordable for dental practice), the availability of LAN technology will have application for dental offices wanting to link multiple sites, to install several terminals, or to tie multiple specialized computer application systems together in one practice. With an increasing number of specialized office management and clinical applications coming to market, interest in connectivity and concern about incompatibility between systems will grow.

Another administrative application of computers is electronic media claims (EMC) for submitting medical and dental insurance claims. In order to file insurance claims electronically, an office needs a computer with a telephone modem and specialized telecommunications software. The data required to complete an insurance claim form is entered directly into the computer. At this point a paper copy of the insurance form could be printed and mailed. However, with EMC the insurance claim information for all patients is periodically transmitted over the telephone lines to an EMC vendor or clearinghouse. The clearinghouse audits and edits the claims received, batches claims by carrier, and then transmits clean, batched claims to the respective insurance companies or payors. The EMC vendor may also provide reports back to health care providers regarding the status of insurance claims submitted. The advantages of electronic submission of insurance claims include faster, more accurate and verifiable transmission of claims to carriers, less administrative paperwork in the office, and postage savings. Electronic fund transfers from payors to providers may soon make prompter payment another advantage.

Processing of paper insurance forms on the free-standing, in-office computer has grown steadily from 46.8% of computer users in 1984 to 73.5% of computer users in 1990. In 1988 the technology for transmitting those dental insurance forms electronically to insurance carriers was made available to dentists. Since that time dental claims cleared through the National Electronic Information Corporation have grown from 3,851 in 1988 to 137,000 in 1989 and over 355,000 in 1990. While the total volume of electronically transmitted insurance claims represents less than 1% of the 160 million dental insurance claims filed in 1990, the number of electronic media claims in dentistry is projected to grow steadily just as it did with hospitals and medical practices when the technology was introduced to those markets. The National Electronic Information Corporation (NEIC) estimates that approximately 20% of the private insurance claims from hospitals today are processed electronically. Transmission of dental insurance claims electronically will represent a quantum leap forward in the sophistication of dental office computer users. This application of telecommunications technology will provide a strong incentive for many dental offices to establish linkages to external data bases for the first time.

Enhanced Administrative and New Clinical Applications

The basic dental office management system typically includes word processing, accounting, spreadsheets, and database management software. Turnkey systems are usually designed to perform more specialized functions that meet the unique needs of medical or dental practices. A number of specialized administrative applications are growing in popularity. Technical exhibits at major dental meetings and a recent survey of trade magazine readers highlight a number of emerging new applications for computers in dental offices. Currently the most popular innovation according to the reader survey is more specialized office management software, performing tasks such as tracking insurance claims (82%), calculating patient insurance co-payments (81%), referral source monitoring (64.8%) and appointment scheduling (33.6%).[8]

In addition to streamlined and enhanced administrative applications, clinical applications are emerging as a new tool in care delivery. Examples of clinical applications cited in the reader survey include computerized health histories and treatment planning (38.5%), periodontal charting (3.3%), and other applications (3.3%) such as computer imaging and occlusal analysis.[9]

Inserted Systems to Integrated Systems

Some of the early installations of medical clinical computing systems failed because the needs of the health care workers were not addressed in the initial design. If a health care worker has to spend more time or effort to perform a patient care task using the computer than is required by conventional methods, the computer will be rejected outright. Designers of health care computer systems must have an understanding of the needs of health care workers and patients if systems are to facilitate rather than impede the delivery of care.

Some of the first generation installations in clinical settings have hardware almost identical to the reception desk. When computer terminals move from the reception desk into the treatment areas, ergonomic considerations and infection control requirements will dictate improved designs for computer hardware used in clinical settings. Computers have been plopped into business offices and treatment areas with little consideration of lighting, space, furniture height or user comfort. As consciousness is raised regarding user requirements for form, function and comfort, computer hardware should become an integrated element of the office design. Software will increasingly accommodate the logical series of steps which should occur during care delivery. New technologies such as voice entry of data and thinner video monitors will allow engineers to design systems responsive to the specified needs of health care providers.

Automation of Current Tasks to New Applications

First generation dental office management systems were designed to automate tasks traditionally managed on paper systems, such as billing, recall notices, and generating insurance claims. The computer industry appropriately responded to demand in the market place by automating routine, time-consuming and troublesome chores. Computers, with their capacity to store and manipulate large quantities of data, can perform functions that were not practical to accomplish with paper systems. For example, as administrative data bases were assembled on dental office management systems, it became possible to analyze trends in practice growth and calculate the profitability of performing various procedures. Dentists now use these features of office management systems routinely. Similarly, it would be possible to build aggregate data bases of patients' conditions and treatments, and over time the outcomes of treatment could be monitored and assessed. However, dentists have not traditionally had access to this type of clinical information, and they are not likely to articulate or demand this capability when purchasing a system today. It is an interesting chicken and egg scenario—will dentists eventually recognize the possibilities for new computer applications and demand them, or will the computer industry identify applications and bring the professional along through marketing efforts? Hopefully both forces will work in tandem, helping computers evolve to their optimum potential in providing informatic health care.

Combining Technologies to Form New Applications

The electronics industry has created new devices and applications by marrying two or three previously existing technologies. The cellular telephone is a hybrid of the traditional, wire-connected telephone and radio waves. The telecopier or FAX is a hybrid of copier machine technology and telephone lines. Similarly, technologies are being coupled to form applications useful in dentistry. The CAD/CAM system, computer assisted design/computer assisted milling, involves linking a laser lighted, miniature video camera to a computer that manipulates digitized images and also drives a robotic milling device to carve inlays and crowns from ceramic blocks. A miniature intra-oral video camera can record a moving picture of a mouth, transmit it across fiberoptic threads to a computer where the image is digitized and stored for display on a video monitor. Radiographs can be digitized and manipulated by computers to enhance the clarity of images. Traditional video cameras, connected to a computer with a specialized graphic program, offer "computer imaging" of projected results after plastic surgery, orthodontic or cosmetic dentistry treatment. By coupling existing and emerging technologies together, an infinite number of new application for dentistry may be developed.

Dental Practice in the Year 2005

In reviewing some routine tasks that are part of dentistry today, numerous administrative and clinical computer applications are possible. The following Table 4.3 summarizes how computers may change the face of dentistry as they become more integral to dental education, practice, and research. Many of these applications are technologically possible or available today—the pivotal question is how quickly these new technologies will be embraced and used by the profession.

The Role of Dental Informatics in the Evolution of Computers

The field of dental informatics is still in the process of defining itself as a discipline. Regardless of how broadly or narrowly one decides to define dental informatics, its primary goal must be to improve patient care.

Health care delivery is information-intensive, but health professionals have been slower than other industries (such as banking and retail) to exploit computers for managing the voluminous amount of data required to make the best decisions. The health care industry, including dentistry, is now poised to play catch-up to technology that has raced ahead. It will require leaders with vision and flexibility to guide the dental profession into the rapidly evolving realm of informatic health care. One of the challenges for dental informaticians is to help new electronic technology transfer into dental practices smoother and more swiftly than it might otherwise happen.

A blueprint for these activities was drafted at a 1989 conference funded by the Westinghouse Electronics Systems Group.[10] Three specific workshop groups addressed issues relating to dental practice, education, and research. The following four recurring themes were identified by the workgroups.

1) The principal focus of dental informatics applications should be on dental practice where they can impact most directly on the delivery of oral health care.

2) The profession needs to support and facilitate the process of planning for both the short and long term. At a minimum planning should take place at two levels: (a) each major dental organization should develop a strategic plan based upon its own mission and needs; (b) each of the plans should be integral to an overall plan for the entire profession.

3) Mechanisms should be developed early to ensure communication and networking among the various components of dentistry including dental professional organizations, dental schools, the dental research community, federal dental services, individual dental practitioners of general dentistry and the dental specialties, dental auxiliaries, the dental trades, other health profes-

Table 4.3. Computer applications for dental tasks.

Tasks in Dentistry	Potential Computer Applications
Dental Education, Dental Licensure Staff Training and Continuing Dental Education	Patient simulation programs to develop decision making skills and encourage life-long, independent learning; exposure to administrative and clinical computer applications available in private practice.
Patient Billing	Billing statements generated at the time of appointment; credit card processing electronically; electronic fund transfers
Dental Insurance Claims	Generate paper forms; electronic transmission of claims to insurance companies; determination of patient eligibility on-line; remittance advice returned electronically from the insurance company along with the electronic fund transfer to the dentists' bank.
Dental Patient Records	Voice entry of examination findings with visual confirmation of entries through graphic display; electronic periodontal probes and intraoral video cameras assist with data collection and store findings directly in the electronic dental record; text, image and sound data is digitized and stored in the computer for later retrieval or transmission to another health provider; patients may carry integrated circuitry health care cards containing information about their medical conditions and medications.
Literature Review	On-line access to National Library of Medicine and other bibliographic data bases.
Clinical Decision Making	Clinical assisted decision support software will selectively provide drug interaction information, differential diagnosis assistance (including color images from laser discs), and abstracts of scientific articles relevant to a specific patient's conditions.
Constructing Prosthetic Devices	Computer Assisted Design/Computer Assisted Milling devices to make crowns and inlays in one appointment. Other robotic devices may assist with surgery or tooth preparation.
Dental Radiographs	Computer enhancement of digitized radiographic images; programs will also assist with interpretation.
Ordering Office Supplies	On-line, electronic catalogs; purchasing of supplies with electronic fund transfers.

Table 4.3. (continued)

Tasks in Dentistry	Potential Computer Applications
Health Histories, Examinations and Treatment Plans	Interactive programs for patients to provide current information; electronic access to patients' medical and pharmacy records to verify past and current conditions.
Treatment Planning and Case Presentation	Computer-generated graphic displays of conditions and proposed treatments; computer imaging of face and teeth showing projected post-treatment results.
Assessing Treatment Outcomes	Aggregate data bases for each practice will be passively constructed in the routine course of filing the electronic dental patient records, making it possible to periodically review patient profiles and outcomes of treatment. Uploading these data to a regional and national aggregate data base will allow for comparisons between different population groups, treatments, and conditions (such as temporomandibular joint dysfunction).

sions, and appropriate members of the computer and telecommunications industry.

4) There is a strong need for the various sectors of the dental profession to achieve agreement on the important issue of standards related to nomenclature, classification and coding of diseases, and the size and number of database fields. There should be consensus on the issue of compatibility of information systems so connectivity can be maximized.

Organized Dentistry's Role

For purposes of this discussion, organized dentistry is defined as the American Dental Association (ADA) and its constituent and component dental societies. Although the ADA formally recognizes and has working relationships with specialty organizations, auxiliary groups, research agencies and dental educational programs, the following discussion will focus more narrowly on the ADA and its affiliated societies.

In August 1990 a Department of Information Science was established at the ADA. This department was created in recognition of the increasing use of computers within the profession and the emerging field of dental informatics. The department has described five general areas of initial activity, most of which will be implemented through existing agencies of the Association.

Monitor the Diffusion of Computers into Dental Practice and the Evolution of Computer Applications in Dentistry

The Bureau of Economic and Behavioral Research regularly surveys all practicing dentists. Questions related to the use of computers have been included on surveys since 1984. As new unanswered questions about computers in dental practices are identified, the answers can be sought through the bureau's surveys of the profession. Focus groups of computer-using dentists will also be conducted to gain insight into how dentists make decisions to integrate new computer technology into their practices.

The Association will monitor technological advances through participation in national and international informatics meetings as well as through exhibits at major dental meetings.

Develop Informational Resources to Make Dentists More Informed Consumers of Electronic Technology

The Council on Dental Practice has responsibility for issues and resources related to dental office management. It has developed written guidelines and publications about selecting dental office management systems, and it also developed a seminar on selecting dental office computers. The Association publications, the Journal of the American Dental Association and the ADA News regularly contain articles about computers in dentistry. These activities will be on-going to keep pace with new technology and applications.

Develop Information Products and Services for Members, while Upgrading Internal Information Management Resources at the Association

Information technology has applications in Association management as well as private dental practices. The Association must keep pace with advances in information technology in order to provide an acceptable level of service to its members. Applications such as voice mail, electronic mail, electronic bulletin boards and networking services will need to be phased in with a sensitivity to user and member acceptance. As dental offices become accustomed to sending and receiving information through on-line computer access, the Association and dental societies will need to make their resources available in that medium.

Review and/or Endorsement of Products and Services

The ADA and several of the state dental societies have endorsed specific vendors' computer systems. These agreements usually include legally binding requirements on the vendor regarding pricing, marketing, servicing and upgrades to the system. Dentists may feel more confident selecting a system which has undergone a review by some agency of the dental society or association. The advantage for the professional association is the potential to generate a non-dues revenue stream if the sales are successful, but the downside could be a loss of member confidence if there are problems with endorsed products or services.

With an increasing number of new, dental-related applications, the Associations and dental societies will have to evaluate regularly the pros and cons of endorsing specific products. The ADA's Council on Dental Materials, Instruments, and Equipment has already been approached by one vendor about expanding the scope of its review activities to include new electronic instruments.

Participate in Standards Setting Activities That Will Impact Practicing Dentists

As noted at the Aspen Conference, there needs to be greater agreement within the profession regarding standards for nomenclature, systems of classification, and diagnostic and treatment codes. This can be thought of as the foundation of a three-tier standards effort that is intimately interrelated. Any lack of consensus between health professions and within dentistry will sabotage all future efforts to take fullest advantage of computers and the aggregate data bases that they are capable of generating. Standardization at this basic level must be an urgent priority since the time lines on such efforts are so long.

Stepping up another level in complexity, measures of treatment outcomes need to be defined and agreed upon in order for the quality assessment efforts to evolve. Without some agreement on what desirable and measurable treatment outcomes are as an end point, it is difficult to establish clinical practice guidelines describing how to get there.

Moving into the electronic age, a third tier of standards related to computer hardware, software applications and electronic data interchange are needed to maximize connectivity and to facilitate the formation of aggregate data bases. Health professionals must become involved in the process of defining and specifying the requirements for electronic technology used in health care. Only through a collaborative effort between engineers, manufacturers and the system users can optimum results in the design of new applications be achieved.

Up to this point the vast majority of dentists have used free-standing, single application computer systems in their offices. Connectivity and compatibility have not emerged as burning concerns. Once attempts are made to connect the primary office computer electronically with other systems—either multiple in-office systems or external data bases—the need for electronic data interchange (EDI) standards will become very apparent. Solutions to these concerns will reside in standardization and specification efforts.

The American Dental Association is currently involved on all three levels of standards development. In relation to codes and nomenclature standards, the ADA's Council on Dental Care Programs maintains the Code of Dental Procedures and Nomenclature.[11] It also participates in the development of dental diagnostic codes contained in the ICD-9.

A new activity was undertaken in 1990 to develop "practice parameters." Practice parameters will attempt to describe the entire range of acceptable treatments for selected conditions, based upon the best scientific knowledge and professional judgement. A special committee on parameter development will integrate dental informatics into its methods as it is timely and appropriate.

Finally, electronic media claims (EMC) processing for dental insurance was introduced to the dental market around 1988. Since then the need for electronic data interchange (EDI) standards in that area has become more apparent. The American National Standards Institute (ANSI) X-12 Committee is the setting where the insurance carriers, provider groups, and system vendors are working on EDI standards for determining patient eligibility, claims submission and claims payment. The American Dental Association has become a voting member of the ANSI X-12 Committee and participates actively in the process. If these efforts are successful, the benefits may be invisible to dentists who take for granted that EMC software on their computers can talk to all dental insurance companies and clearinghouses.

The only thing certain in the fields of health care computing and dental informatics will be change. As computer-using dentists become a majority in the profession, and as computer applications become more sophisticated and complex, issues and concerns related to the use of computers will be identified and directed to the professional associations for action. The challenges ahead are great, but so are the opportunities.

References

1. American Dental Association, Chicago, Il: Dental Practice Outlook (Vol. III, No. 10, October 1990, p. l).
2. ibid, p. 2.
3. American Dental Association, Chicago, IL: 1988 Survey of Dental Practice.
4. ibid.
5. American Dental Association, Chicago, IL: Dental Practice Outlook (Vol. III, No. 10, October 1990, p. 2).
6. ibid, p. 4.
7. ibid, p. 2.
8. Dental Products Report, December 1990, p. 83.
9. ibid.
10. Salley, J.J., Zimmerman, J.L., Ball, M.J. eds. Dental Informatics: Strategic Issues for the Dental Profession, 1990, p. 75.
11. Report from the Council on Dental Care Programs, Journal of the American Dental Association, January 1991 (Vol. 122 No. 1:114-134)

5
Dental Informatics and the Delivery of Dental Care

Howard L. Bailit

Introduction

Computer-based management information systems are bringing about fundamental changes in many industries. Some well-known examples include American Airline's SABRE reservation system,[1] Otis Elevator's computer diagnostic repair service,[2] and Frito Lay's electronic inventory retrieval system.[3] These companies have used information in new ways and have gained a major competitive advantage in the market place. Indeed, the innovative use of information is now a critical success factor in business, and many companies have appointed Chief Information Officers to develop and implement information strategies.

The innovative use of computers to collect, process, retrieve, analyze, and present information is also certain to have a profound influence on the structure of the health care delivery system. Health care organizations such as hospitals, large group practices, and their suppliers are already heavily invested in computers for fiscal administration, general operations and increasingly, patient care.

This is just the beginning. The health care system is undergoing rapid restructuring in an effort to control the rise in costs. This is seen in the dramatic growth of managed care programs, such as Health Maintenance Organizations (HMOs), and the increasing government control over provider fees and medical technology. The success of many of these efforts are dependent on the effective use of information technology.

In addition, some companies such as Spectrum Systems, a joint venture between IBM and Baxter, and National Data Corporation are developing electronic connections among providers, payers, suppliers, and other components of the delivery system so that information can be quickly and cheaply transferred among these units.[4] These interconnections increase the efficiency of the delivery system by decreasing administrative costs (such as claims processing).

Of even greater importance, the data collected in these online systems has great heuristic and economic value and is leading to a "re-engineering" of the health care system. For example, a new industry is developing to collect and analyze health data and sell it back to practitioners, managed care companies, medical equipment and service suppliers, and others as information. The connections among delivery components may also lead to the formation of new types of organizations that are linked by a common information system as a network of hospitals and associated medical practices may be in the future.

To date, the dental care system has had little involvement in the information revolution, but for reasons that will become apparent, this is about to change. The purpose of this chapter is to examine the current trends in the delivery of personal dental services, to explore the implications of these trends for computerized dental records, and to speculate on the future of electronic dental practice systems.

Trends in the Dental Delivery System

The successful application of information technology to the dental care delivery system depends, in large part, on having a fundamental understanding of how dental care is provided in the United States. Emphasis is on delivery system features that will influence the establishment of electronic practice information systems. This section also focuses on the basic differences between the dental and medical care systems in relation to how services are financed, organized, and delivered.

Financing Care

The financing of dental care in the United States comes mainly from private funds. Of the $29 billion spent in 1988 for personal dental services, less than 3 percent (ca. $700 million) was publicly financed (mainly Medicaid).[5] Thus, unlike medicine, federal and state governments have little direct influence on the purchasing or delivery of dental services. As long as government faces severe budgetary restrictions, dental care can be expected to continue as a predominantly privately financed service. This also means that dentistry, in contrast to medicine, will not be affected by the regulatory and financial restrictions that are now being imposed on the Medicare and Medicaid programs.

Americans pay for dental care all or partly out-of-pocket.[5] Approximately 110 million people have group dental insurance as a benefit of employment. This compares to 182 million people with private hospital insurance. Although there is a large untapped market for dental insurance, with the problems of rapidly growing medical costs, most employers are not interested in expanding employee benefits. Indeed, they are having great difficulty just keeping up with the 15 to 25 percent premium increases for current health insurance programs seen in the last few years.

To deal with this problem, employers are giving employees financial incentives to join HMOs and Preferred Provider Organizations (PPO)s, increasing employee cost sharing (often with higher deductibles), and reducing the services covered by health plans. In fact, the numbers of people enrolled in dental plans has declined somewhat in the past few years.[5]

For those with dental benefits, insurance pays approximately 44 percent of charges.[5] This percentage is actually increasing and may reflect some modest expansion of dental benefit plans to cover new services such as adult orthodontics.

Organization of Delivery System

Almost all dental care is delivered in owner-run, solo or small group practices.[6] Although many hospitals have dental departments, these are usually limited operations, staffed with volunteers and residents.

Approximately 66 percent of practices consist of one dentist.[6] Another 21 percent of practitioners are in two dentist offices, and the rest are in groups with three or more dentists. There are very few large groups with five or more dentists.

Unlike medicine, the growth of dental group practice is quite slow, so that solo practices will predominate for the foreseeable future. The reasons for this are not really known, but a few explanations seem plausible. First, group practices may not offer substantial economies of scale in delivering dental care: larger practices do not appear to be more efficient, therefore they do not have a competitive advantage over solo offices.[7] Second, the cost of starting a solo practice is rather modest - less than $100,000 - and therefore, affordable to individual clinicians. Finally, most dentists may prefer to be "their own boss" and work alone.

Of course, this propensity for solo practices could change as dental technology evolves. That is, if starting a dental practice required purchasing a million dollars of equipment, then dentists could not afford to practice alone. With the recent development of expensive and complex computer-assisted systems to prepare teeth for restorations and to mill replacement fillings and crowns, the cost of developing and operating dental practices could change. This technology is still experimental but shows great promise and if successful, could lead to the growth of group practices.

So far, managed care has had little impact on the organization of the dental delivery system. First, few staff/group-model HMOs, such as Kaiser, have established large group practices to provide dental services. Second, although several major insurers and state and local dental societies have started dental health maintenance and preferred provider organizations, it is estimated that less than 10 million people are enrolled in these plans.[8] Further, the plans are usually made up of networks of solo or small group practices: any one provider may belong to several networks, and most continue to spend the majority of their time treating non-managed care patients. So far, managed care has not led to the development of larger dental organizations either by linking solo dental offices to form new practice units or by organizing group practices.

The insurance industry is watching the dental managed care business very carefully. Two large carriers, Prudential and CIGNA, have invested heavily in dental HMOs and have been successful in enrolling customers from their indemnity plans into these new delivery organizations. However, managed dental care capacity has not led to significant shifts in dental market share among insurers. To date then, managed dental care is a relatively small business for most major insurers. Whether or not it eventually becomes the predominate method for delivering dental care remains to be seen.

Dentists and Dental Practice

Number and Types of Dentists

There are approximately 147,000 dentists in the United States, and 90 percent of them work in private practices that they own by themselves or with other dentists. The total number of practices is about 110,000.[6]

Starting in 1978, the number of applicants to dental school began to decline, and this has continued until the present time. As a result, 37 percent fewer students graduate from dental schools now compared to 12 years ago. In several areas of the country the dentist-to-population ratio is declining, as fewer dentists enter practice, and by the year 2000 this will be common-place.[9] This means that the dental delivery system is beginning a major contraction, and there will be thousands of fewer dentists over the next 20 years.

Eighty-five percent of dentists are generalists.[6] The percentage of specialists is increasing slowly and will not exceed 20 percent within the next 10 years. This is in direct contrast to medicine where 80 percent of practitioners are specialists. So, the great majority of dentists will continue to be solo, general practitioners.

Practice Income

The income generated from the average solo, general practice was $254,000 in 1988.[6] With 65 percent of revenues going to overhead, the average general dentist had a pretax practice income of $87,000 which is substantially less than the $117,000 earned by the average physician.[10] For the past few years the rate of increase in dentists' incomes has approached those of physicians, and in the future may even surpass physicians' as government and managed care programs focus on controlling medical care costs.

The net income generated by practices is almost entirely dependent on the dentists' business and clinical abilities and personal ambition. Dentists have little opportunity to improve their efficiency by substituting technology, capital, or labor (beyond the use of the usual support staff). However, as noted previously, the introduction of new dental technologies and the associated growth of large group practices could change this. As the size of dental firms increase, the efficiencies gained from computerized information systems could well be significant.

Staff and Facilities

The average owner practitioner has a staff of 3.5: one or more secretary, dental assistants and a part-time dental hygenist.[6] The support staff have a high turnover rate with the average dentist losing 48 percent of his/her staff in 12 months.[11] Most solo practice facilities consist of two operatories where the dentist and part-time hygenist provide care, and a reception and business area.[6]

Use of Computers

The percentage of dentists using computers is estimated to be between 20 to 30 percent with slow but steady growth.[12] Computers are used primarily for fiscal administration such as billing, accounts receivable, and accounts payable. There are many regional software vendors of dental practice packages, and no one vendor appears to have a large share of the market. Most vendors have adapted small business systems for application in dental offices.

The use of decision-assist systems to guide dentists or their staff in making better fiscal and clinical decisions is just beginning. There are a few such programs, but they have not had wide distribution.[13,14,15] In large part, this is because most operate as stand-alone systems and therefore are not convenient to use.

Demand for Care

The demand for dental care appears to be increasing and this will accelerate after 1995 and continue well past the turn-of-the-century. The primary reasons for the increasing demand are:

- With a marked reduction in the dentist to population ratio, each practitioner will have more patients.
- The elderly without teeth are low users of dental care. Now, fewer senior citizens are becoming edentulous, and those with teeth are using care as frequently as younger cohorts.[16] In addition, the elderly are becoming more affluent and educated, two factors commonly associated with greater use of dental services.
- Patients are seeking new and more expensive tests and procedures. Examples include new dental materials, diagnostic tests for microflora, and tooth transplants and implants.
- The attitudes of the American people about oral health appear to be improving, and they are demanding higher levels of oral health. This is seen in the growing percentage of people visiting dentists one or more times per year and the greater number of visits for those going to dentists.[17]

With greater demand and fewer dentists, the rate of increase in dental incomes will grow, and dentists will be more affluent. This also suggests that dentists will have less interest in joining managed care plans, since they will not need to reduce prices to gain adequate numbers of patients.

Implications for Computerized Dental Record Systems

This analysis of current trends in the dental care delivery system has several important implications for the development of electronic dental records, especially for the industry that develops to sell and support these systems and the specific features of dental practice information systems.

Electronic Dental Record Industry

1. Size of Potential Market

The dental delivery system is relatively small and will decrease in size over the next 20 years. Even if one software vendor were to capture a large percentage of the dental market, say five percent, it would mean some 5,000 practices. This is a relatively small number and few companies may want to invest a great deal of money developing software and associated distribution systems that are unique to dentistry. This suggests that a successful computerized record system for dentistry is likely to be adapted from a medical record system and distributed by a vendor interested in several health professions. This would greatly enlarge the potential market for software vendors.

2. Marketing Costs

The cost of marketing software to dentists will be very high. This is because most dentists are in solo practice and will only buy one copy of a program. Each sale will require considerable time and effort from sales people. An attractive alternative might be to sell dental record software by mail or from local software retail stores. The problem with this solution for most dentists is the need for local support to install and maintain systems.

3. Installation, Training, and Support

The installation and training costs for electronic dental records will be relatively high, and dentists cannot afford to spend a great deal of money on this technology. With solo offices predominating, the installation will require a team of people going to each office and converting paper records, fiscal and patient, to electronic. Further, dentists and their staffs need to be trained, and once the programs are operating, they need continuous support. The latter will be a substantial problem since most dentists and their staffs do not have a strong background in computers, and the average tenure for staff is less than two years.

Considering that solo dentists have modest incomes and that they need to have computers in at least three rooms (two operatories and a business area) to use this technology efficiently, many practitioners may not be able to pay for the installation and continued maintenance of a fully electronic record system based on three microcomputers and a local area network.

Perhaps, as hardware and software costs decrease and as a local software support industry develops for all health practitioners, these problems will become less important. In addition, dentists will become more affluent and may be able to afford more expensive computer technology.

It may also be that conventional thinking on how electronic record systems will operate for solo providers will need to be re-examined. One alternative is discussed later.

4. Relation to Managed Care

Managed care companies could become a vehicle for distributing and servicing computer technology and decision-assist systems to practitioners. Indeed, this appears to be happening in medicine. However, this is unlikely to happen in dentistry.

With the increasing demand for dental services, managed care programs may not have much impact on the dental delivery system. This is because dentists will be in a very strong position negotiating with managed care companies and will not be willing to significantly discount prices, accept restrictions on referrals to specialists, or comply with stringent utilization management requirements.

This scenario could change under some circumstances. For example, the government has tried (and so far failed) to tax employee health benefits beyond a certain level as income. Thus, employer contributions for health premiums of more than some level, say $250/month per family, would be taxed as income. If this were to happen, many employees would opt out of dental and pharmacy plans in favor of medical/ surgical plans. The net effect would be reduced demand for dental care, and with reduced demand, interest in managed care plans would increase.

Another possibility that would decrease the relative demand for dental care is changing state laws to expand the practice of dental hygenists to restore teeth or to function as independent practitioners. This would greatly expand the supply of dental services and therefore, decrease absolute demand.

The interest groups that are against the tax on health benefits and the expansion of dental hygenists' duties are so formidable that these two changes in the dental delivery system are improbable at best. This suggests that managed care is unlikely to capture a significant share of the dental market in the foreseeable future.

Features of Electronic Dental Record Systems

Setting aside all the market place constraints in developing electronic dental records, there are a number of features that must be included in the record system to have it acceptable to dentists.

5. Integration of Fiscal and Clinical Records

It is unreasonable to expect that dentists and their staffs would accept clinical record systems that are separate from fiscal programs. Separate systems would require double key entry of basic patient demographic data, and many files are needed for both clinical and fiscal management (e.g., treatments planned and received). On this basis an acceptable record package must include fully integrated clinical and fiscal management programs.

6. Clinical Record Content

The accounting profession has established a standard data set needed for effective review of the fiscal operation of businesses including dental practices. This is not true when it comes to the clinical treatment of patients. There is no such thing as an American Dental Association recommended clinical record or data set that should be collected on each patient or types of patients. It is no surprise then that there is great variation among practices in the types and amount of data collected and stored.

This means that it will be very difficult to get the average dentist to adhere to one fixed clinical record format. A successful record will allow customization of the record format and the types and amount of data collected.

7. Practice Efficiency

Dentists will be unlikely to make a large investment in computer hardware and software unless there is strong evidence that this technology will result in higher practice incomes. Incomes can increase as a result of reducing the cost of producing technical dental services or the cost of administering the practice.

At this time, it is not at all clear that an electronic fiscal and clinical information system will reduce the cost of producing services. That is, the time and effort needed to insert an amalgam restoration is unlikely to change with the use of computerized patient records.

Further, electronic systems are unlikely to save much money by reducing the inefficiencies associated with paper records. This because dentists take radiographs on all patients and plaster casts on many. These have to be physically stored and retrieved. Perhaps, over time, the radiographs and casts will be stored electronically, but this will be many years in the future.

Some savings may come from the processing of dental insurance claims electronically with direct linkages between the computers of dentists and insurers. Online electronic checking of patient eligibility and adjudication of claims are now commonplace in hospitals and retail pharmacies and will soon be seen in most medical and dental practices. Insurers and other managed care companies are moving aggressively ahead in this area. Still, dentists are not going to achieve major efficiencies through online claims processing.

Also, as previously noted, incomes from dental practices are very dependent on dentists' ability and ambition, and this will not change with the introduction of computers. The question then becomes, how will electronic records make dental practices more efficient? As long as the majority of dental practices are solo and current dental technology continues, there is no obvious answer to this question.

This also suggests that a successful electronic information system will have to have other features that make it advantageous for dentists. As will be discussed next, the major advantage of computerized record systems may well come from the use of decision-assist systems and the electronic linkages among practices and their payers, suppliers, and even patients.

8. Decision-Assist Systems

For both fiscal and clinical decision-making solo dentists must rely on the knowledge they have obtained during their training and from continued education once through training. This problem takes on two dimensions: knowledge needed for the care of individual patients and knowledge needed to assess the fiscal operation of the practice and care provided to aggregates of patients.

Individual Patients

In a busy solo or group practice it is difficult to stop in the middle of treating patients and to seek advice from colleagues or check the latest literature. Decision-assist systems that are fully integrated within computerized patient records have great potential for solving this problem. These systems will provide dentists immediate access to information that is directly related to the care of a specific patient. Some of these systems are passive and require dentists to purposively seek assistance. Others actively read the information collected and offer recommendations on the care of patients.

When fully developed, these knowledge-based systems are expected to assist dentists in making better decisions for almost all areas of clinical practice. Examples include deciding what information to collect on patients with a history of serum hepatitis, the differential diagnosis of white lesions on the dorsum of the tongue, the preferred antibiotic for the treatment of a chronic periapical abscess, and the design of a partial denture.

Clinical decision-assist systems are relatively advanced in medicine and at least one is fully integrated with an electronic medical record. It is only a question of time before these knowledge-based systems are available to dentists.

Aggregates of Patients

Dentists have very little fiscal and almost no clinical data on aggregates of patients. This is because the cost of collecting and analyzing data from paper records is very expensive. A related problem is that most dentists have never been trained to use data on groups of patients.

On the financial side, dentists use accountants and other business specialists to assist them in collecting and interpreting aggregate data such as cash flow, production costs, taxes, and more generally practice efficiency. These specialists have to gather data from practices manually in order to assess the fiscal health of practices and to make recommendations. This is an expensive process, because of the time needed to collect and analyze data.

Interestingly, there are no counterparts to accountants on the clinical side; no consultants are employed to evaluate practices and make recommendations that will improve the quality of care provided to patients.

With access to a computerized fiscal and clinical data-base, decision-assist systems can help dentists analyze their practices and to solve administrative and clinical problems. On the fiscal side the decision-assist system substitutes to some degree for accountant services. On the clinical side decision-assist systems can provide dentists with insights on the effectiveness of their care of patients. Examples include the longevity of different restorative materials, the long-term impact of preventive programs on plaque levels, or the types of patient complaints following root canal treatment.

This suggest that electronic practice information systems that incorporate fiscal and clinical decision-assist systems might be quite attractive to practitioners. These systems could reduce the use of accountants and be of great value to dentists in diagnosing and treating patients and in assessing the effectiveness of their treatments, retrospectively. Indeed, computerized record system are likely to have a major impact on improving the quality of care provided to patients.

9. Query Systems and Normative Data

A related issue is the need to have simple query systems that will allow dentists to quickly and efficiently generate customized reports on the fiscal and clinical operations of their practices. The value of query systems would be greatly enhanced if dentists had access to normative data from other practices nationally or from the same general geographic area. Currently, dentists have little information on their own practices and even less on others. Without access to comparative data, it is difficult for them to evaluate the meaning of their own information.

10. System Reliability

A successful system must be very reliable, since dentists cannot afford to have their systems down for more than a few hours. This also means that hardware and software vendors must have local and easily accessible maintenance and repair systems that can respond quickly when systems do go down.

11. User Friendly

It is obvious that the complex fiscal and clinical information system just described must, at the same time, be very easy to learn and use. This is because with a small staff and high turnover, most dentists are not in a position to spend hours training new staff to use electronic record systems. Further, most dentists may not take the time to master a very complex system, let alone teach their staff. This also means that practices need to have immediate access to program experts to assist them in dealing with technical problems.

Future of Electronic Dental Record Systems

The previous section raised problems that must be overcome for computerized record systems to become established in dental practices. These obstacles will be overcome, but no one can predict exactly how this new technology will become established in dental practices. However, some predictions are possible.

The development and distribution of electronic dental record systems may be taken over by companies that are in the electronic transfer of information business. Many of these companies are large and well-known such as American Express, National Data Corp, and GTE. An excellent example of how these companies may impact dentistry is now seen in the retail pharmacy business.

Approximately 70 percent of the 55,000 pharmacies in this country are electronically linked to payers. This permits electronic checking of patient eligibility, transfer of claim information, transfer of payments, and some utilization management. It is only a question of time before the electronic link from physicians to pharmacies takes place, further increasing the efficiency of the system.

Some of the companies doing the electronic hook-ups are also selling pharmacy management systems at low cost to pharmacies. These companies also provide the training and service needed to support pharmacies in their use of these systems.

The reason that these companies are able to offer services to pharmacies relatively cheaply is that in addition to the charges to the pharmacies and the payers for transferring the information and adjudicating claims, they also make money from selling the information captured from the pharmacies. In addition, they use "expert systems" which they have developed to analyze the data, allowing them to increase the value of the information when sold to others.

Those interested in the data include drug manufacturers who need to understand how their products are being used which, in turn, enhances their ability to market them. This is also true for other suppliers of goods sold in the pharmacies. It may be surprising, but the pharmacies themselves want access to the data especially after sophisticated data analyses that allow them to run more profitable operations.

The point is that the key to making computers cost-effective in dental practices may be the secondary use of the information generated from these systems. This will allow companies to install and support the technology in solo practices at relatively nominal costs to dentists.

Indeed, a new industry is developing in the United States to electronically link all major components of the delivery system, to install and service practice management systems, to undertake extensive analyses of the data captured from the clinical and fiscal management programs in order to increase its value, and to sell the enhanced data.

It is only a question of time before dental practices are involved in these electronic networks. The long-run impact of these networks and the general information revolution on the practice of dentistry is unknown, but it is certain to be profound.

References

1. Hopper, M. New ways to compete on information. Harvard Bus. Rev. May/June 1990;118-125.
2. Ives, B. and Vitale, M. After the sale:Leveraging maintenance with information technology. MIS Qtrly. 1988;12(1):7-21.
3. Winkler, C. More sales, fewer "stales". Comput. Decis. 1988;20(11):26-27.
4. Kennedy, O. Info systems head toward central decision-making. Modern Hlth. Care 1990;20(27):32-37.
5. Office of National Cost Estimates. National health expenditures, 1988. Hlth. Care Fin. Rev. 1990;11(4):1-41.

6. Bureau of Economic and Behavioral Research. The 1989 Survey of Dental Practice. American Dental Association, 1990.

7. Douglass, C. and Lipscombe, J. Are larger dental practices more efficient: an analysis of dental services production. Hlth. Serv. Res. 1986;21:635-661.

8. Personal Communication with Kent Nash, American Dental Association, 1991.

9. Solomon, E.S. Dentists and dentist-to-population ratios. Manpower project. Washington, DC, American Association of Dental Schools, 1988.

10. Owens, A. Earnings: are you one of those losing ground? Med. Econ. Sept. 1989;4:131-150.

11. Bader, J. Auxiliary turnover in 13 dental offices. JADA. 1982;104:307-312.

12. Abbey, L. Dental practice for the twenty-first century. Unpublished paper presented at the National Conference on Dental Informatics. Aspen Institute Wye Center, Wye, MD, 1989 August 14-16.

13. Hyman, J. Doblecke, W. Computerized endodontic diagnosis. J. Amer. Dent. Assoc. 1983;107:755-758.

14. Abbey, L. An expert system for oral diagnosis. J. Dent. Educ. 1987;51(8):475-480.

15. Bailit, H. and Truax, T. Dental Clinician: A computerized patient record. J. Dent. Prac. Admin. July/Sept. 1990.

16. Evashwick, C. and Douglas, L. Factors related to utilization of dental services by the elderly. Amer. J. Publ. Hlth. 1976;72(10):1129-1135.

17. National Center for Health Statistics. Department of Health and Human Services. Data from the National Health Interview Survey, 1966-1987.

6
The Use of Information Technology for Continuous Improvement of Patient Care

Ina-Veronika Wagner

Introduction

In spite of the fact that in many countries dental care has reached a high standard, much can still be improved in regard to optimal care for patients. Extensive analyses of dental practice have revealed that the development of an appropriate computer-based workstation could contribute to improved patient care. The main purpose of introducing such a workstation should be to support the dentist in the domains of diagnosis, therapy, and prevention.

Dental care can further be enhanced by improved continuing dental education. It is well known that too often the desired outcome of conventional continuing education is difficult to measure and unrelated to the large amount of organizational, professional and economic effort required. The development of continuing dental education programs using computer-assisted interactive multimedia technology appears to be a major breakthrough.

Work Analyses in the Dental Practice

Extensive work analyses performed by the author in a number of dental practices[1] have revealed that there are four main problem areas in dental care:

1. The specialty-specific, selective design of the dental patient record in most cases does not allow an integrated approach to diagnosis and treatment of orofacial problems. In addition, the different elements of the patient record are not easily available.

2. Lack of decision support for diagnosis and therapy.

3. Inadequate monitoring of continuous patient recall.

4. Insufficient psychological and pedagogical guidance for patients.

Today we know that these problems can be solved to a large extent by an adequately designed computer based workstation for the dental unit.

The Dental Patient Record

3.1. The Conventional Dental Patient Record

Medical and dental history, anatomic, functional and radiographic status, treatment plans, and daily treatment and progress notes are the key parts of the patient record. A precise and complete medical record is also a necessity from a legal "standpoint". A look at daily practice, however, reveals that deficient patient records are rather common. The reasons for this unsatisfactory situation are manifold.

In order to handle patient records properly even in a busy practice, the following requirements must be fulfilled:

- Updating of the medical record must be simple and straightforward.
- The various parts of the medical record (including X-rays) needed for the treatment must be immediately available and accessible in a synoptic, comprehensible and easily managable way.

Updating the patient record by the dentist at the chairside is not appropriate from both a time and ergonomic point of view. The dental work sequence would be: disinfect, examine, disinfect, note, disinfect and so forth. Such a sequence would be impossible in a well run practice.

Ergonmically it is much better if the notation into the patient record is performed by the dental assistant or secretary by writing from dictation. This mode has two disadvantages:

- When taking dictation, the dental assistant is confined to the desk and can, therefore, not work at the dental unit.
- Due to the many detailed findings, errors are inevitably introduced.

The multiplicity of status sheets and billing forms hampers integrated thinking during diagnosis and therapy in dentistry. Tracing the sequence of treatments is especially difficult when patients are seen frequently. Many of these problems can be eliminated, to a large extent, by a well organized, well-tuned dental team. This system is out of tune when an experienced dental assistant gets sick or the dentist must be replaced temporarily. Consequently there is a problem with reliability and continuity that must be addressed when new approaches to the patient record are contemplated.

The Concept of a Computer-Based Dental Patient Record

Until now, one of the greatest obstacles to computer use during the treatment was the problem of data entry. Using conventional computer techniques, information is dictated to an assistant keying the data into the keyboard of a standard computer terminal or a PC. Thus the above-mentioned disadvantages of data registration in the case of conventional record keeping remain. To some extent, they are even worsened by handling the keyboard and adaptation to a rigid, sequential computer dialogue which often is more cumbersome and time consuming than using paper and pencil. Data entry with a digitizer reduces the use of a keyboard and has been shown to be much better suited for the assistant (Figure 6.1).

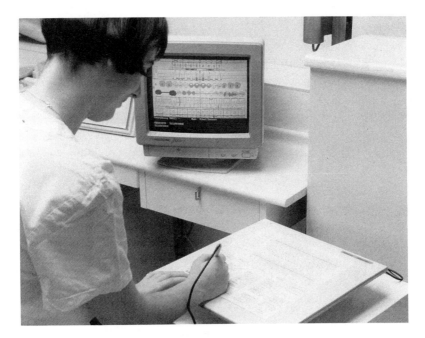

Figure 6.1. Data updating by digitizer.

By far the ergonomically effective solution to the data entry problem would be one which allows the dentist to dictate the data directly into the computer and receive instant verification, thus allowing full concentration on the patient and manual clinical tasks. It is possible to attach a microphone unobtrusively on the frame of eye glasses or even on an ear attachment (Figure 6.2). In order to avoid constant interruption of examination routines by the examiner viewing the screen to ensure correct data, a so-called earphone (voice repeater) should be used. This allows the dentist to verify the data captured by the computer without having to interrupt the examination and refocus the eyes on the screen.

A workstation that addresses the four problem areas in dental care must include an appropriately large presentation area with high resolution. The clinical circumstances and work habits determine the actual layout of the presentation area (Figure 6.3). The exhibiting oral status graphics as well as the X-rays should therefore always be presented on the upper part of the screen throughout the treatment session at the dental unit. The lower part of the screen must allow room for diagnosis, therapy planning, and progress documentation. If, in addition, visual decision support (as described later in this chapter) is required, it can be viewed on the right half of the screen, including the area reserved for X-rays.

Based on recent results in the field of human-computer interaction research[2] the patient's name, age, and risk factors should always be displayed and remain displayed in the same place on the screen, preferably in the horizontal margin at

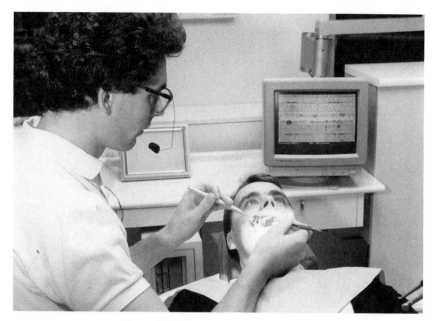

Figure 6.2. Data updating by voice input.

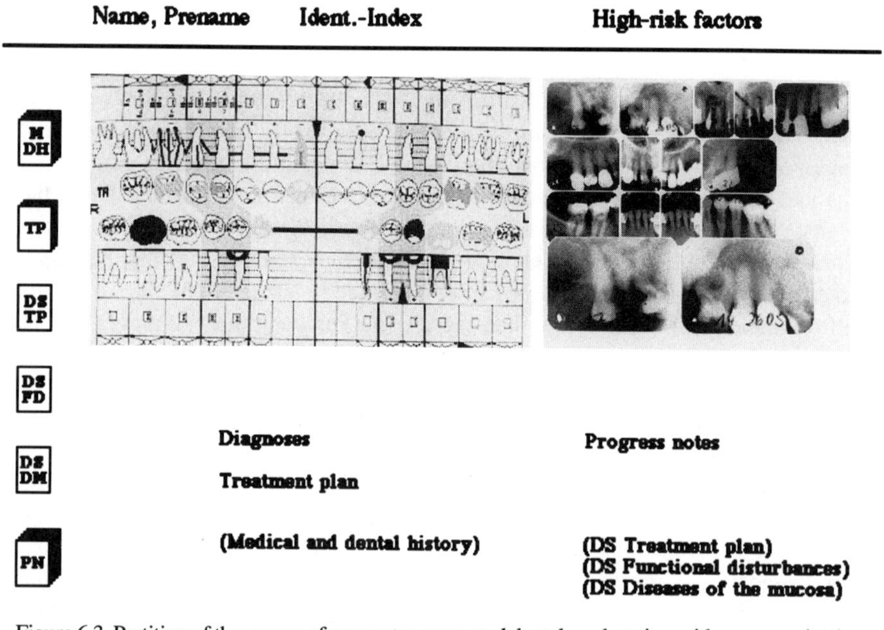

Name, Prename   Ident.-Index   High-risk factors

Diagnoses   Progress notes

Treatment plan

(Medical and dental history)   (DS Treatment plan)
(DS Functional disturbances)
(DS Diseases of the mucosa)

Figure 6.3. Partition of the screen of computer supported dental workstation with a appropriately large presentation area with high resolution as prerequisite. Calling functions of the modules not constantly presented on the screen. MDH - patient history; TP - former treatment plans; DS TP - decision support treatment plan; DS FD - decision support functional disturbances; DS DM - decision support diseases of the oral mucosa; PN - progress notes.

the top. In the left margin of the screen, icons can be placed for activation by voice input or digitizer. These icons are for presentation of additional patient information and other workstation functions.

Medical and Dental History

This part of the dental patient record should include a comprehensive summary of data concerning the patient's general health that is directly relevant to the care delivered in dental practices:

- drug regimen
- cardiovascular diseases
- coagulation problems
- allergies
- liver and kidney diseases
- immuno-compromised states
- sexually transmitted diseases (AIDS)
- infectious diseases
- pregnancy

Of course it must be easy and convenient to add and retrieve additional data (such as data concerning serious illness). The selection and presentation of the medical and dental historical data must be done in such a way that the patient's chief complaint, the reason for the visit, past dental experiences (frequency of visits and previous treatments), dental phobia and family history can be adequately considered in regard to dental treatment planning.

The dentist should further be able to classify a patient as "at risk" by marking specific history data with the label "watch". This should cause an automatic display of these data by the system in the horizontal margin at the top of the screen whenever data concerning such a patient is presented in one or another way.

Graphical Presentation of the Oral Status

The documentation of oral status in the form of graphic symbol markers is a method that has been used in most practices. Empirically, the synoptical comprehensibility of the complete medical status is facilitated by the use of different colors and easily-understood symbols. It has also been shown that complete presentation of coronal, periodontal and radiographic status in graphics promotes integrated, clinical thinking and simplifies the treatment planning. Use of conventional computer techniques implies an alphanumeric (not graphic) presentation of oral status on a monochrome screen or on computer printouts and the use of formal language coded expressions. The consequence for the clinician is a cognitive decoding effort combined with loss of information. Thus an alphanumeric presentation hampers the dentist in getting an overview of the oral status. The use of such a presentation technique encourages selective, tooth-referenced thinking, particularly among less experienced dentists.

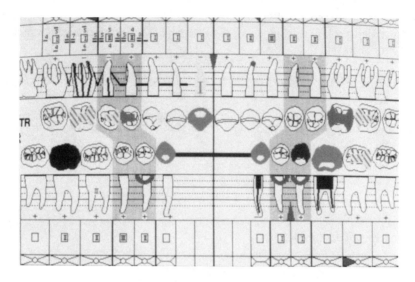

Figure 6.4. Graphical documentation of the oral status.

A computer-supported workstation for dental practice, therefore, should emphasize human information processing performance by building upon people's genuine perceptual ability.

Visualization of the oral status can of course be done in many different ways. A thoroughly elaborated and well assessed form is the one recommended by a special working group within the German Association of Dentists (Arbeitsgemeinschaft für Funktionsdiagnostik, Deutsche Gesellschaft für Zahn-, Mund- und Kieferheilkunde). Of course it had to be subject to partial modification in order to derive the full benefit of computer graphics. Missing teeth are, for example, simply removed from the graphics instead of being crossed out. Other modifications were made in order to further improve the comprehensibility and to include presentation of the periodontal and mucogingival status (Figure 6.4). It should be possible to indicate the probing depth and bleeding by a 2-, 4- or 6-point scale. The registration of plaque should be possible in a 2- or 4-point scale of the area. The graphics detail the following:

- coronal status (caries, restorations, vitality)
- periodontal status (plaque, bleeding, probing depth, tooth mobility, furcation classification)
- mucogingival status
- radiographic status in which the bone loss is also visualized

Handling and Presentation of Radiographs

Radiographs present special handling problems especially when serial films are to be viewed with long term treatment-intensive patients. A computer workstation

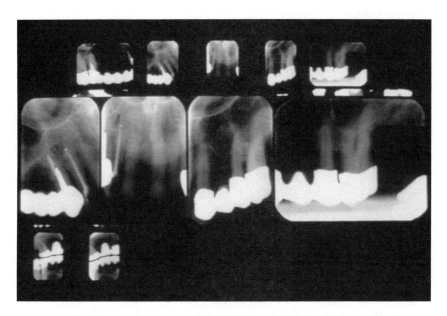

Figure 6.5. X-ray presentation with selective magnification for comparison.

should realize improvements in this area. Thus, in a clinical view, it is desirable that alongside the oral status graphic, all the relevant X-rays be displayed on the screen during the consultation or treatment of the patient. Through such a simultaneous presentation, a quick review of the clinical picture is possible and the treatment planning becomes easier as well. In addition, routines should be available for magnifying single pictures and for comparing groups of pictures side-by-side (Figure 6.5). With a scanner camera, it is readily possible to digitize conventional X-rays into the computer, without loss of quality. The time, equipment, and economic investment for the input of the X-rays is low. The practical relevance of this method for X-ray presentation and handling can readily be assessed. Of course, the image handling should be controlled by voice input.

Handling and Presentation of the Progress Notes

An important and extensive part of the patient record are progress notes, the sum of all the progress data that is relevant from a medico-legal point of view. This data also serves as a basis for billing. Thus, computer-supported billing systems should be subordinated as subsystems of the medical documentation. Unfortunately, up to now the situation has been the opposite, since billing is the foremost purpose of most current dental computer systems. Thus the aim of a computer-supported workstation must be both to document patient treatment in accord with the needs and duty of the dentist and to link up with various billing systems. Under no circumstances should progress notes be dictated from the billing system, since the data used is too sparse to be useful.

The data for daily progress notation should be entered by voice input or by the digitizer. The module for progress documentation should be designed so that after designating a specific procedure, a menu (such as "bridge" or "extraction") appears on the screen with sub-menus that include all steps for proper documentation (professional and business). The data for billing can be generated from the treatment documentation by connection to a billing system.

Patient Recall

At the completion of therapy, the dentist should place the patient on an automated recall system. A graphic presentation of the patient's status at completion of treatment should serve as a basis for aftercare. Furthermore, prevention-oriented recall schedules, that take into consideration individual risk for caries and/or periodontal diseases, can contribute to optimal aftercare. Such recall schedules can be generated from the system's clinical parameters and should be simultaneously available with the graphics detailing the dental and periodontal condition and the treatment plan.

Computer-Based Decision Support in the Dental Practice

Extensive analyses of dental practice have revealed a number of situations where the dentist is severely hampered in making decisions due to the unavailability of reference material. These situations arise in diagnosis, treatment and preventive phases of care.

Modern computer scientists enthusiastically promulgate application of AI techniques as the salvation for problems related to decision-making. Thus in most areas of human activity so-called knowledge-based systems, especially expert systems and expert critiquing systems, are increasingly available. There is no doubt that AI techniques are of great potential value for the construction of tools for decision support. As will be shown, however, they are not the only techniques. Of even greater importance is the fact that, independent of the technique eventually applied, any successful solution to a problem related to decision-making requires careful analysis of the problem situation in regard to what information is needed to make a decision and how that information should be handled. It is necessary to delineate the human and the computer's role according to respective strengths and weaknesses. The dentist should be able to work and communicate with the computer in a human way, which would not interfere with his/her need to concentrate on the actual task and which allows full use of unique human information handling and processing capabilities.

What are the areas where an improvement in the decision-making process would be useful? Which technique(s) are best for solving the various problems encountered?

From a scientific point of view, the design of advanced, domain specific computer and electronic media based decision support systems is by far the most interesting. It must be pointed out, however, that the most important step in improving decision-making in dentistry is to make the different parts of the patient record immediately available and accessible in a synoptic, comprehensible and easily managed manner.

A Decision Support-Oriented Patient Record System

A prerequisite for making adequate decisions is that all the needed data (including X-rays) be available in a comprehensible and easily manageable way. Today, with an ever expanding information base, this prerequisite is not fulfilled by conventional patient records. A transition to electronic records seems, therefore, clearly indicated. Up to now, attempts to computerize medical and dental records have made the situation worse. This is because conventional methods of information analysis and alphanumeric computer technology were applied with no real consideration of the present and future needs of the dentist. It almost seems as if current computerized dental records and charts were produced with the only objective being to automate conventional paper systems. This objective renders the electronic record very "familiar" to the practitioner but it fails to take the additional capabilities of computers into account. A new concept of a decision support-oriented patient dental record was described earlier in this chapter.

Decision Support for the Diagnosis and Treatment of Functional Disturbances of the Masticatory System

It is well known that diagnosis and treatment of functional diseases of the orofacial system is one of the more problematic areas in dental care. The main reason for this is the large variety of devices and procedures available for diagnosis and treatment of specific disorders. Dentists not specialized in this area clearly need some kind of additional decision support. On the basis of easily observable clinical symptoms, we are therefore developing an image-based decision support system for the diagnosis and treatment of functional disorders of the orofacial masticatory system (see Körber, E., Körber, A., Schneider, W. et al. for a more detailed description).[3] Careful psychologic and pedagogic planning is a prerequisite for the design of such a system.

Decision Support for Diagnosis and Treatment of Diseases of the Oral Mucosa

Decision support for diagnosis and treatment of oral mucosa diseases is especially dependent on the availability of relevant, high quality image material. These images must be easily accessible and manageable in a form compatible with the needs of the dentist. The system must provide for simultaneous image display of a variety of lesions of different degrees of severity, with both typical and atypical appearance, as well as other similar diseases that would be included in a differential diagnosis. Using computer-based interactive multimedia technology, an image-based decision support system has recently been developed by Wagner and Schneider[4] which seems to fulfill all relevant requirements.

By calling upon the decision support system, the dentist is asked three questions about the color, surface structure and location of the lesion in question. After answering, the computer will choose characteristic clinical pictures/diseases that are consistent with the features described and simultaneously present them on the screen (Figure 6.6). As a rule, there are 12 different images available per disease/clinical picture (Figure 6.7). These images can be presented simultaneously or one at a time magnified on the entire screen (Figure 6.8).

Furthermore, the system includes a support structure to aid in delineating the differential diagnosis. In this case, the dentist suggests in the first step a specific diagnosis. In the second step the system presents the image stack (a file of specific images) illustrating the corresponding clinical picture on the left side of the screen. In the third step the system selects those diseases which are included in the differential diagnosis and makes each corresponding image stack available on the remainder of the screen for comparison (Figure 6.9). Artificial intelligence-based decision routines are employed to support the image-based system at specific points in choosing the images to be displayed and to lead the dentist to the appropriate decision.

It is not the aim of this decision support system to make a specialist in oral mucosa diseases out of every practitioner. Quite the contrary, the aim is to make him/her secure in regard to the further management of the patient by giving access to specific data and information often only found in the specialist's domain. All too often, practitioners are left at the mercy of memory or reference books that are not conveniently available or easy to use. Basically the practitioner should, within the limited time of the treatment session, make the right decision regarding:

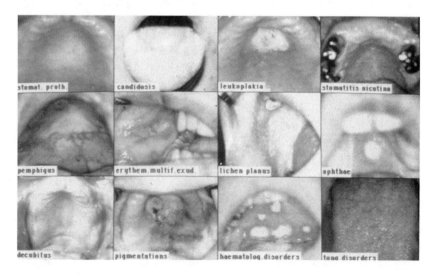

Figure 6.6. Image-based decision support for diagnosis and therapy of oral mucosa diseases.

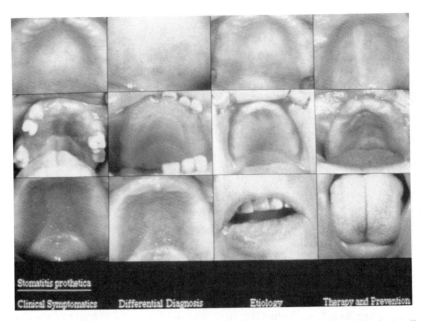

Figure 6.7. Presentation of all images concerning one disease (stomatitis prothetica)—dictionary part included.

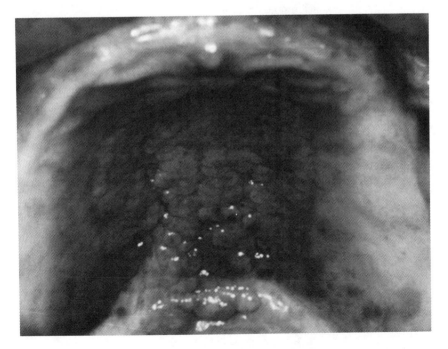

Figure 6.8. On the same screen, a magnified image of a stomatitis prothetica (hyperplasia).

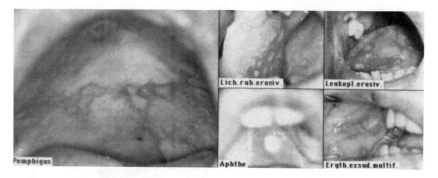

Figure 6.9. Image-based decision support for the differential diagnostic clarification of a clinical picture.

- immediate referral to a specialist, since the symptoms require specific treatment or a definite diagnostic clarification
- begin treatment
- make a new appointment as soon as possible to clarify the diagnosis and/or the exact treatment plan. Of course this might lead to a referral to a specialist at a later date

The dictionary accompanying the decision support module is based on similar principles as the parent module. The dictionary briefly defines the clinical symptoms, etiology, differential diagnosis and therapy of a disease. This decision support system will be operated by voice input.

As a further aid, one should have a video camera which allows direct projection of live images of the patient's oral mucosa onto the screen of the workstation. This function would considerably simplify the comparison between the actual clinical picture and the images prepared and presented by the computer. It would also allow transfer of the digitized live image over phone lines through a modem to a specialist for immediate consultation. Digital cameras producing images of the quality required in this context are not yet available at practical cost. It is safe to say, however, that they will evolve the way of most technology and will be available in the foreseeable future.

Decision Support for Treatment Strategy in Complex Clinical Situations

For the support of treatment planning in complex clinical cases a specific AI-technique, the so-called expert critiquing method[5] is particularly appropriate. This method allows the dentist to receive, if requested, alternative therapeutic approaches, including cost estimations. First the dentist must propose a treatment plan, then alternative solutions are offered from the computer. Such a system provides immediate support and continuous education. Thus, the computer is experienced as a desirable tool for the assessment of decisions in a professional consultation. This system helps avoid the "tutoring" phenomenon of traditional expert systems.

Continuous Dental Education

The Actual Situation

The development and practice of continuing dental education has for many years been hampered by the lack of adequate technical means to deliver individual, on-site education. As a consequence, the format of continuing dental education programs still consists mainly of conferences and courses. This format implies restrictions due to such organizational problems as the difficulties of long term and sometimes long distance displacement of practitioners. Evaluation of classroom continuing medical education clearly indicates the low level of effectiveness of this format on actual measurable professional behavior in medical practice.[6,7] Exceptions are programs focusing on very well-defined objectives[8] such as special training courses in specific prosthodontic procedures.[9] Improvements in the effect of classroom continuing education on professional behavior in practice can be observed in dentistry if individual practical exercises are included.[9] In general, however, the outcome of conventional classroom continuing dental education seems, even in dentistry, to be restricted to making the practitioner adequately aware of the problems, diagnoses and treatments addressed by the actual continuing education programs.

Obviously the foremost goal for continuing dental education programs must be improved patient care. Alteration of the professional behavior of the practitioner through continuous dental education programs is therefore a condition *sine qua non*. Although many attempts have been made to achieve individual onsite re-education and training using methods such as videofilms, telephone interviews, and chart audits, the results are rather poor. There appear to be three main reasons for this situation:

- The difficulties encountered by the practitioner when attempting to comprehend a problem addressed by a continuing dental education program in the context of his/her own patient material.
- The lack of decision support when the dentist intends to apply the diagnosis or treatment procedures acquired by continuing dental education in an actual patient situation.
- Deficiencies of the available continuing dental education methodology.

It goes beyond the scope of this chapter to survey the known deficiencies of conventional continuing dental education methods. It is necessary, however, to point out two crucial issues:

- The difficulty of delivering a variety of audiovisual educational material (such as images and films with or without spoken, textual, or visually animated comments).
- The practical impossibility of delivering self-administered interactive continuing education.

Although videofilms might be considered a partial solution to the first problem, this medium does not provide for an interactive mode. In addition, the low quality presentation of still frames by videofilm equipment severely restricts the use of this medium for overcoming both of these problems, since it would be difficult to review and study a particular image.

Future Possibilities

A prerequisite for the development of interactive multimedia technology-based, continuing medical and dental education programs is the availability of a powerful software package comprising advanced tools for:

- high resolution scanning, handling, and processing of color images and slides
- high fidelity sound recording
- the manipulation and mixture of sound records
- videofilm recording
- animation
- the composition of interactive video sessions
- voice input technology.

Obviously the use of interactive multimedia technology reveals new possibilities for teaching and for producing teaching programs in continuing dental education.

For a broader use of interactive multimedia technology, it is equally important that the development tools—in spite of their obvious complexity—be easily handled by teachers or researchers without programming experience.

As described elsewhere[10,11] interactive multimedia programs are composed of a collection of videoclips, images, texts, and digitalized soundclips. They should be constructed in such a way that parts of them can be used independently in modules for self-examination, ex-cathedra education, dictionary search, decision support at the dental unit, and also in selected situations for patient education in preventive dentistry.

Of special interest is the inclusion of regularly updated parts of multimedia continuing dental education programs in interactive decision support systems used chairside with real patients. This method, recently introduced by Wagner and Schneider[10] provides for a continuous reinforcement and review of education and underlines the educational nature of practice. Thus, continuing education becomes truly "continuous."

References

1. Wagner, I.V. Work analyses in dental practices. Sweden. Uppsala: UDAC, Unpublished data, 1988.
2. Lind, M., Pettersson, E., Sanblad, B. et al. Computer-based workstations in health care. Amsterdam: Elsevier Science Publishers B.V. (North-Holland), IFIP-IMIA, 1988.
3. Körber, E., Korber, A., Wagner, I.V., et al. Decision support for the diagnosis and treatment of functional disturbances of the masticatory system. Unpublished.
4. Wagner, I.V., and Schneider, W. Computer-based decision support in dentistry. United States, June 1990. Alexandria, VA: Symposium on Second Generation Clinical Databases and the Electronic Dental Record.
5. Miller, P. Expert critiquing systems. Berlin:Springer Verlag, 1986.
6. Manning, P.R. and Petit, D.W. The past, present, and future of continuing medical education, achievements and opportunities, computers and recertification. JAMA. 1987;258:3542-3546.
7. Haynes, R.B., Davis, D.A., McKibbon, A. et al. A critical appraisal of the efficacy of continuing medical education. JAMA. 1984;251:61-64.
8. Stein, LS. The effectiveness of continuing medical education: eight research reports. J Med Educ. 1981;56:103-110.
9. Wagner, I.V. Evaluation of continuing dental education in prosthodontics. Germany 1986. Dresden: Medical Academy Internal Report, Unpublished.
10. Wagner, I.V., and Schneider,W. The use of interactive media technology in continuing education of dentists concerning the biological adaptation of removable dentures. In: Salsmon, R., Protti, D., Moehr, J., eds. Proceedings of the international symposium on medical informatics and education. Victoria, Canada: The Queen's Printer, 1989:p. 374-377.
11. Johnson, L. The dental diagnosis and treatment project. In: Salsmon, R., Protti, D., Moehr, J., eds. Proceedings of the international symposium on medical informatics and education. Victoria, Canada: The Queen's Printer, 1989: p. 367-370.

7
What Renders Dental Informatics Specific?

Werner Schneider

The Peculiarities of Dental Informatics

"Micro, mini, megamini - minisuper, gigapico and so on - gateways, fiber, LAN and WANT-knowledge bases, robotvision, PACS - Email, fax and teletex - laservision, CD-ROM and videotext. Forget the books and folders, throw away your pencils, staplers, clips, erasers. Avoid the human ways of working and of thinking, 'human factors' are too dangerous. Hyperknowledge, expert systems, robots make life easy and yet better, more productive, stimulating, innovative." That is the song of the computer sirens. An ever increasing number of hesitants are starting the hazardous journey towards the enticing sea-nymphs dwelling on the islands of the electronic digital world. Sayings such as: "the transition to the computer era is sooner or later a must, better go through it right away than before it is too late" or: "my colleagues have it, I must have it too" are typical. There is, in other words, a solution, one has just to find the appropriate problems. In case there are no such problems one has to change both the work and organizational contexts in such a way that appropriate problems arise. Because this way of change does not intrinsically relate to or come from the needs and possibilities for improving actual procedures and organization at a specific work place, experienced actors at the work place cannot themselves invent and design this change. Instead this is made by informatics consultants who in the best case have some prior knowledge of the activities they are going to change.

How to adapt the large variety of traditional, domain specific ways of handling and processing information to the enlarging assortment of increasingly powerful products of the computer industry, has, unfortunately, been the main stream of activities in the field of medical informatics. Ever since this new field of human endeavour emerged the scientific programs of the steadily increasing number of conferences devoted to it basically consist of pseudo-scientific papers such as: "The use of the hardware and/or software tool XYZ in the YZX procedures in the clinic ZYX". It is obvious that there is nothing really specific and/or scientific in the mere replacement of manual routines by information technology-based procedures. An evaluation of the activities in the newly created field of dental informatics reveals a considerable risk of falling into the same trap.

What makes dental informatics a scientific field of study? The basic requirement is that electronic-based methods of information handling and processing be specifically designed and applied solely for the sake of

- expanding the knowledge and understanding of the biological and biomedical processes of the orofacial and stomatological system,
- improving prevention, diagnosis, treatment and follow-up of the diseases of the orofacial and stomatological system, and
- refining dental education.

Obviously a prerequisite for success is that as many experienced researchers, educators and practitioners as possible, representing all dental specialties and professional disciplines, become motivated and engaged in an appropriate integration of human and electronic-based methods of information handling and processing. Unfortunately this fact is still essentially overlooked in medical informatics. Thus the driving forces are basically informaticians and young, clinically unexperienced medical doctors, nurses, and laboratory assistants. As a consequence the results of too many projects are of no or little biomedical or clinical relevance. The whole area is characterized by overpromises and underachievements and a vast array of pseudo-scientific activities.

In launching dental informatics, dentistry has a unique chance to learn and profit from the experiences and mistakes made in medical informatics. The most important lesson to be learned, it must be stated again and again, is that a prerequisite for success is motivating and engaging as many experienced researchers, educators, and practitioners as possible, representing all dental specialties and professional disciplines. This requires education in strategic and tactical issues of informatics as well as in basics of human specific skills and competencies [1], especially in regard to the particular skills and competencies that characterize the dental profession.

Basic Aspects of Informatics

It is well known that in spite of its short history informatics has become a vast and rapidly evolving field. A complete description in even the most general terms goes far beyond the scope of this chapter. There are, however, some basic aspects of informatics which are relevant to what is said in the remainder of this chapter. In spite of its multifaceted character, informatics can be considered to consist of two basic domains: the development of tools for the application of formal languages on one side, and the support and refinement of human ways of expressing thoughts and feelings on the other side.

Formal Languages

The aim of being able to grasp at least parts of the "eternal truth" has led to the invention of formal languages by philosophers, especially philosophers of ancient Greece. In a more general context, the objective for constructing formal languages is to be able to describe and understand parts of reality in such a way that the ambiguities and human cultural dependencies inherent in natural languages are eliminated. The most characteristic elements of a formal language are the set of symbols, the available rules for constructing expressions with these symbols, and the methods for interpretation of such expressions.

The geometry of Pythagoras is rather well adapted to human ways of perceiving and processing information, since its elements to a large extent are represented in an analogue form. To exploit the full power of other formal languages, however, goes beyond the human capabilities of interpreting expressions formulated in terms of such languages. Thus special tools are required. The first tools of this kind were the mechanical calculators invented during the 17th century by Schickart, Pascal and Leibniz. Programming languages represent one specific category of formal languages. It must be pointed out, however, that most programming languages do not fulfill all the requirements set forth for classifying as a "pure" formal language.

Since Leibniz (1646-1716) invented calculus, the formal methodology of interpreting logical expressions, logic became the formal language, two thousand years after it was created by Aristoteles. Tools for the execution of the various forms of calculus had to await modern electronics. When the first electronic computers were presented, only a few understood that the most essential breakthrough was not that huge computational power had suddenly become available, but the fact that it was the successful automation of a specific calculus which rendered the realization of these machines possible. The calculus in question was Boole's algebraic calculus of the numbers **1** and **0**, where **1** represents the set of all objects in the universe and **0** the set to which no object belongs.

Considerable progress has been achieved in regard to automation of various calculi such as the relational calculus as the basis for relational database management systems, and the Lambda calculus and predicate calculus for different disciplines (such as expert systems and robotvision) of artificial intelligence (AI).

In the context of this chapter, the primary question is not whether computers should be used in dentistry, but whether the application of formal languages (such as predicate calculus) is indicated in the field. Which kind of dental knowledge can and which can not be represented in terms of formal languages? Where are rule-based representations indicated, where are representations by semantic networks or frames preferable? Where are simulation techniques suitable and where not? These are of course very difficult and complex problems. How can they be overcome? Should the dental professionals acquire all that competence? It must be clearly stated here and now that this would be the wrong way to go. These problems can only be solved by interdisciplinary teams of expert dental professionals, informaticians, psychologists and human-computer interface specialists.

Multimedia Technology

Throughout history people have been inventing tools and methods to record and distribute various types of human expressions. The first recordings were drawings and/or written text engraved on objects such as gravestones and cave walls. Distribution of such recordings became possible by the use of bricks. Recording and distribution of drawings and written text was significantly improved by the invention of papyrus and ink. The printing press invented by Gutenberg in the middle of the 15th century made it possible to "mass produce" this kind of recordings.

Significantly improved means for distribution became available, however not earlier than during the 19th and 20th centuries, when the means for physical transportation were dramatically improved.

The invention of photography, cinematography and phonography, and their integration into sound-film widened the scope of available media dramatically. Suddenly it became possible to record and distribute all modes of human expression that can be perceived by the senses of hearing and sight (such as plays and dance).

A further dramatic breakthrough was the transition to electronic means of recording and distribution. Of special importance is the enormous, actually ongoing progress in regard to the digital form of representing such recordings. This provides not only for interactive handling of sound, images and sequences of images but also for interactive processing of such material by digital computers. This technology is called interactive multimedia technology.

There is no doubt that interactive multimedia technology will play a major role in dental informatics and dentistry at large.[2] It provides e.g., innovative ways for improving dental education, especially private study and examination by pract-Hioners. Further, new approaches for advanced decision support in different care contexts become possible. Last but not least, a more adequate human-computer interaction can be accomplished.

Computer-Based Workstations

In spite of the amazing progress in the field of computer technology the basic architectural structure of almost all commercially available digital computers has not been changed during the last three decades. Examining the technological progress in the frame of this structure, the von Neumann model of a digital computer (Figure 7.1), reveals that until a few years ago most of the development efforts had been devoted to the processor and storage components, whereas the input and output components were of much lesser interest. Improvements in the input/output area have been basically restricted to refinements of printers and the "24x80" alphanumeric visual display unit. The rather rudimentary selection of available peripheral devices did not require local "von Neumann" capacity in an office, ward, or other working place. The justification of such capacity was merely a question of cost, performance and reliability of the existing communication network facilities as well as the pricing of central computer services in relation to the costs for acquiring and operating local equipment. Other aspects of major importance were issues such as data protection, vulnerability of operations and needs of organizational independence. In this restricted context centralized versus non-central computing[3] was and often still is a theme for debates and emphatic discussions which tend to be more like a religious war than a part of a pragmatic problem solving process.

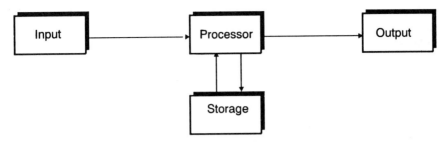

Figure 7.1. The "von Neumann"-model of a digital computer.

Although during the second half of the sixties the need for graphical presentation of intermediate and final results was important, only a few could afford a real-time display of such information. This was due to the fact that considerable, costly computing power was necessary to maintain even the rather poor graphic terminals of that time. Thus the results which should be presented graphically had in most cases to be recorded on magnetic tape for later output via an off-line plotter. A broader use of graphics for presenting information was therefore severely hampered. During the seventies the problem of being able to afford the computer time needed for interactive work with graphics soon became much less accentuated. Instead the lack of adequate line transmission capacity between the computer and remote graphic terminals became the major problem even though most of these terminals only could produce vector graphics. Consequently there was an increasing need of local computing facilities for the real-time creation and display of graphical information in a number of rather well-defined application areas such as computer-aided design in industrial environments and dose planning systems in the field of cancer treatment. The need for application-specific graphic workstations thus arose.

A quite similar development can be observed in regard to the input component of the von-Neumann model. Because of the limited data transmission capacity of existing computer communication networks, automatic collection and preprocessing of larger amounts of data from measurement equipment required local process-control computers. In the field of medicine this leads to an increasing need for a variety of custom-designed laboratory workstations.

In summary, the need for improved input and output techniques, in the absence of adequate data transmission capacity, created the need for workstations and thus local computer equipment even in otherwise rigid centralistic environments. On the other hand the success of the first generations of workstations created the demand for dramatically improved input and output devices such as high-resolution monochromatic and color graphic displays, a variety of input tools, and devices for voice input and output. These leading-edge technologies do not come cheap.

The rapidly increasing availability of low price "micro-von Neumann's" in the form of so-called PC's during the last decade has, however, dramatically changed the scene. Due to the enormous market potential and the sizable established market base the availability of advanced input and output facilities is rapidly improving. Thus suddenly computer graphics-aided analysis of data using monochromatic or color screens is on the way to becoming a broadly usable, cost effective tool. Together with more and more advanced hardware and software tools for word and text processing, electronic mail services, terminal emulation, database handling and file transfer, very versatile and powerful PC-based general purpose workstations are now broadly available at an affordable price. Most important is the availability of increasingly advanced tools for design of appropriate human-computer interfaces on this kind of workstation (such as multimedia technology-based interfaces).

The problem of inadequate line transmission capacity remains in spite of the availability of workstations. This is due to the fact that very often the data that should be processed interactively in these workstations have to be imported from other computer systems. In cases where rather large amounts of "external" data (for example, a collection of digital images) are needed, the transfer by magnetic or optical storage devices still is the only reasonable choice and this will be the case for some time to come.

A thorough presentation and discussion of how to select adequate workstation equipment would go far beyond the scope of this chapter. If human competence and skill are to be preserved in computer-assisted work environments, workstations have to be designed for the specific work environment in which they will be used. Thus it is impossible to define universally applicable human computer interfaces. What can be done is to create a selection of more and more powerful computer-aided tools for the design of adequate interfaces for each specific work environment.

However, almost any computer based workstation should fulfill some basic requirements:

- the availability of communication facilities for the main internationally-accepted transmission protocols (such as X.400, TCP/IP, and OSI).
- the availability of compilers for C, C++, Lisp (Common Lisp), Prolog and in specific cases still Fortran.
- a relational database management system with SQL must be available, if possible with facilities for handling image and sound records, both in analog and digital form.
- the availability of tools for the development and implementation of various kinds of decision support systems (for examaple, different AI- as well as simulation model-based approaches).
- a broad selection of input and output devices should be supported, such as high resolution color graphic screens, and voice input/output devices.
- a number of input and output devices must be operational simultaneously.
- the availability of high quality tools for the development and maintenance of multimedia technology-based human-computer interfaces on human terms.

Typical dental-specific requirements include the availability of tools for voice input and response, the capture (digital cameras), handling and presentation of high-resolution color images as well as for the generation and presentation of high-resolution graphics (see Chapter 6). Of equal importance is the availability of high quality tools for the development and maintenance of educational programs using simulation and multimedia technology.

Human Information Handling and Processing

Many people consider themselves to be "computer ignorant" and they suffer feelings of inferiority, especially watching young hackers in the electronics division of a department store. It is, however much more serious that almost everyone, especially computer people, are ignorant about human information processing. And what do we really know about human competence?

What is human competence? And if there is something like human competence, is it or will it not be obsolete in the era of computers and artificial intelligence? Many people pessimistically heed the statements of some leading AI-researchers that it is not anymore a question of whether or not computers and robots will fully replace the human being, it is just a question of when. Reality is, however, quite different. It goes beyond this chapter to discuss this issue in more detail. Let us just note that one of the basic reasons for this kind of miscomprehension of human competence and skill lies in the fact that in the field of cognitive psychology, information processing machines are increasingly used as metaphors to conceptualize human information processing. This leads to a model of a person as a constantly consciously active, basically sequential thinking machine; a machine which can be evaluated in relation to the performances of existing or planned computer systems. To reveal the limitations of people is of course the main purpose of this kind of "computer glorification" behavior. It is exactly people's awareness of their very poor computing and logical inferencing capabilities that has been the driving force behind invention of mechanical calculators and other data processing tools, long before the birth of cognitive science.

However, people are primarily neither a computing machine nor an inference engine but a system of extremely advanced and complex perception. It is, to a large extent, because of the integration of all these modes that in many domains people will forever be superior to formal language based electronic machines.

Human perception is among other things highly specialized for processing spacial information. It is also extremely powerful in regard to the recognition and analysis of similarities between different sensory input patterns (such as form and Gestait of a certain physical object in relation to other physical objects) as well as between different control contexts. If one takes these aspects into consideration one gets quite a different image of the human-computer relation. It is true that we are almost unable to accomplish even a single addition per second whereas computers are performing at a rate of billions per second. However, people are faster than any supercomputer in the direct recognition of images and similarities and will remain so due to the specific, intrinsic characteristics of the human biological system.

"Humans forget, computers do not" is a widely known and accepted statement. However, the reverse statement "computers forget, humans do not" is true as well. Or is there still somebody who has not heard about or even been affected by a "computer virus" or "Trojan horses,"? It is, by the way, still better if the computer forgets than if it processes falsified data with falsified programs due to undetected manipulations of the stored data elements. On the other hand, is there somebody who does not remember the first airplane flight or the first love affair? Such memories comprise not just an alphanumerical character string but "emotional film clips," meaning a huge number of "pixels" and other sensory data, amounts which go far beyond the best of what digital storage technology can offer in a long-range perspective. Additionally, on the basis of similarities of some details humans can associate directly to the image sequence in the "film" where the details are present. In the "computer world" this will not be possible for a long time to come.

The immediate recognition of non-standard, sometimes incomplete alphanumeric characters (and words formed by such characters) is another area where human perception is enormously powerful. Computers are in general still far away from acceptable performance in this respect, especially concerning the recognition of spoken language. In those special cases where acceptable solutions are available, the related costs are of a magnitude which makes human work costs look rather modest. One has to keep this in mind when confronted with the news of Human Factor Research Laboratories revealing humans' almost ridiculous reading speed of only 6-8 characters per second as compared to the "super performance" of digital computers. Humans do read character by character, but only in childhood when the skill of reading is being trained and if the text is badly printed. In addition, humans get most of their information through means other than written text.

There are many more examples of how human competence and skill is disregarded, underestimated or misunderstood. For the purpose of this chapter it is sufficient to state that an optimal use of computer technology is only possible if humans can give their best. Human competence and skill must not be replaced but supplemented. Why, where, and how this should be done must be the object of careful analysis.

The Appropriate Integration of Human and Electronics-Based Methods of Information Handling and Processing

Methods of Work Analysis

There are two strategies for design of computer-based support for a specific work place. The first emanates from introducing an existing method of computer-based problem solving into a specific work domain. This implies not only re-organization of staff and work procedures, but also involves a change in regard to the required professional competence and skill. In many cases essential competencies that can only be acquired by experience through real work in health care, and that are based on genuine human capabilities, are "side-stepped".

Instead, priority is given to the ability of handling formal languages (such as query languages) and command procedures. Due to the fact that this kind of activity is genuinely "non-human" much effort is made to "humanize" it. Visual programming languages, menu techniques, icons, voice input and other techniques are increasing in popularity in order to achieve acceptable "user-friendliness".

The second strategy takes an opposite approach.[4] First the existing problems at a working place are identified and analyzed with respect to the goals to be achieved within the framework of the overall goals of the organization. The analysis is made on the basis of the identified expectations in the work performed expectations that can be identified by each group of individuals involved in, addressed, or affected by the work. Thus the expectations of the customers on the kind and quality of the services to be delivered are explicitly introduced and treated.

In the second phase different methods of solving the problems are investigated involving (in an integrated perspective) development of organization and work organization, alternative staffing, enhancement of the competence of the staff, optimal planning of premises as well as organizational and technical means.

Only in the third phase can the required computer-based tools be specified. The specifications arise from the genuine human competence and skill of handling tools out of and in a specific work context. In the case that information technology-based tools must be part of the solution chosen for solving actual problems and/or improvement of the work performed at a specific working place, it is of great importance that they are designed on the basis of genuine human competence and skill specifically related to that work context. Thus, advanced means for human computer interaction have to be available. This requires local computer capacity in the form of advanced workstations. As described earlier they must be designed specifically for the particular work environment in which the computer techniques will actually be used.

Human-Computer Interaction

In the following we will presume that, based on a careful work analysis, an appropriate work distribution among humans and computers has been achieved. There are still two important problem complexes: How can humans work with the computer-based tools and how can they communicate with the computer?[5] Unfortunately this is the area where we meet such serious problems that human performance is severely reduced in spite of an adequate work distribution.

Ever since the first computers were constructed, one was simply dealing with input and output: one feeds the computer something and out comes something, the faster the better. Of what the input may consist and where, when and how the input can take place is determined by the limitations of technology and to what degree computer industry is willing to invest in innovative products. The same holds for the specification of what the output may consist of, where and in what form. The consequence of this bias in favor of the computer and computer-based robots is, however, a serious loss of user productivity. Let us consider some examples:

The most commonly used input and output device is still the 24 x 80 character CRT. This format is a consequence of the fact that at the time when the first CRTs were constructed, the computer input was almost exclusively based on the 80-column punched card. The transition from off-line punching to on-line "punching" had therefore to preserve this input format in order to avoid huge and costly reprogramming efforts. Today the limitations of this type of CRT are very serious. The size of the presentation area as well as the repertoire of characters are definitely too limited, the graphic resolution is insufficient and, of course, any kind of image is excluded. This leads to undesirable means of expression (such as "cryptic" shortenings and "artificial" verbalizations) and considerable fragmentation and sequentialization in the work process. In other words, the computer forces people to conform to its means of working instead of the other way around.

In the non-computerized work environment the entire sensory space, especially the audiovisual space, is "the menu". Anything positioned within the physical range can be touched or seized. Books, documents, folders, card-indexes, the agenda and technical tools can be directly recognized and seized. However, the computer can be "anything" (such as a book, a document, or an agenda), depending upon the momentary status of the actually executed application. Thus we have first to recognize what the computer actually "is" and then to manipulate it to "become" what we want it to be. This has to be accomplished through cumbersome menu hierarchies and by a formal language-based dialogue. As desired earlier, formal languages have been invented and designed in order to dispose of "non-human" means of description. They are therefore totally inadequate for being used by humans for communication with computers. As a consequence, the internationally standardized query language (SQL) is not an end-user language. Being "non-human" it is "un-human" to use it in this context.

In order to make use of the above-mentioned unique human perceptive capabilities, everything of importance in the context of a specific work situation must be accessible by direct manipulation. The use of multimedia technology together with high-resolution color screens, digitizer tablets, multiple screen setups (for achieving a sufficiently large presentation range), voice input devices, and ergonomically positioned touch screens opens the way to design and construction of significantly improved human-computer interfaces, a human-computer interaction on human terms. In the future one can imagine a desk surface consisting of a number of flat, high-resolution color screens of different sizes, and task-specific image and sound generating and recognizing devices placed on that desk.

Browsing books and folders, overlooking or just glancing over several document pages together with writing, drawing, and calculating are the usual activities at many work places. The conventional 24 x 80 alphanumeric character CRT provides very rudimentary capability in this respect. The resulting fragmentation and sequentialization of work leads to considerable time loss. Moreover, some human intellectual activities cannot take place due to some associative processes being confined to items which are simultaneously perceived.

Conventional CRTs create still another important problem: the limited size of the screen restricts the amount of information that can be preserved on the screen in parallel to the dialogue between the user and the computer. This should be compared to a scenario of a manual work situation where after each work step both desk and bookshelves are cleaned. Using multiwindowing techniques can help solve this problem. In any case it is essential that the presentation of results can be done in parallel to the user-computer dialogue, which in some cases can even be achieved with conventional CRTs.

One of the genuine human competencies is that we continuously can and do create dynamic models of "what could and/or should happen next", for example, what we expect our collaborator(s) to do next. On the basis of these very advanced and complex anticipation processes our consecutive behavior is planned and controlled, mostly automatically, since we delegate these activities to some kind of an internal "autopilot". Unfortunately, most computer applications are constructed in such a way that users cannot create adequate dynamic models of system behavior and of the interaction between them and the system in the context of their intentions. If they, nevertheless, try to (or unconsciously do) anticipate this most often leads to a series of frustrations because the system makes things happen differently by conforming to the system's own "logic". The result is that people become reluctant to engage themselves in the work process. In order to avoid frustration they adapt to play a passive role by just awaiting the system's next step. It is therefore of utmost importance that application systems are constructed in such a way that their usage can be compatibly integrated into the complex human mental control system, and that provision is made for maximum transparency even in unforeseen situations.

Finally some words about communication between humans and computers. In most cases communication is based on a formal language-based dialogue. This is, as already mentioned, a real yoke for man since most of the necessary formal language expressions can not be created through recognition, but must be generated "out of memory" using the rather poor human means for creating and handling such expressions. The use of formal languages requires in addition that the user strictly adheres to rules and rigid sequential work procedures. Still only written communication is possible. Low cost voice input and output devices with sufficient performance and reliability will not be available in the near future. As long as the dialogues are formal language-based there is no real use for these gadgets, due to the fact that it is very difficult to pronounce formal language expressions and to understand synthesized formal language talk.

Obviously natural language-based voice input will, sooner or later, be a reality. There is, however, still a long way to go until a decent human-computer dialogue can take place in natural language. It is very important to note that the availability of natural language communication would solve only some of the problems concerning human-computer communication. This is due to the fact that much of our communication is non-verbal. We do not talk to our tools and most of us do not talk to ourselves, especially not for issuing a sequence of commands to ourselves.

Improved Decision Making in Dentistry

It is the purpose of this section to demonstrate how decision making processes in dentistry could be improved by appropriately integrating human and electronics-based methods of information handling and processing in which specific requirements on information technology and human-computer interaction must be fulfilled.

Work Analysis

Dentists, dental assistants, hygienists, technicians, and administrative assistants are primarily concerned with the problems they encounter when performing their work both as individuals and as members of the dental care team. Their main interest is to get help in identifying and analyzing the problems at the work place relative to the goals to be achieved. From their point of view solutions which are based on the use of information technology are not preferable. They want to choose among different ways of solving problems involving (in an integrated perspective) alternative staffing, enhancement of staff competence, optimal planning of the premises, as well as organizational and technical means.

It is in connection with the design of these alternative solutions and in such an integrated perspective that the possibly required information technology-based tools can be specified. Dental care professionals assume of course that those assisting them in solving their problems are using the term "information technology" in its very general sense. Therefore nothing existing or soon to be available within the field of information technology should be excluded from being considered.

On the basis of work analysis in dental practice as well as clinical settings in dental schools Wagner has identified some important domains of decision-making in dentistry where different kinds of computer-based support are needed (see Chapter 6).

Some Dentistry-Specific Requirements on Information Technology and Human Computer Interaction

One of the most important outcomes of the work analysis mentioned in the previous section is that AI-based decision support tools are not of primary interest in this context. Contrary to common opinion within the scientific community and computer industry, the role of standard AI-techniques is limited to a few essential refinements of other decision support techniques. Although the so-called expert critiquing systems approach is of major importance in the case of perioprosthetic problem cases, even here this powerful Al- technique must be embedded in a more extended decision support tool.

Analysis of the basic decision processes at the chairside has revealed that a significant improvement can be achieved if the dental patient record can be presented in such a way that the human way of decision making is optimally supported. This requires the design of a synoptic and comprehensible graphic presentation of oral status. How this is optimally done requires further research into the way the dentist perceives and cognitively represents the clinical facts in regard to appropriate clinical management of the patient. The graphic presentation of the oral status presented in Chapter 6, reflects the actual state of the art in this respect.

The analysis of the decision processes involved in diagnosis and treatment of diseases of the mucosa clearly indicate that major improvement requires a special image-based decision support approach. (A first realization of this approach is described in Chapter 6.) Special presentation techniques with high-resolution color images had to be designed and developed based on the results and experience from earlier research and development work in the field of human-computer interaction.[6]

In regard to diagnosis and treatment of disturbances of the masticatory system, the work analysis revealed not only a serious need for improved decision making but also that such improvement requires design and development of advanced multimedia technique-based decision support tools. Existing commercially available technology is not yet sufficient. In order to produce a prototype system special software is under development at the author's institute.

Finally, work analyses have clearly led to the conclusion that voice input is the only appropriate way for entering data and commands in connection with the use of computer assisted methods at the dental unit. In specific cases this must be combined with voice response from the computer. In any case human-computer dialogue must be based on use of advanced multimedia technology (as described earlier) in order to fully benefit human professionals' perceptive skill and competence.

References

1. Schneider, W. Teaching informatics to health professionals. In: Salamon, R., et al., Medical informatics and education. Conference Proceedings, School of health information science, University of Victoria, 1989: p. 135-142.
2. Wagner, I.V. and Schneider, W. The use of interactive multimedia technology in continuing education of dentists concerning the biological adaptation of removable dentures. Conference Proceedings, School of Health Information Science, University of Victoria, 1989: p. 374-377.
3. Schneider, W. Strategies for future systems architectures and development. In: Hansen R., et al. Medical Informatics Europe '88, Germany: Springer-Verlag, 1988: p. 42-48.

4. Lind, M., Pettersson, E., Sandblad, B., et. al. Computer based workstations in health care. In: Bakker, A.R., et al., eds. Towards new hospital information systems. Amsterdam: Elsevier Science Publ., 1988.

5. Peterson, H. and Schneider, W. Human-computer communications in health care. Amsterdam: Elsevier Science Publ., 1986.

6. Sandblad, B., Lind, M., and Schneider, W., Requirements for human computer interfaces in health care. In: Peterson, H., and Schneider, W., eds. Human-computer communications in health care. U Amsterdam: Elsevier Science Publ.,1986: p. 99-110.

7. Schneider, W., Lind, M., Allard, R., et. al. Human cognition and human computer interaction. In: Van der Meer et al., eds. Readings on Cognitive Ergonomics - Mind and Computers. Germany: Springer-Verlag, 1984: p. 76-80.

Section 2
Integrating Technology into the Dental Environment

8
Nosology: A Critical Link Between Computers and Dental Education, Practice and Research

Brian D. Monteith

Nosology is a word, it is said, that most clinicians are unlikely to have heard of,[1] yet it describes a process that has occupied the attention of medical scientists since the time of Hippocrates: *the systematic classification of diseases.*[2] The word itself is likewise not a new one. It derives in part from *nosos,* the Greek word for disease, and was in common use in centuries past — as is typified by its presence in the title of the first published attempt to enumerate diseases, the *Nosologia Methodica* of François Bossier de Lacroix (1706-1777).[3]

The resurgence of interest in nosology after a century or more of neglect can be largely attributed to two factors: the first arising from the need for a scientifically precise classification that would be able to accommodate rapidly increasing computer applications in the health sciences; while the second pertains to an increasing awareness of the inadequacies of the *International Classification of Diseases* (ICD), the main nosological system in world-wide use today.

The scientific implications of the first of the above factors were addressed recently by Feinstein,[1] who outlined three fundamental requirements that a nosology laying claim to a scientific basis would need to satisfy. They are the following:

1. the classification must have a suitable organizing principle;

2. use must be made of standard terminology;

3. agreement must be reached on standard operational criteria.

At first sight these might seem to be self-evident; yet it is only when one sets out to unravel the historical circumstances that have shaped nosologies over the years that it becomes apparent that much of the taxonomic tangle that persists today can be ascribed to the dereliction of one or more of these three principles.

Taxonomic Turmoil in the Chronicles of Medicine

As shown on the left of Figure 8.1, the organizing principle of choice by the middle of the nineteenth century had become as urgent as it was self-evident: *a Classification of the Causes of Death.* The need for a "a uniform statistical nomencla-

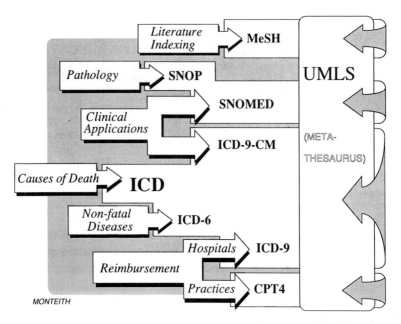

Figure 8.1. Originating from a primary preoccupation with "causes of death", subsequent changes in organizational needs have given rise to a host of differing classification systems in medicine.

ture...for...enforcement in Bills of Mortality" was being voiced at this time by the English nosologist-statistician, William Farr (1807-1883);[4] and it was perhaps fitting that it was to Farr that the First International Statistical Congress (Brussels, 1853) should have turned, in conjunction with d'Espine of Geneva, with the task of preparing *"un nomenclature des causes de décès applicable a tous les pays"*.[5] Appropriately, it was Farr's efforts in this field, together with the subsequent work of Bertillon (1851-1922), that eventually resulted in the "International List of Causes of Death" out of which ICD was born.

With *Causes of Death* firmly entrenched as the predominant organizing principle, the situation remained static for decades. In the meantime, other nosological requirements — such as the need to classify non-fatal diseases — began to assert themselves. Incredibly, it was only with its sixth revision in 1948, that ICD was at last extended so as to make provision for morbid conditions. Although ICD could now at last be justifiably construed as standing for the *"International Classification of Diseases"*, it still remained less than suitable for addressing general clinical applications. Consequently, when the ninth revision was due, the U.S. Department of Health and Human Services, seeking to redress this, released the new version in modified form as ICD-9-CM,[6] where the CM signified a "Clinical Modification".

Pathologists in the U.S., meanwhile, had also long been mindful of the shortcomings of ICD. They had been devising their own systems for some time and indeed, had a particularly successful one already in place: the *Systematized Nomenclature of Pathology* or SNOP.[7]

The organizing principles of SNOP ranged around four simple and rational axes: 1) *Topography* - the site affected; 2) *Morphology* - the observable pathological changes involved; 3) *Etiology* - the cause of the disorder and 4) *Function* - a descriptor that has been termed "...a generous basket of 'physiological or chemical' disorders".[8] Encouraged by SNOP's widespread acceptance, the College of American Pathologists saw it as a promising starting point for expanding the area of application from mere Pathology to something that might successfully serve the broader needs of Medicine as a whole, and thereby provide a suitable alternative to ICD. The result was SNOMED - the *Systematized Nomenclature of Medicine*[9] — an ambitious venture, organized around no fewer than seven organizational axes.

There were, however, other organizational imperatives seeking alternate solutions. For example, the need for easy access to the body of medical literature gave rise to MeSH, the index of *Medical Subject Headings*.[10] Unfortunately, the very qualities that enable MeSH to serve so admirably the objectives for which it was designed render it generally too imprecise to act as a taxonomic model for any other application.

Turning to what is probably the most powerful organizational imperative of them all, reimbursement, the standard, for hospital applications in the U.S., and indeed throughout the world, remains uncompromisingly vested in ICD. However, for the private sector, where procedures rather than pathologies tend to dictate the scheme of things, the American Medical Association has provided its *Current Procedural Terrninology*, or CPT4.[11] Like MeSH, it is more than adequately suited to the purpose for which it was designed; however, being directed specifically to billable items, its design is too specialized to accommodate any broader purpose.

Finally, in seeking a concept that might give holistic expression to all of these disparate organizational imperatives, The National Library of Medicine instituted the *Unified Medical Language System* (UMLS).[12] As demonstrated to the right of Figure 8.1, the intention of UMLS was not to provide yet another classification. Instead, it was meant to serve as a Meta-Thesaurus that would provide a structural model for linking and mapping amongst the existing systems.

Although the evolution and establishment of clear organizing principles that could successfully reflect a range of changing circumstances was at best difficult, it was the violation of Feinstein's second point - the need for a common nomenclature - that was to sow the greatest taxonomic confusion. Indeed, it is less for historical interest than its implications for databases and other electronic applications that the following review is given.

The Problems of Nomenclature in Medicine

It isn't difficult to understand why nomenclature problems should have arisen. Medical terms in any era have always tended to reflect the conceptual understanding of that era; however, given the natural reticence for change, and the sanctified inertia of tradition, many terms have persisted long after the philosophies that spawned them had disappeared.

There are three factors that have been available for centuries as foci for medical classification: the observed clinical manifestations of human illness (signs and symptoms); the entities believed to be causes of those manifestations (etiological factors); and the evolving patterns of events likely to follow such manifestations (sequellae). All three have served latterly - as organizational axes within SNOP, for example, where they contributed fundamentally to the system's success. Each has also at various stages in history, enjoyed an extended, if at times bizarre, vogue. Witness the predictive value of the *Hippocratic facies* in discerning impending death; the criteria of appearance embodied in descriptors such as *cyanosis* and *scarlet fever*; and the notion that disease was due to an imbalance of a patient's four body "humors" - blood, phlegm, black bile and yellow bile (with their respective "treatments" of bloodletting, blistering, purging and puking).[1]

The terminological chaos that ensued from such philosophical confusion over such an extended period of time was hardly surprising, so that by the middle of the nineteenth century, a plethora of conflicting medical terms and classifications had evolved. At this time, however, increased understanding of the derangements seen at necroscopy prompted greater emphasis upon a more rational appreciation of etiology. Consequently, new terminologies began to emerge that were better able to give expression to the new levels of understanding. Thus, the use of terms describing clinical perceptions of an observational nature such as *angina pectoris*, began to be challenged by new terms like *coronary artery disease* that were more descriptive of the underlying cause. Each of course had its advocates, and with the forces of conservatism and change inevitably ranged against one another, the old and the new terminologies were eventually obliged to assume a state of uneasy co-existence. The unfortunate result however, was that "causes of death", as entered on death certificates, tended to be given different names by different practitioners, with the ensuing statistical chaos being sufficient to prompt the cry for a nosology and nomenclature that would permit greater epidemiologic precision.

The use of imprecise nomenclature on death certificates had prompted Farr to complain in 1856 that "...each disease has, in many instances, been denoted by three or four terms, and each term has been applied to as many different diseases".[4] What Farr has alluded to here, in modern terms, are the twin taxonomic traps of *redundancy* and *ambiguity*; factors as problematic today as then, but harbouring additional hazards for database design. In view of their implications for this and other electronic applications, it would be well to review each of them briefly.

Redundancy is said to occur when a database's design permits a single concept to be accessible via more than one term or code. Apical granuloma provides a particularly suitable dental example: it is referred to in various textbooks by a number of different names,[14,15] five of which have been used in Figure 8.2 to illustrate the problem. The main anomaly that arises is that allowing more than one term to refer to the same concept will greatly reduce query sensitivity.[16] Thus, a

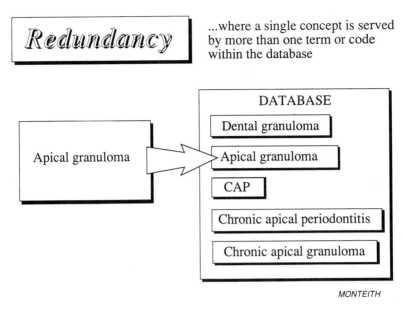

Figure 8.2. The problem of redundancy arises when a single concept within a data base is served by more than one term or code, with consequent reduction in query sensitivity.

query for all cases of apical granuloma in the database depicted will miss case data that has been entered as Chronic Apical Periodontitis, CAP, or any of the other variants listed.

One way of avoiding this in database design would be to make use of synonymy, and it would probably be helpful at this point to draw a distinction between this concept and that of redundancy. This distinction centers on the means of data entry in the database; for while it is important that only one term be used to access data within the database (a state of non-redundancy), synonyms of that term can be very useful in accessing the controlled term outside of the database particularly in the face of terminological conflict.

Turning now to the problem of *ambiguity*, this describes the situation that arises when different concepts are stored in a database under the same term or code. As depicted in Figure 8.3, ICD code 528.9 illustrates the point nicely, while at the same time highlighting one of the major flaws in the way ICD has been structured. The hierarchy of ICD permits only nine variations of a term at each level, with anything beyond that number having to be accommodated in a tenth category entitled "other". Such an arrangement patently has no place in a classification that lays any claim at all to being scientific, because by such forced bundling of distinct clinical entities under a single code, individual entries will become inaccessible, and a query concerning any one of them rendered totally meaningless.

It has been pointed out that ICD was intentionally designed as a means of classifying a heterogeneous set of discrete disease entities into homogeneous lumps so as to provide data categories suitable for statistical analysis.[5] The rules of

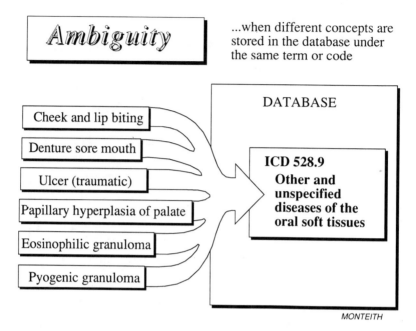

Figure 8.3. Attempting to access different concepts under a single data base code constitutes ambiguity, and gives rise to a loss of query sensitivity.

procedure of ICD would certainly seem to support this idea; which immediately draws into contention Feinstein's third point,[1] the importance of having *standard operational criteria*. In the electronic context, these criteria mean that the rules for coding data should be consistent with sound operational principles.

In a hard-hitting editorial in the Archives of Internal Medicine, Mullin[13] delivered a withering indictment against ICD, stating that "rigid adherence to the ICD mortality coding rules is having a devastating effect on health care statistics". The example he gives concerns an ICD coding convention that requires even "suspected" myocardial infarcts to be coded as *de facto* infarcts - one of many inconsistencies which across the board, are "...wreaking havoc with health data".

Constructing a Nosology for Dentistry

In addressing this task, the prime objective is to formulate a rational concept-framework for organizing and coding dental knowledge in a way that will make it readily accessible for purposes of education, patient care, quality assurance and research. However, in selecting a suitable organizing principle upon which to build a dental nosology, one must recognize the double identity crisis that dentistry is experiencing today as regards both its structure and mission.

Outmoded Structures and Tomorrow's Needs

As described earlier, it was the persistence of *causes of death* as an organizing principle in the face of altering circumstances that led to much of the nosological confusion in Medicine. Dental classifications, by contrast, have remained fairly rudimentary, which is hardly surprising, seeing that dentistry's structures continue to reflect its historical preoccupation with the process and sequellae of caries. Moreover, attempts to accommodate broadening perspectives have (as in medicine) been characteristically inconsistent, as typified by the unpatterned accretion of clinical dental specialties: some are deemed to be domains (like prosthodontics and operative dentistry), others are named according to site (like endodontics and periodontics), and still others according to the age of the target group (pedodontics).

Indeed, the only clearly defined organizing principle to emerge in dentistry so far has centred on *treatments* - with the remunerative factor as an attendant yet significant incentive. Unfortunately, fiscal formulae are patently not of sufficient substance upon which to base a nosology. This is even more true if one considers the future role such a structure would be required to play in the upcoming era of electronic patient records, quality assurance, decision support and electronic curricula.

Outmoded Premises and Tomorrow's Philosophies

Even more disturbing than lack of structure is the apparent lack of mission which dentists would appear to have acquired. Morris and Bohannan's assessment of private dental practice[17] compared recent with less recent graduates and found that dentists who qualified after 1974 scored lower than their predecessors on every component except operative procedures. In a word, although dentists continue to place fillings, they are not recording medical history, not examining soft tissues, not recording periodontal disease, not taking full mouth radiographs, and not drawing up treatment plans.

Recognizing that the source of any anomaly in dental attitudes should be sought in the dental schools, Morris and Bohannan were led to conclude that "a wide gap exists between the way faculty believe dentistry should be practiced and the way it is practiced, and that if our teaching is not carried over into practice, then something is wrong. *Either we are teaching the wrong things or we are teaching the right things the wrong way* [italics added]."

There is little doubt that educators urgently need to redefine the emphasis in dental education until the ability to compound a patient problem-list, using computer-assisted knowledge-couplers,[18] receives equal emphasis and the same reward as the ability to create elegant confections of gold and porcelain. However, to succeed in this will require that a dental nosology be evolved whose organizational axes will give proper expression to these objectives, and which will serve as a framework whereby the needs of dental education, patient service and quality assurance might be optimally served.

New Nosological Axes for New Premises of Problem Management

Mullin[16] has suggested that "since the patient is the ultimate unit of data, it would seem reasonable to assume that a system which accurately describes the patient's or individual's problems would be useful to all users". Consequently, the most rational classification would seem to be one that approaches dental endeavour from the perspective of the patient's problems, with technical procedures relegated to their proper role of serving, rather than constituting that end. Thus, the focus of dental practice ought to be concerned with addressing a broad spectrum of dental diseases, *with the ultimate goal of restoring and maintaining a state of optimum oral health in all individuals within the community.*

A Holistic View of Disease as the Key to Achieving Zero Defect in Oral Health

To achieve total oral health requires that one be in a position to exclude all oral disease; the corollary being that one requires a broad perspective of all possible problems one is likely to encounter to be able to achieve this. A synoptic model that might well prove suitable for this purpose is illustrated in Figure 8.4. It is based upon the natural history of disease, as first described by Leavell and Clark in the mid-fifties,[19] their intention having been to provide a basis whereby a common strategic pattern might be applied to the prevention and management of any medical condition both at the community and individual levels. Being equally applicable to dentistry as to medicine, the use of such an axis would seem to provide an ideal means of achieving a holistic perspective of dental diseases, and thus counter the fragmented speciality orientation typical of traditional dental thinking.

As depicted in the upper portion of Figure 8.4, the natural history of a disease follows a generic axis that is made up of *prepathogenic* and *pathogenic phases.* Prepathogenically, the interaction of a causative agent upon a susceptible host within a predisposing environment triggers a stimulus that elicits the inception of the disease process within the host. Initially, in the early pathogenic phase, disease development remains imperceptible and at a subclinical level; however, it eventually emerges above the clinical horizon to enter a phase of early discernibility. At this stage - if diagnosed early enough - it is frequently still capable of reversal without residual disability. This is approached either through enhancing host resistance, suppressing agent virulence or both. Unchecked, however, the disease will frequently progress into an advanced phase in which it is no longer reversible, and where permanent disability will almost inevitably result. Thereafter, and depending upon the particular disease, death, recovery, chronicity or other complicating sequellae will ensue.

As originally envisaged, this model enables disease management to follow a generic pattern that permits application at both community and individual levels. Initially, the aim of PRIMARY PREVENTION is to apply *Specific Protection* measures while pursuing strategies of *Health Promotion.* Such measures are aimed

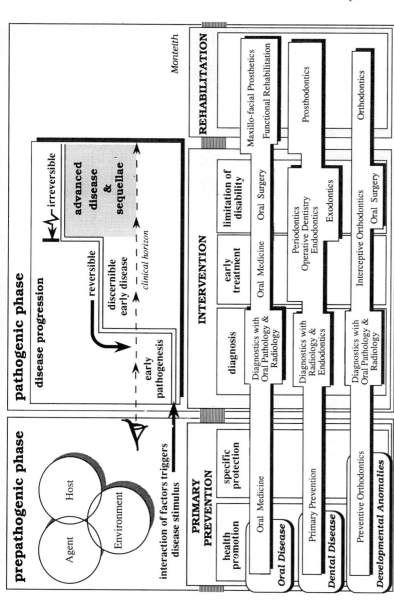

Figure 8.4. The Natural History of Disease as a holistic organizational principle for dentistry. The various phases reflect an interplay of etiological factors, and progress through an initial state of possible reversal to ultimate disability and sequellae of varying gravity. Management is designed to be applied broadly at community level, as well as individually. The latter is illustrated as it applies to the three main axes of dental concern, showing how the various dental disciplines are distributed along the axes.

at achieving a balance between host, agent and environment that will preclude the stimulus arising that will typically initiate the disease.

Once the disease has started, however, management enters a secondary phase of INTERVENTION. This phase aims at combating the disease first by ensuring its early detection; second, by instituting early treatment while the disease is still reversible; and third, by applying strategies to arrest the disease process once it has progressed into its advanced stage, thereby attempting to limit the degree of disability it will cause. It is only once limitation of disability has been achieved that disease management passes into the final tertiary stage of REHABILITA-TION. This ideally consists of a phase of post-curative rehabilitation in which efforts are instituted to repair damage and effectively restore function, morphology and aesthetics.

Using Disease Axes in an Integrated Approach to Achieving Oral Health

The application of the above management categories as they pertain to dentistry is illustrated in the lower portion of Figure 8.4. This recognizes three major categories of dental involvement - *Oral Disease, Dental Disease* and the *Management of Developmental Anomalies* - and demonstrates how the various dental clinical disciplines can be arranged as a continuum along these axes.

If one takes dental caries as a means of demonstrating the model, PRIMARY PREVENTION would involve attempting to enhance host resistance, minimize agent influence, and create an environmental imperative that would preclude the balance of factors arising that would act as a stimulus for pathogenicity. At the level of community management, *Specific Protection* might involve fluoridation of water supplies, while *Health Promotion* would involve various community programs aimed at engendering oral health education through the promotion of individual selfcare. The aims are similar when applying the model at the individual level. Here, *Specific Protection* might involve topical fluoride treatments, application of fissure sealants and the like; while *Health Promotion* would be concerned with inculcating awareness and commitment in the individual patient such as will ensure selfcare through the practice of successful oral hygiene.

Moving on along the disease axis to the secondary phase of INTERVENTION, the brief phase of initial decalcification in the disease's early stage is capable of being successfully reversed through recalcification, and underlines the importance of a clinical horizon having sufficient acuity as to ensure an early diagnosis. Undetected, this phase quickly enters the advanced phase of permanent disability. In its earliest stage, the aim of removing affected tooth structure and subsequent obturation of the defect by placing a restoration should be viewed essentially as a means of limiting the disability and preventing the disease from recurring. Further progression of the disease with attendant pulpal and subsequent periapical sequel-lae requires the application of endodontic principles, with in its advanced final stages, the possibility of exodontic intervention.

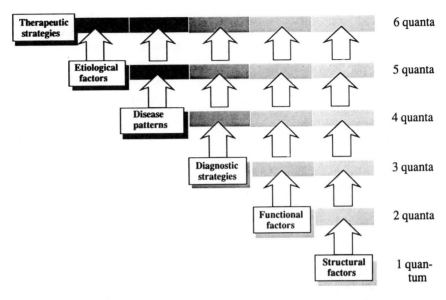

Figure 8.5. The six conceptual layers of Gabrieli's Nosology: Semantic quanta (or packages of meaning) are summated within each successive layer.

The Disease Axes and the Representation of Dental Knowledge

The essential purpose of a nosological classification is to enable one to gain a better understanding of an ensemble through the grouping of related entities.[4] Indeed, within the context of knowledge representation, Luger and Stubblefield[20] have stated that objects take on meaning only "...through their relationships with other objects...something that is equally true of the facts, theories and techniques that go to make up any field of scientific study."

The idea of using "meaning" relationally as an organizing principle has already been tried in medicine; for, when Elmer Gabrieli[8] drew up his nosology, he chose as his "key" the fact that every medical term has a *meaning-load*, or *semantic-load* that can be fitted into a hierarchy of organizational principles at six successive levels. These semantic layers make use of the fact that most medical concepts are only meaningful when seen in the light of other pre-existing concepts; and as can be seen from Figure 8.5, the ascent through the six conceptual layers involves an additional quantum (or package) of implied information being added as a prerequisite for each successive layer.

Gabrieli named this system the *Quantum Theory of Medical Terms*, and used it to construct a vast nosological tree, made up of a hierarchical network of nodes that serve as electronic addresses for more than 120,000 primary medical terms.[21] The implications of such a structure for dentistry, particularly for dental education, are exciting; for if one conceives of a *cognitive-load*, analogous with Gabrieli's semantic-load, as a prerequisite of each successive quantum layer, the Nosology emerges as a framework that should be capable of accommodating the full canon of dental knowledge. However, because the meaning-load of each of Gabrieli's stored terms is present only by implication, the envisioned dental nosology would require that the resident concept at each node be "fleshed out" through the inclusion of additional descriptive detail.

The way in which such a structure could be applied to dental needs is illustrated in Figure 8.6, which demonstrates how vertical associative links would need to be forged over the six conceptual levels, to form a cohesive *Knowledge Web* of cognitive information.

As envisaged for dentistry, the *basic* (one quantum) *cognitive level* would embody descriptions of all dentally relevant structures, encompassing both regional and gross anatomy, as well as histology and ultrastructural detail. The descriptive material at this level is static and essentially three-dimensional, but would need to be available as a given before one would be in a position to comprehend related *functional* information at level two.

The *second* (two quanta) *level* has a greater cognitive load than the first, in that it includes *time* as an additional dimension, and deals with the normal functions of the stomatognathic system and the human mind. This would typically include physiology, psychology, biophysics and related preclinical sciences; and together with material imported from level one, would be instrumental in establishing *criteria of normality*.

Having established what is "normal", in terms of the physical structures and phenomena of the first two levels, the common goal of the third and fourth-quanta levels is to store information relevant to differentiating health from disease through the establishment of clinical patterns of abnormality.

Here, the role of the *third cognitive level* concerns the actual strategies and methods of data capture, and the normal qualifying and quantifying criteria necessary to separate and delineate the abnormal. Information at this level, therefore, is devoted to all the various diagnostic tests needed to reach a dental diagnosis, and would include information dealing with biopsies and sample collection (together with their various normal values), as well as material relevant to microbiology, dental radiology and the like. The *fourth quantum level*, on the other hand, builds on the strategies of third level data-capture through the interpretation of the diagnostic patterns established there, such as signs, symptoms, diagnoses and syndromes.

The *fifth quantum level* involves information relating to the interplay of the etiological factors of oral and dental disease and developmental anomalies, as was described earlier in the Leavell and Clark[19] model. Included here would be information pertaining to microorganisms, as well as to chemical, social, genetic and environmental factors.

Considering the notion, presented earlier, that effective treatment involves the manipulation of the etiological factors relevant to host, agent, and environment, the *sixth quantum level* involves the therapeutic strategies whereby this might be best accomplished, both at the community and individual levels of application. In

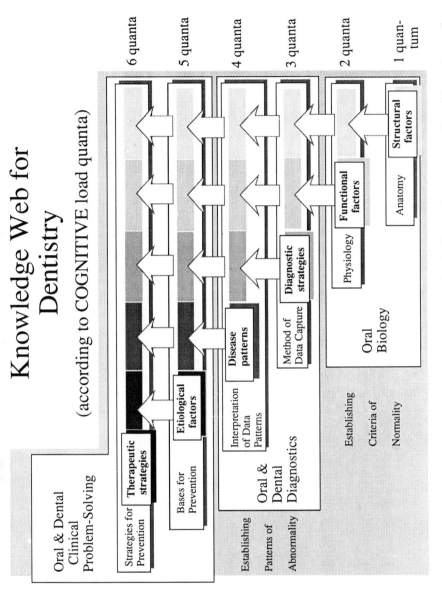

Figure 8.6. A proposed dental nosology after Gabrieli's model, showing how analogous quanta of cognitive understanding would need to be in place as a prerequisite for comprehension at each successive layer.

addition to primary prevention, strategies relating to the phases of therapeutic intervention as well as rehabilitation would also be included here, encompassing details of drug therapy, as well as surgical, operative and prosthodontic procedures.

The organization of these diverse concepts within the nosology can be visualized in terms of discrete packages of cognitive information arranged within a tree-like, hierarchical structure. Each package constitutes a distinct knowledge node, with the nodes being grouped together conceptually in domains so as to ensure close sibling neighbourliness at each level of the tree. This arrangement lends itself to electronic navigation amongst related matters, by permitting lateral browsing within a domain; while vertically, organization of the hierarchy is such as to permit one to proceed from the general to the specific — an arrangement that is consistent with Aristotle's ancient yet compelling principle of ranking entities from the simple to the increasingly complex.[5]

Figure 8.7 provides an example of how the sixth level tree, pertaining to *Oral and Dental Procedures*, might be developed so as to accommodate the three conceptually distinct domains of *Oral Disease Management*, *Dental Disease Management* and the *Management of Developmental Anomalies*. The actual strategies of problem managment within each of the three disease areas have been arranged in accordance with the Leavell and Clark model,[19] with the domain of *Dental Disease Management* further developed to demonstrate the way in which the traditional dental disciplines might be accommodated.

The strength of using an electronic environment for such an application is the ease with which the information at each knowledge node can be accessed. Furthermore, by using the mechanisms of *Hypertext*, pointers can be set at each node which will permit access to related information at any number of other nodes throughout the tree. The actual electronic connections involved are referred to as *arcs*, of which there are two main types. The first is used to link nodes within neighboring domains at the same level (as in establishing concept links between *gross anatomy*, *histology*, and *ultrastructure* within Level One); the second provides the means of forming the associative links with nodes situated within other quantum levels of the nosological tree, as depicted by the vertical arrows in Figure 8.6. In this way the *knowledge web* allows quick location of all information relevant to a specific need. The required mix of knowledge nodes and arcs will obviously differ according to the dictates of the need. Generically, such a contextual grouping is termed a *State Space*;[20] however, in specified applications, such as problem-based learning, it is more specifically referred to as the *Problem Space*.

Nosology: The Key to Competency in Dentistry

The competencies required to practise dentistry emerge as a significant focus in the Strategic Plan that was issued by the American Dental Association in 1983.[22] This document states that "a clear-cut description of the competencies...would provide a sound basis for curricular design"; but as no one has yet described them, recommends that an urgent study of these competencies be made as a basis "for

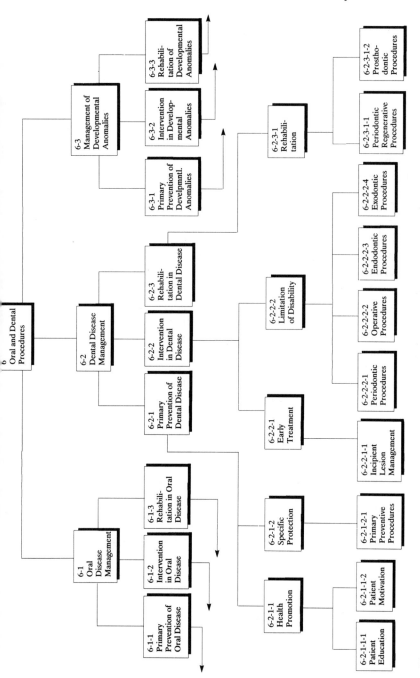

Figure 8.7. The sixth level of the nosological tree, demonstrating the nodal arrangement of concepts relating to strategies of dental and oral problem management. Related domains are juxtaposed permitting lateral conceptual browsing; whilst vertically, downward progression takes one from the general to the particular.

the practice of dentistry in the future". With this in mind, *competency in clinical problem-solving* should be regarded equally as the primary goal of dental education, the primary focus of patient and community care and the chief concern of quality assurance strategies - all sustained, maintained and fortified through the ongoing efforts of dental research.

The Role of Nosology in Competency Development

In dentistry, the inculcation of clinical competency imposes burdens of didactic responsibility that transcend those of most other health professions. The reasons are not hard to find, being vested mainly in the need for considerable finger-skill development, that must conform to exacting quality criteria: this in addition to the constraints of rigorous decisionmaking protocols, and a knowledge base that stretches from the biological to the metallurgical.

By using the Leavell and Clark based model as a conceptual framework, a comprehensive range of a dentist's expected competencies can be defined and circumscribed in terms of a set of *competency development units*. As illustrated by Figure 8.8, each of these units comprises two basic components. First, there is a skill development module, which might apply equally to either psychomotor or reasoning skills. Of necessity, the skill development process must be linked to a specific methodology of performance, as well as to a set of criteria against which the standard of performance will be measured through the assessment of outcomes.

The second component within the unit is a knowledge base. This represents the cognitive content essential to the rational performance of the particular skill and is made up of a series of knowledge nodes, which in an electronic environment, would be linked by *arcs*, so as to permit exploratory navigation of all relevant areas of supporting knowledge. These components can all be conceptually accommodated, at various levels, within the nosological knowledge web; while interactive links with ancillary databases containing *glossary definitions*, *graphics*, and *literature references*, enhance the relevance of the textual material at each node.

In *problem based learning*, the above material constitutes the *problem space* which a questing student is required to traverse in search of solutions. Typically, the problem itself would be presented in the form of diagnostic observations, set out on a representation of a patient's record, on the computer screen. This means that in terms of Gabrieli's six quantum levels, entry into the problem space occurs at Level Four: the student then being required to explore the implications of the displayed data pattern, by arcing from node to node in a cognitive exploration through the lower levels.

This process is illustrated in Figure 8.9, using the example of the superficial enamel lesion of incipient caries. The problem space for this portion of the exploration is represented by the nodes and connecting arcs contained within the stippled area.

Once information has been gleaned sufficient to enable identification of the problem, the quest moves upwards through the fifth layer of etiologic possibility, to a finally evolved treatment strategy at Level Six.

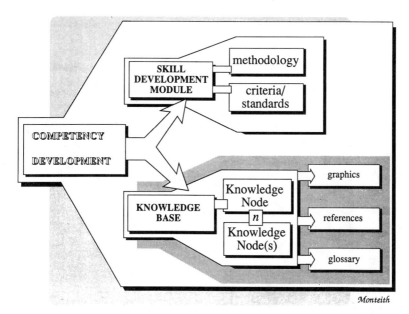

Figure 8.8. The anatomy of a competency development unit. The process of skill development relies upon a circumscribed methodology together with a set of criteria to determine
the quality of outcomes. The associated knowledgebase is defined strictly in accordance with
its relevance to the skill development process, and can be linked to separate databases
containing references, a glossary and pictorial material.

Competencies in Practice: The Role of Nosology in Patient Care and Quality Assurance

The educational imperatives embodied above are intended to engender a
philosophy of dental care that encompasses all aspects of patient evaluation,
diagnosis, treatment planning and treatment. Equally important, however, is that
this problem-solving protocol find practical expression in the field of real-time
patient care and service.

Previous tendencies to equate the *quality* of dental care with technical quality
of dental work are no longer appropriate. As stated by Jerge and Orlowski,[23] the
primary concern of patient care ought to be with the progress of oral and dental
disease; and the quality of care should be equated with the effectiveness of the
measures used in counteracting that progress.

The general inadequacy of record-keeping practice, documented by Morris and
Bohannan[17] in their survey of dental practices, indicates that the paradigm here
remains firmly vested in the technical. Indeed, in the U.S.A. there would seem to
be little likelihood of its shifting as long as the present remuneration policy as
enshrined in the A.D.A. treatment codes continues to color practitioners' perceptions.

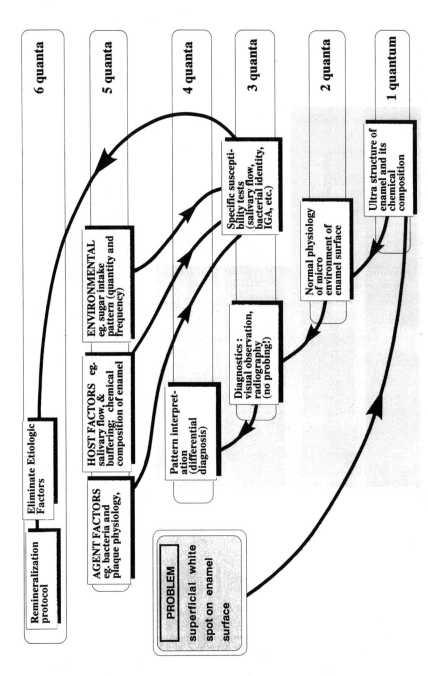

Figure 8.9. The Nosology in use for problem-based learning. The problem is presented as diagnostic detail in screen format. In a search for a solution, the student is guided through the relevant *problem space* by means of arcs that electronically link the nodes.

In expanding the paradigms, the four clinical functions identified as essential to the proper documentation of patient care have been stated as being 1) the *data base* (history and clinical findings), 2) *clinical problems or diagnoses*; 3) *the plan of treatment* and 4) the *treatment rendered.*[23] In terms of the nosology, these concepts can be accommodated sequentially within levels three, four and six; and although the coding here would differ from that of the present A.D.A. listing, electronic cross-referencing would render the distinction functionally transparent.

With regard to quality assurance, the ability to construct arcs linking nodes at various nosological levels would materially benefit the conduct of an *analytical audit*. This type of audit is employed "to evaluate the judgement, clinical decision-making and overall clinical performance of the provider",[23] and deals with questions concerning the adequacy of the database; whether the diagnoses were correct (given the available information); whether the treatment plan was well-founded and whether the treatment itself was properly prioritized and carried out in an appropriate sequence and manner. According to Jerge and Orlowski,[23] such assessments are by their very nature subjective - even though they do provide a high level of validity for auditing purposes, when completed by an experienced clinician. However, arc linkages between definitive criteria within the nodes of the knowledge web might serve as an effective audit trail, providing both consistency and objectivity in the evaluation of individual providers. Moreover, specific pointers, founded on research, can be incorporated within the nosological knowledge web, which could provide longitudinal assessment of treatment efficacy over a broad front. Even *focused audits*, which concentrate on particular procedures or modalities, will be capable of objective assessment: this being made possible through the availability of a set of standards as part of each competency statement, as illustrated in Figure 8.8.

Setting the Paradigms for Competency: The Role of Nosology in Research

Weed[24] has highlighted the observation that there is defective linkage between bodies of knowledge and the use of that knowledge, and as evidence of this has pointed to the large "voltage drop" that occurs from what is known from research to what is eventually done on the average patient.

These comments were of course directed towards medicine; however, much of what Weed had to say is equally applicable to dentistry — the prime example being the steady demise of dental caries. Central to this phenomenon was the successful application of strategies of prevention, established in response to research; the supreme anomaly being that dentists all the while continued to immerse themselves in operative procedures that in essence had very little bearing upon the conspicuous success of the campaign.

It has been emphasised already that dentists need to liberate themselves from a limiting preoccupation with "treating teeth", and that they acquire a holistic concern with the need to address all oral problems. The nosology, by permitting wide-ranging exploration of all aspects of patient care, will fulfill a cardinal role simply by acting as a continuing reminder of the full scope of a dentist's clinical responsibility. Because the nosology is designed to accommodate all aspects of dental endeavour within a rationally arranged structure, it will facilitate the ready categorization of new knowledge as it emerges from dental research. This in turn will facilitate keeping knowledge and skill bases within the nosology up-to-date, permitting it to continue as a relevant reflection of current research findings.

Weed has sounded the *caveat* that "real problems in the real world - practical or theoretical problems - do not fit neatly into academic boundaries". However, by constructing a nosology that will assist the development and implementation of professional competencies, and by maintaining its relevance through research, the structural transition towards the electronic applications of the future will be assured. Thus empowered, one will be in a position to answer with confidence Weed's plea for "...an information system...that rigorously couples the fruits of scholarly effort and research to the everyday actions of us all".

References

1. Feinstein A.R. ICD, POR and DRG: Unsolved scientific problems in the nosology of clinical medicine. Arch Intern Med 3;148:2269-2274.
2. Onions C.T. ed. The Shorter Oxford Dictionary. Oxford, The Clarendon Press. 1959.
3. Knibbs G.H. The International Classification of Disease and causes of death and its revision. Med J Aust 1929;1:2-12.
4. Farr W. Registrar General of England and Wales: Sixteenth Annual Report. Appendix, 1856:75-76.
5. Gabrieli E.R. The medicine-compatible computer: A challenge for medical informatics. Med Inform 1984;9:233-250.
6. International Classification of Diseases, Ninth Revision, Clinical Modification, publication (PHS) 80-1260. US Dept. of Health and Human Services, 1980.
7. Systematized Nomenclature of Pathology, 1st ed. Chicago: College of American Pathologists, 1965.
8. Gabrieli E.R. A new electronic medical nomenclature. J of Medical Systems 1989; 13:355-373.
9. Cote R.A., ed. Systematized Nomenclature of Medicine (SNOMED), 2nd ed. Chicago: College of American Pathologists, 1979.
10. Medical Subject Headings. Bethesda, MD: National Library of Medicine, Library Operations, 1989.
11. Clauser S.B., Fanta C.M., Finkel A.J., eds. Current Procedural Terminology, Fourth Edition - CPT4. Chicago: American Medical Association, 1984.
12. Barr C.E., Komorowski H.J., Pattison-Gordon E., Greenes R.A. Conceptual modeling for the Unified Medical Language System. In: Greenes RA, ed. Proceedings of the Twelfth Annual Symposium on Computer Applica-

tions in Medical Care. Washington DC: IEEE Computer Society Press, 1988; 148-151.

13. Ingle J.I., Beveridge E.E., eds. Endodontics. Philadelphia: Lea & Febiger,1976:398.

14. Jablonski S. Illustrated dictionary of dentistry. Philadelphia: W.B.Saunders Company,1982:367.

15. Cimino J.J., Hripcsak G., Johnson S.B., Clayton P.B. Designing an intro-spective, multipurpose, controlled medical vocabulary. In: Kingsland CK, ed. Proceedings of the Thirteenth Annual Symposium on Computer Ap-plications in Medical Care. Washington DC: IEEE Computer Society Press, 1989:513-518.

16. Mullin R.L. The nosology of clinical medicine. Arch Intern Med 1988;148:2114-2115.

17. Morris A.L., Bohannan HM. Assessment of private dental practice: Im-plications for dental education. J Dent Ed 1987;51:661-667.

18. Abbey L.M. An expert system for clinical teaching in a school of dentistry. In: Salamon R, Protti D, Moehr J, eds. Proceedings of the International Symposium on Medical Informatics and Education. Victoria BC: Univer-sity of Victoria, BC., Canada, 1989:364-366.

19. Leavell H.R., Clark E.G.: Preventive medicine for the doctor in his com-munity: an epidemiological approach, ed 3. New York, McGraw-Hill Book Company, 1965, pp 14-28.

20. Luger G.F., Stubblefield W.A. Artifical Intelligence and the Design of Ex-pert Systems. Redwood City, CA: The Benjamin/Cummings Publishing Company, Inc,1989:23.

21. Gabrieli E.R., Murphy G. Computerized medical records. Journal of AMRA 1990;61:26-31.

22. American Dental Association, Report of the Special Committee on the Fu-ture of Dentistry: Issue Papers on Dental Research, Manpower, Education, Practice and Public and Professional Concerns and Recommendations for Action. Chicago:American Dental Association, 1983,43-44.

23. Jerge C.R., Orlowski R.M. Quality assurance and the dental record. Dental Clinics of North America 1985;29:483-496.

24. Weed L.L. New premises and new tools for medical care and medical education. In: Salamon R., Protti D., Moehr J., eds. Proceedings of the In-ternational Symposium on Medical Informatics and Education. Victoria BC: University of Victoria, BC., Canada, 1989:23-30.

9
Informatics in Dental Education

John E. Eisner

This chapter begins with a general review of computer use in dental education. It is a short review, as the primary application of computers in dental school has been directed toward clinic management systems. Several other educational applications are also reviewed.

The chapter concludes with a discussion of how the informatics trends which are now evident in dental practice will likely impact on dental education in the future. Concepts and proposals described in this section include:

- an electronic dental patient record
- a "second generation" clinical database which includes decision support and quality assessment tools for tomorrow's practitioner and promises an improved research perspective for future clinicians
- the electronic dental patient record as a focal point for tomorrow's problem-based curriculum
- a design for a "problem-based, informatics-mediated" dental curriculum, the electronic component of which could be available before the year 2000 and could include:
    1. a 'discipline' axis
    2. a 'disease' axis, and
    3. a problem or 'case' axis
- a plan for gathering the national resources needed to develop an informatics curriculum in dentistry.

Introduction

The task of discussing computer applications in dental education is, at the same time, both an extremely broad and extremely narrow assignment. It is broad in the sense that dental education, by its most general definition, includes clinical, research, teaching, and administrative applications. It is narrow in the sense that compared to the development of general trends in information science and particularly medical informatics, dental education has focused on only a few applications, with limited progress, during the past two decades.

Although medical informatics fellowships and training programs have been in place since the mid 1970s, only a few dentists have had the opportunity, or encouragement, to pursue both dentistry and informatics training, or careers in dental informatics. Similarly, few schools have had the opportunity to collaborate in application development of much use beyond their own walls. As a result, we have many "one of a kind" applications, born out of necessity, or perhaps curiosity, and which have extended one individual, or one institution, to the current limits of their available local resources.

This chapter will offer the reader an overview of several of the more important applications of informatics in dental education. This overview will be very brief as the broader challenge is to engage the reader in an exploration of how informatics could apply to curriculum development for the year 2000. The approach taken is broad and holistic. The chapter projects a significant change in the profession's approach to record keeping and information access as dental practice becomes more complex, and as dental offices become increasingly computerized. The chapter also redefines curriculum, learning, and teaching in the health professions, and describes what might become known as the "problem-based, informatics-mediated" dental curriculum.

A Brief Review of Computer Applications in Dental Education

To date, the most obvious, and most successful, application of computer technology to dental education has been in the dental clinic. As early as the mid-sixties, mainframe computers were engaged in tracking "student requirements" and billing patients.[1] The seventies witnessed the expansion of these clinical computing efforts to almost all aspects of clinic management, and the migration, in most institutions with computers, from mainframes to mini-computers. Also in the seventies, many Dean's offices developed financial applications, frequently on micro-computers, allowing them to have a better grasp of their budgetary situation. Databases have also simplified applicant records,[2] the preparation of acceptance letters, curriculum schedules, grade reports, and other administrative tasks. In many dental schools, word processing has also facilitated the writing of many papers by faculty whose secretarial support has diminished.

Early evidence of a broader interest in educational computing came from Nebraska with the development of some 30 dental patient care simulations. They were equal, at the time, to "state-of-the-art" medical simulations, but were restricted in their access and general acceptance by the fact that they were tied to a single mainframe computer manufacturer. Additionally, they relied on slow media including random access videotape and slide projectors which further detracted from their excellent educational design. Had these simulations, which were fifteen years ahead of their time, been designed this year they would have been able to take advantage of a number of recent advances in microcomputer technology, including better authoring software, videodisc technology and digital imaging, all of which would have produced a highly desirable product.

In the mid 1980s, The University of Iowa picked up the dental simulation gauntlet, using videodisc technology.[3] Second and third year students now complete a number of simulations during their oral pathology clinical rotations, and other departments, including dental hygiene, are now developing simulations which are specific to their individual disciplines.

Individuals at other dental schools have developed a handful of small, single-concept programs focusing on topics such as oral radiology[4] and partial denture design[5], while other software companies have produced programs of interest to dental education, such as those in nutrition.[6] Such efforts, isolated as they now are, will surely continue. Indeed, until there is a national "critical mass" of individuals who have attempted to develop their own single-concept software, and who can perhaps see the need for larger software programs which are integrated across disciplines, we will not be able to make any significant informatics breakthroughs in our approach to dental education.

Recent evidence of the search for a critical mass among dental educators has come through the Section on Operative Dentistry within the American Association of Dental Schools. With the approval of the section membership, individuals from the Operative Dentistry departments at six dental schools recently combined their efforts in 1988 to produce a "training" videodisc for dental anatomy.[7]

Additional evidence of the need for collaborative efforts can be seen in the formation, in 1990, of a consortium of more than 30 US and Canadian dental schools to pursue the development of software which could be used to analyze both the content and process of the dental curriculum.[8] The concept of analyzing a school's curriculum as if it were a database, has been attempted at several medical and dental schools during the past decade.[9,10,11] By entering course outlines as well as keywords collected from every teaching session (lecture based or problem-based) and by cross-referencing these data with curriculum goals or clinical competencies, a school has the opportunity of conducting a curriculum analysis at four distinct levels. These include:

1) an analysis of individual session content and learning behaviors,

2) the analysis of courses by objectives, texts, reading assignments, content and evaluation strategies,

3) the contribution of courses and disciplines to school-wide curriculum goals and/or clinical competencies, and

4) the analysis of the curriculum by national yardsticks such as the American Dental Association's Curriculum Standards. The field test version of the software is expected in 1991, with a final version to be released in 1992.

For those in dentistry who are interested in more detail about the development of informatics in both medical and dental education, perusal of the Subgroup Report on Medical Information Science Skills in the GPEP report,[12] the proceedings of a medical education symposium titled *Medical Education in the Information Age*,[13] the dental education chapter in *Dental Informatics: Strategic Issues for the Dental Profession*,[14] a recent article on hypermedia in the life sciences,[15] or the medical education chapter in *Medical Informatics: Computer Applications in Health Care*[16] would provide an initial foundation. For the most part however, these and other volumes decry the absence of leadership, the absence of faculty skills in informatics, and fragmentation between software, hardware, and approach within our ranks. No doubt this will continue throughout the nineties as it will take time to realize the most appropriate directions and approaches to the integration of computer-managed instruction in dental education.

The remainder of this chapter focuses on one approach, one vision, the aim of which is to maximize the potential for informatics in dental education.

The Development of The Dental Curriculum

After its turbulent beginnings in the mid-nineteenth century, dental education was offered in both non-profit and proprietary settings through the 1920s. The reform that the Flexner Report[17] brought to medical education after the turn of the century finally arrived on dentistry's doorstep with the Geis Report in 1926.[18] It called for an increased emphasis on the relevance of the basic sciences and more obvious efforts to integrate the basic and clinical dental sciences. During the four decades following the Geis Report, curricula in US and Canadian dental schools were relatively stable and almost exclusively followed the "two plus two", or "vertical", model, with two years of basic science courses, frequently in the company of medical students, followed by two clinical years. In the late sixties there began a movement toward earlier clinical experience and, as one response for the continuing lack of correlation of basic and clinical sciences, a number of schools created departments of Oral Biology which, it was hoped, would extend the impact of the oral basic sciences into the third and fourth years. The result of these earlier clinical experiences and the extended basic sciences was often referred to as the "diagonal" curriculum.

With only a few exceptions,[19] the "diagonal" model has continued into the 1990s as the dominant format for the dental curriculum. Within this model, the most prevalent form of teaching is the discipline-based lecture, or "lecture with slides", and the most widely utilized form of testing is the multiple choice examination. These methodologies generally require the student to memorize as many facts as possible in preparation for the examinations. In this passive, teacher-centered environment, student retention is questionable, as are clinical judgement, problem-solving, and continuous learning skills.

In the 1970s, several medical schools began experimentation with problem-oriented, or the even more demanding, problem-based curriculum mode.[20] These models were born of the philosophy that medical knowledge was changing so rapidly that it was more important to offer students a good grounding in problem-solving and information retrieval skills, both of which would insure an active, inquiring approach to the practice of medicine. Independent study, group study, and problem-centered small group tutorials are the predominant teaching/learning methodologies used in the problem-based curriculum. Lectures are usually restricted to orientation and overview functions, and examinations rely increasingly on Objective Structured Clinical Exams (OSCEs) or on the use of simulated patients rather than the exclusive use of multiple choice testing. In the 1980s a number of computer-based patient simulations were also introduced to medical students, in part by the National Board of Medical Examiners. The Board has indicated that the format of their Part III Clinical Examination will eventually change to include computer-based simulations.

In the late 1980s, a large number of medical schools initiated,[21] and a few dental schools began to explore, problem-based learning and, in the process, initiated a series of major curriculum changes. The course of studies and, by extension, students or practitioners were no longer repositories of facts. Indeed, the goal was to learn the skills of problem solving and the acquisition of relevant knowledge in the context in which it is needed. In this information-gathering process, the value of computers and their large clinical databases, as well as their regularly maintained knowledge and image bases soon became evident. Thus, with the parallel maturation of both problem-based learning and medical informatics at the turn of this decade, the potential for combining the problem-based curriculum with computerized knowledge bases could now be fruitfully explored. The remainder of this chapter offers such an exploration, beginning where curriculum reform should begin, with a discussion of the real world of dental practice and the impact which computers will have on that environment and its educational precursor in the near future.

Dental Practice: Already Changed and Going Further, Faster

Before focusing on the changes being brought about in general practice by the computer, it is important to realize that many changes in dental practice are occurring quite separately. The increasing age of our patient population, their improved capacity to live with chronic disease often with the assistance of several different medications, the explosion in the number of such medications and their possible adverse interactions, the new requirements for working with patients with auto-immune diseases, as well as insuring infection control and occupational safety in the office, are but a few examples of the constantly changing problems facing the profession. Additionally, the increased number of specialists in dentistry and in medicine has lead to the increased sharing of care among health professionals as well as the increased need for the dentist to be able to converse intelligently with these colleagues. Finally, concern for litigation and the increasing interest in patients participating in the determination of their own care, requires dental health personnel to be excellent communicators. The combination of a) increased problem-solving skills within an ever-expanding universe of facts, pharmaceuticals, and regulations, b) increased communication with medical and dental colleagues, c) improved communication with the patient, and d) no decrease in the patient's expectations for high quality and constantly improving technical skills are potent "patient-driven" factors to consider when designing new methods for teaching our developing professionals.

Turning now to the computer itself, in the late 1980s, many clinicians and some academicians were becoming aware of the potential for computers to positively impact on dental practice in an unprecedented variety of applications. A short list of in-office computing power now includes sophisticated office management programs, electronic data interchange for the transmission of insurance forms and payment, cosmetic imaging for projections of dental and facial treatment, in-office milling of crowns and restorations, on-line access to both drug information databases and the medical literature, and the potential for the digital exposure and storage of radiographs.

In late 1989 a survey in one of the dental trade magazines suggested that nearly 50% of all dentists then used a computer in their offices. While only a small number were pursuing the above innovations, the availability of both technical computing power and information processing power, plus an awareness of the increasing complexity of patient diagnosis and treatment, was having an impact on the way younger dentists approached their patient care responsibiiities. Let us now continue to project where this association with the computer might lead the profession through the remainder of the 1990s.

Educational Implications of Projected Change in Dental Practice

Quite apart from the improved learning opportunities which accrue from problem-based learning (mentioned earlier in this chapter) there appear to be real needs for this type of learning based solely on what is happening in dental practice. A grounding in dental informatics, both from the point of information acquisition (for problem-solving) and proficiency with in-office software applications, data communication, and hardware capabilities appears to be essential, as does the ability to communicate effectively with patients and colleagues while maintaining technical proficiency. The curriculum we will propose is based in problem-solving and informatics skills.

The Electronic Dental Patient Record: Focal Point for Dental Practice in the Future

Although the move will not be a speedy one, practitioners will gradually expand their current dental office practice management systems to include the electronic storage of diagnostic information in addition to the currently stored treatment and billing information. Once this occurs, two new opportunities open up for the practitioner. The first involves the addition of decision-support systems to their current software and the second involves the incorporation of quality assessment measures into their practice management reporting programs. These advances will be discussed further, in the section on clinical database design, but first we need to look in some detail at the functionality, display characteristics, and data entry requirements which arise with the capture and use of diagnostic information in an electronic dental patient record.

Functionality

Although there are several initial products now on the market[22] which illustrate some of the concepts of an electronic dental patient record (EDPR), the "complete" version is still several years away. Therefore any beginning discussion of the EDPR must offer a listing of the various features one must assume will be present. To start broadly, an empty EDPR would be the receptacle for all patient information which can be easily captured in digital format. This includes all data now in the paper record such as patient demographics, chief complaint, medical and dental history, extra-oral, oral, periodontal, dental and home care charting, diagnostic tests and results, problem list, diagnoses, treatment plan, treatment record, progress notes, medical or dental laboratory prescriptions, letters of referral or consultation, and a record of patient education, instructions and acceptance of treatment. It also includes the possibility for digitized photographs of the patient and relevant casts, digitized radiographs, and the actual prosthodontic designs ready for transmittal directly to the dental lab. A rough visualization of the EDPR we are working with (reduced from a 19" screen to the size of a book page) is shown as Figure 9.1.

Data Capture

In April of 1990, a number of presenters at a symposium[23] on "The Second Generation Clinical Database and the Electronic Patient Record" confirmed that all such elements of the proposed electronic record could now be captured, digitized and stored in a relational database. The technology for the electronic record was not the issue. What was, and still is, under debate is the preferred dentist/machine interface and the preferred method(s) of data entry. From work in other fields there is considerable evidence that the most successful forms of data entry, at least from the point of view of provider acceptance and cost, are those which occur at the first point of possible data capture. In dentistry, electronic periodontal probes and digital radiographs are the best examples of direct capture. Another example of capture at the time of "first encounter" would be the use of voice entry, done at the time of charting and when generating progress notes. While this is not direct, as the clinician must "speak" each step of the charting activity, it is no different than if the dentist were dictating the charting information to a dental assistant. Other methods which are being explored involve the use of a touch screen, light-pen, or graphics tablet by other office personnel at the time the dentist is describing patient findings or treatment procedures which are in progress. Each of these methods include one additional step from the voice entry process described

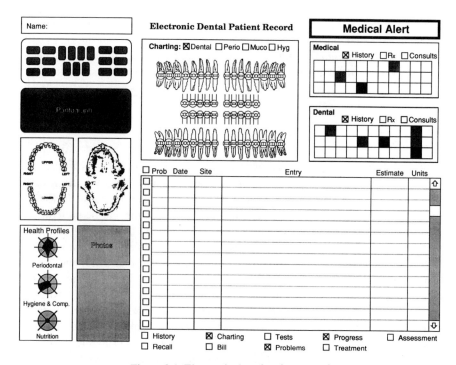

Figure 9.1. Electronic dental patient record.

above, where errors can occur; that being the (usually unseen) transcription of the dentist's words to the paper chart by the assistant.

Except for the initial recording of patient demographics by the office staff, typing will be minimized through the use of patient data entry where appropriate, pre-programmed menu selections and simple voice commands. For the dentist, keyboard input will likely be eliminated altogether, particularly if voice input is adopted and, where necessary, the use of digitized and compressed voice-notes, spoken and recorded by the dentist, then electronically attached to the EDPR, becomes feasible.

The Health History: A Vital Connection to the Medical Record

The capture of health history information about a given patient deserves separate discussion. Some offices now ask patients to enter their own health history directly into the computer. Alternatively, if the history is taken by the dentist or another member of the office staff, it could be entered by that individual at the time of the patient interview. In either situation, an electronic record of the patient's responses and the practitioner's follow-up questions and analysis are generated at the initial appointment and can be added to as necessary at subsequent appointments. This method is far from ideal.

At some point in the future, when both the dentist and the physician are using electronic records, one would hope that the "dentist's version" of the patient's health record will simply be a subset of the patient's medical history containing those relevant portions of the patient's medical record which the dentist should have access to, as an involved provider. Consequently the dentist, as the first observer of a number of conditions which have a broader medical relevance, will be able to transmit new findings to the "full" electronic medical record for review by the physician or other appropriate health care workers.

When the electronic records of the physician, dentist, and other health care professionals are dynamically linked, all involved providers will have access to a single electronic health history. This will be much better than the current situation where each member of the team is required to create a separate, and perhaps erroneous, "mini-history" for their own special use. Therefore, as we close this discussion on the capture of health history data, one can see that the eventual widespread use of the electronic patient record will greatly change the way we collect and update this most critical entry in the patient record.

Design of the User Interface

Turning to the question of the dentist/machine interface, it is difficult to represent the "look and feel" of an electronic record on paper, but one should be able to envision a "home base" screen from which any aspect of the patient's record should be accessible with a single click of a button, a voice command, or other means of selection. From this home base, other views would "zoom" or emerge into the foreground displaying the needed information. As computing in general moves to graphical interfaces it is likely that the electronic dental chart will take full advantage of this simplified form of navigation through the use of icons, which are pictorial representations of information. Icons will likely become most heavily used on the home base screen to allow quick "point and click" selection as well as to signify whether or not a given data element is present. For example, if an icon depicting a panographic radiograph was highlighted (by display of a dark image) it would indicate that there was such a radiograph in the record and that if the icon were clicked, the radiograph would be shown. Similarly, if the icon were "dimmed" through the use of gray patterning, it would indicate that no such radiograph was in the chart and the practitioner should not even bother to select the icon.

Other graphic display techniques, particularly methods of pattern recognition, will surely be developed which will make navigation among the various elements of the record a matter of considerable ease. Two forms of graphics used in similar graphical interfaces include a simple matrix and a polar cap. For example, a 50 question medical history might be represented in a 5 x 10 cell matrix with each cell representing a specific question in the health history. A neutral or green colored cell could indicate a "normal" or healthy response to the question, where as a grey or orange cell might suggest caution or occasional follow-up and a black or red cell, while not yet a medical alert condition, might suggest that the patient should be questioned about the progress of this condition at each appointment.

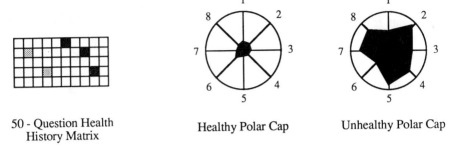

50 - Question Health History Matrix

Healthy Polar Cap

Unhealthy Polar Cap

Figure 9.2. Electronic chart pattern recognition examples.

A polar cap is simply a circle in which four to eight different indices (such as the Periodontal Index, Gingival Index, Bleeding Points, and Mobility) are represented on different lines or spokes running out from the center of the cap. All indices are scaled such that a measurement at the center of the cap, on on any of the axes, represents a healthy condition, whereas measures at the outer edge of the cap represent an unhealthy situation.

The purpose of such graphic representations is to take advantage of the computer's ability to collect and combine a variety of information and represent that information in the most compact and visually meaningful way possible. With the use of a consistent display technique, clinicians will begin to recognize certain "patterns" as being unimportant allowing a quick focus on those which deserve more attention. Examples of this pattern recognition technique, using a matrix and two polar caps, are shown in Figure 9.2.

Display

We now assume that there will be a large (at least 19"), true-color (24-bit) screen, easily visible to both patient and dentist, in every dental operatory in the practice, and that there will be an identical screen in the patient education or counselling office(s) as well as in the dentist's personal study, whether this is at home or in the dental office. Slightly smaller monochrome screens would also be available to the office staff in the reception and business office locations in the practice, as is now the case in offices which use computers for practice management. The final aspect of "display" technology involves the use of color printers which will be able to produce excellent patient education materials such as dental charts or graphs of patient progress, and photographs from the patient's own mouth. These images will be captured by digitizing "still" cameras or, when more affordable than at present, by miniature videocameras which take freeze frame intra-oral photos.

Educational Implications of the Electronic Dental Patient Record

Perhaps the most obvious impact of the increasing use of an electronic dental patient record in practice will be the value of teaching students how to use such a "chart" while still in school. While it would be exciting to think that the EDPR could be the focal point for clinical students as they treat each of their patients, this would be done only at a considerable cost either to the institution or students. Most dental schools could not afford to place a microcomputer at each student operatory, and it is unlikely that more than a few schools will attempt to do so in this decade. However, it would likely be possible to set up a bay of 4 - 8 units which use an electronic chart in their daily activities and then have students rotate through the bay at regular intervals in order to become familiar with this approach to dental records, decision support and quality assessment. On the other hand, many universities are now requiring engineering and business students to come to school having already purchased a microcomputer. Should the health professions be that far behind?

Beyond this obvious training benefit for clinical students, we believe that access to an electronic patient record will be even more critical for first and second year students as it will provide the means for moving beyond the methodology of "lecture with slides" and directly into a computer-mediated problem-based learning environment. The EDPR could provide students (and practitioners in the form of home-based continuing education) with a clinical window through which they can study the patient "cases" available within their problem-based curriculum materials. (See Figure 9.3.) From these cases they will be able to navigate easily to the other dimensions of the problem-based, informatics-mediated curriculum proposed here, which will contain a "reasonably complete" knowledge, skill, and image bases important to the field of dentistry.

Later in the chapter we will return to a description of how these knowledge bases and their navigational media might be developed, but let us now continue with a discussion of the complex relational database that underlies the appealing graphic interface of the EDPR.

The Second Generation Clinical Database: The Key to Dental Office Decision Support and Clinical Quality Assurance

The dental office computer system of the future must contain not only the relatively static summary of treatment codes, which has been the case for many years, but also the shifting oral status, diagnostic, and treatment assessment information. This expanded set of information must now be housed in what has been described previously by this author as a "second generation" or procedural clinical database. Such databases were designed primarily for administrative or financial reasons and focused on what treatment was performed so that patient statements and insurance

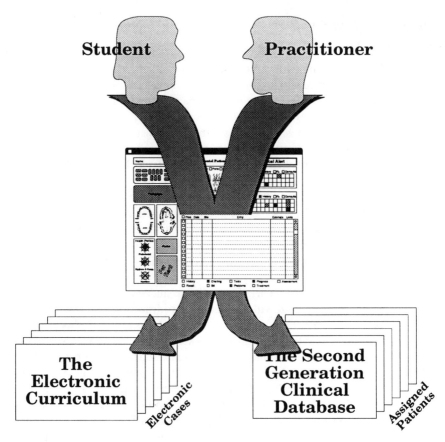

Figure 9.3. The electronic dental patient record: window to the curriculum and to patient care.

claims could be processed as rapidly as possible. The twin focal points of such databases were the demographic databases (patient name and address as well as insurance company names and addresses) and the listing of treatment rendered by procedure code, fee, and date. To be sure, some systems added space for planned treatment, recalls and appointment scheduling, while others added in word processing and sophisticated financial and productivity reporting capabilities. In all cases however, the focus was on practice administration.

Very recently we have begun to see the development of "stand alone"[24] diagnostic applications which house the oral status and diagnostic information for a given patient. True "second generation" or comprehensive dental patient databases will have been achieved when these stand-alone programs become fully integrated into the dentist's computer system. Other chapters in this volume will describe the work being done on the design of these new databases. In this chapter it is our purpose to show how this development will impact on the education of dentists. To do this, we will briefly reflect on how these comprehensive databases enable two other important aspects of health care, decision support and quality assessment, to emerge in ways that have been impossible in the past, at least in dentistry.

Decision Support

Decision support is discussed in several chapters of this book, but for our purposes suffice it to say that health care can be improved if a computer system can automatically provide appropriate diagnostic or treatment reminders to busy practitioners who must look after thousands of patients each year. The programming of these reminders is best accomplished if the data used to generate the reminder is in the computer prior to the time a decision is made which relies on that data. Ideally, a practitioner who was planning to administer a local anesthetic with epinephrine would be alerted if the patient had an allergy to the medication. Paper records offer only rudimentary reminders such as color coded stickers and red ink, whereas the computer could be programmed to include a wide variety of such reminders. The important point is that these reminders will only be functional if the patient record is in an electronic format and if they are allowed to operate in the background. In the preceding example, the dentist did not stop to ask the computer if the patient was allergic, but the computer did the check automatically (in the background) when informed of the treatment plan, and alerted the dentist when it found conflicting information.

Quality Assurance

The second feature which the electronic patient record allows is the ability to pursue the clinical research component of future dental practice, as was mentioned earlier in the overview of the informatics curriculum of the future. While the analysis of an electronic record for a single patient is a routine aspect of health care, the analysis of the electronic records of many patients becomes the basis for clinical research and, more specifically, the basis for "personal" quality assurance. A practitioner of the future will be able to narrow down a dental practice of 5,000 patients quite quickly by selecting those patients who, for example, at the time of their first oral examination were over 45, had a history of diabetes, and presented with periodontal pockets of greater than six millimeters in two or more quadrants. This sub-population would take only a few seconds to identify. Now the practitioner can begin to compare and contrast this population with a similar sampling of a "control group" of patients in the practice without diabetes. Alternatively, the practitioner could look at the success rates of the various treatment modalities offered to one or both groups. In time, these same practitioners will be able to dial into regional or national databases to see how similar populations of patients have responded to various treatment alternatives.

Serious attempts to conduct quality assurance research will not only require the integration of diagnostic data into present day clinical databases, it will also require the collection of new data elements, which are usually not recorded by practitioners unless they are involved in specific clinical trials. These new data elements include the regular recording of qualitative information regarding the clinical quality and function (outcomes) of previously completed treatment and/or the status of previously identified conditions. At the time of each recall appointment, one of the "stock" reminders which will automatically be presented to the practitioner will be a listing of those previously completed procedures and previously documented conditions for which an evaluative assessment should now be recorded in the electronic record. The timing of each such assessment should have been previously set out on a time line so that the computer would know when to list the needed assessments. (For example, partial denture assessments, after initial insertion recalls, might be every two years, plus or minus six months.) In this way only selected items are recorded during a given appointment. Further, one assumes that there will be a protocol (a standard set of characteristics or criteria to be assessed) which should be followed for each treatment or condition so that when qualitative assessments are to be made, the appropriate data will have been recorded. For example, if the presence of wear or chipping on porcelain fused to metal crowns is important in a later assessment of the crown's longevity or serviceability, this data must be recorded at regular intervals.

Educational Implications of Second-Generation Clinical Databases

Some observers will argue that the introduction of decision support systems into the undergraduate dental program will lead to an unreasonable reliance on a machine to do the thinking for the student. Others will argue that the student must become accustomed to the benefits and limitations of several different decision support systems, as well as the value of common sense and reasoning, while under the tutelage of the educational institution. We recommend the latter approach.

Some observers will argue that in the hands of anyone less than a trained epidemiologist, both the accuracy of quality assessment data and the analyses which would be forthcoming might be very misleading. Others would suggest that this new, and higher, level of "science" should pervade dental practice in the future and that our graduates should be able to generate and analyze such hypotheses as easily as they now offer their empirical opinions as to which form of treatment is best in a given situation. Without informatics training and access to the electronic dental patient record and its accompanying database, the point is moot as there is no vehicle for such analysis. With them we can at least debate the question and decide what level of training in the analysis of quality assessment indicators we wish to require of our graduates and offer to practitioners as a means of discovering their "personal" practice profiles. Assuming their use becomes accepted, their value will continue to be questioned if those practitioners who use them a) do not appreciate the critical importance of complete and accurate data entry, b) have not been trained to do the data collection, and c) do not have sufficient research design and hypothesis generation skills to conduct and interpret the necessary analyses.

To accommodate this we will propose a strong research design component as one of the *modus operandi* of, the pre-clinical technique labs, as well as the addition of a quality assurance lab which runs in parallel with the clinical years as direct manifestations of the quality assurance aspects of dental practice in the future. The design of both the electronic record and the clinical database, as well as their reinforcement and application within the problem-based, informatics-mediated curriculum, must offer a user-friendly approach to data capture, decision support, hypothesis generation, and the analysis of clinical quality.

Summary of Dental Practice Indicators for Curriculum Change

This concludes our discussion of the factors which are influencing the "informatics" future of dental practice. Standing alone, the demographic, epidemiological, and regulatory changes are substantial and they are only compounded by the expanding popularity and functionality of the computer. These changes, as well as the parallel emergence of both problem-solving educational techniques and the accessibility of powerful informatics tools, have guided the design of our problem-based, informatics-mediated curriculum research described in the remainder of this chapter.

A Problem and Informatics-Based Dental Curriculum for the Year 2000

To begin a discussion of how informatics and a problem-based curriculum might be fused at some point in the future, we have chosen simply to lay out one possible design which contains the elements that best support our view of the future. In this view of future dental curriculum, which is depicted in Figure 9.4, there are ten key activities, each of which is summarized below.

1. **Orientation Lab:** A four to six week orientation program focusing on the acquisition of skills for independent study, information retrieval, problem-solving, computer literacy and hypermedia navigation, electronic patient record retrieval and inspection, as well as an introduction to the problem-based informatics curriculum, criterion-referenced assessment techniques, student/faculty dialogue methods used to improve thinking and judgement, generic perceptual and motor skills, and a review of rudimentary research design and biostatistics.

2. **The Weekly Class (Town) Meeting:** (Class and Curriculum Administration, Special Lectures, Student Assessment, and Program Maintenance) One half-day per week for a) orientation and special lectures, when needed, b) regular assessments of student progress (both formative and summative), c) regular assessment of curriculum organization, learning effectiveness, and teaching effectiveness, and d) other class activities.

3. **Small Group Problem-based Tutorials:** Group problem-solving activities, supported by assigned cases from the electronic curriculum and through bi-weekly tutorials with faculty facilitators working with eight to ten students per team.

4. **Elective and Remedial Studies:** This aspect of the curriculum can be seen as either elective (completely optional) or selective (a selection among available choices is required). Students with basic or clinical research interests, or those with instructional interests, will be encouraged to pursue them through a mentoring system. Similar opportunities will be available for students wishing to engage in library research or additional patient care activities within a particular discipline, perhaps in anticipation of advanced study. Also, at either the student's or faculty's request, time will be made available for remedial study and assessment.

5. **Rounds:** The presentation of patients, by both full and part-time faculty, to reasonably small student groups (10 - 20 students per faculty member), occurring twice weekly in all years of study, and offered both in the dental school setting and in the hospital or other remote settings.

6. **Computer-based Patient Simulations:** Daily computer-based patient simulations of 15 - 30 minutes in duration, with individual responses to be filed electronically to their "self study" database, on a daily basis.

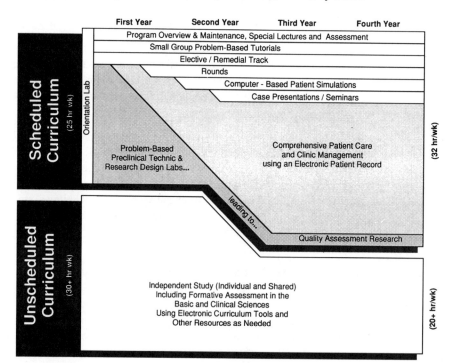

Figure 9.4. An informatics curriculum for the year 2000.

7. **Case Presentations and Seminars:** Case presentations, occurring in small groups at least twice weekly in the second through final years of study, encouraging the preparation and analysis of simple through more complex cases. Case reports, including the electronic patient record and videotaped student-patient highlights, would be brought to the seminar by each student for viewing by the facilitator and group.

8. **Problem-Based Pre-Clinical Technique and Research Labs:** Integrated, pre-clinical laboratory courses which focus on developing perceptual, motor, postural, clinical judgement, and clinical research design skills.

9. **Comprehensive Patient Care and Clinic Management:** Integrated clinical experiences which focus on comprehensive patient care, ethics, quality assurance, and the analysis of patient databases for the assessment of treatment outcomes.

10. **Independent Study:** Individual and Shared: Problem-based independent study, supported by an electronic curriculum which includes relevant information about all dental and basic science disciplines, all oral and systemic diseases encountered in dental practice, and a wide variety of assigned cases used to guide the study of a given class.

The most controversial aspect to this design will surely be the absence of any "traditional" courses in either the basic or clinical sciences. Such courses are replaced by a single course, the integrated, problem-based tutorial, which will be accompanied by extensive independent study (both individually and in informal small groups) which, in general, should occupy about 30 hours (approximately one half) of the combined scheduled and unscheduled curriculum time of 65 - 65 hours per week during the first two years of dental school, with this number dropping to 20 hours per week during the final two years of study in order to allow for an increase in the time devoted to patient care.

An Overview of the the Problem-Based Aspect of the Future Dental Curriculum

Before addressing the informatics aspect of the future curriculum being discussed here, it is important to establish the conceptual framework for the problem-based aspects of the curriculum. The simplest framework is one in which there are no discipline-based didactic courses. These would be replaced with a series of cases, the exploration of which would cause the student to study, and to learn in a relevant clinical context, the necessary information which pertains to the various disciplines. In medical schools where this is now accomplished, the cases are cross-referenced with a master discipline-based content listing, assuring that all important aspects of a given discipline are covered by the cases. Generally, the cases are discussed in a twice weekly problem-based tutorial where faculty act as facilitators, not as sources of knowledge.

The relinquishing of discipline-based lecture courses accomplishes three important curriculum changes. These include: a) the release of content as the driving force behind the curriculum and its replacement by a focus on problem-solving, b) a shift in responsibility for learning from the content-driven teacher to the case-driven student, and c) a freeing up of time in the dental students' schedule which allows the shift to self-study and also creates new opportunities for the coordinated scheduling and integration of pre-clinical lab and early clinical activities.

With the single exception of the Elective/Remedial option, all other scheduled activities, as displayed in Figure 9.4, are of a cross-cutting, integrative nature. To be sure, there will be the occasional overview lecture given by a specific discipline, and among the interdisciplinary pre-clinical technique labs there will, no doubt, still be a number of technique labs offered by a specific discipline. However, it is also suggested that the pre-clinical laboratory course, as a whole, should adopt a problem-based approach to the learning of technical skills, the solving of technical dilemmas, and the assessment of clinical quality. The pre-clinical lab of the future should become a second source of problem-solving skills, beyond that of the problem-based tutorials.

In addition to the shift toward a patient-based, problem-based focus in each of the tutorial and laboratory courses, a movement toward the daily challenge of a new 15 - 30 minute patient simulation,[25] or simulated patient[26] should also be promoted. Such simulations will provide an ongoing form of both formative and summative assessment of the skills being developed in the tutorial and laboratory courses.

Beyond the projected shift from a fact-based to a problem-based approach to learning, it is also suggested that there should be a second major shift in curriculum during the 1990s, the inclusion of clinical research skills. One of the underlying concepts of a problem-based curriculum is hypothesis generation and testing. Up to this time, dentistry has been data poor, or at least poor in data that was organized, reliable, and accessible. Earlier in this chapter it was argued that this will change in the 1990s with the development of clinical databases and their accompanying analytical tools.

The first focal point for the inclusion of research methods in the curriculum described here is in the Orientation Lab where appropriate focus can be offered on the need for practitioners to create their own clinical databases, as well as be able to access larger or disease specific databases, in order to investigate various hypotheses which they will develop. The second focal point would be in the pre-clinical lab where exercises in hypothesis generation and testing can be carried out at the time they are learning to measure the clinical quality of the various techniques they are learning. Finally, as an extension of this research-based laboratory activity, these skills can be put to the test on either "dummy" or real databases during the students' clinical years through the design and conduct of quality assessment studies focusing on specific clinical questions.

Surely, during the decade of the nineties, there will be a wide variety of transitional scenarios developed as few, if any, schools will want to adopt such a radical change to their lectures and laboratories in an abrupt, "cold turkey", fashion.

Some schools have already asked departments (disciplines) to reduce their lecturing in favor of the insertion of several problems, whereas other schools have reduced time for all courses across the board, and added a number of cross-discipline, problem-based tutorials. While such modifications only partially acknowledge the importance of the shift to a problem-based approach, they usually represent the limits of change which an organization can realistically accommodate within a given period of time.

In summary, movement toward a problem-based curriculum in dentistry can be best accomplished by 1) the shift from a lecture-based, content driven program to one which is grounded in problem-based, case-driven independent study supported by tutorials, 2) the offering of patient simulations as both formative and summative assessments of developing problem solving skills, 3) the design of pre-clinical laboratory courses to include an active problem-based approach to the solution of technical problems and the development of manual skills, and 4) the inclusion of clinical research skills into the pre-clinical laboratory so they can be learned in concert with clinical evaluation skills and can later manifest themselves in quality assessment research in dental practice.

An Overview of the Informatics Aspect of the Future Dental Curriculum

Since computer literacy and computer use are not yet wide-spread in dentistry or in dental schools, most discussions of dental informatics continue to rely on belief rather than acceptance. With this in mind it should be stated that this author's belief is that medical care, and consequently dental care, will be greatly influenced by the computer over the next decade, principally through the acceptance and widespread use of the electronic patient record. Similarly, the educational environment will become increasingly dependent on the power of the computer as a clinical patient care tool, an information resource, a hypertext and hypermedia navigator,[27] a problem-based learning coordinator, and also as a repository for patient simulations and other individualized student or continuing education materials. If one believes this scenario, and one accepts the shift to problem-based learning as being inevitable, the dental curriculum must be viewed through new eyes. This new view could become known as the "Problem-based, Informatics-mediated Dental Curriculum" (PIDC) and, as a model, it can be applied just as easily to any of the health professions as it can to dentistry. The informatics, or computer-based, portion of this curriculum has generically been referred to as an "electronic curriculum" and is a dynamic extension of the electronic syllabus and electronic textbook metaphors which have been used in other settings for several years.

In its broadest sense of acquiring "dental" or "biomedical" knowledge, an electronic curriculum should allow learners to sit down at a computer and learn as much as they wish to know about dentistry, and when the local knowledge bases they are exploring have reached their limits, the learners should be offered direct gateways into the medical literature or national clinical databases which should be able to provide them with the answers they seek. Such learning should be intuitive with one concept leading to another and yet another, all in the search for a wide variety of solutions to a particular research hypothesis or patient problem.

Similarly, on the clinical side, students should be able to explore computer-based simulations in order to discover the preferred solutions to realistic patient problems. These same computer-based simulations should carry students directly to the analysis of the problems and needs of each of their assigned clinic patients. By extension, students should also be able to analyze the problems and needs of a larger population of patients, either within their own school's clinical database, or by accessing regional or national databases. The curriculum proposed here offers such an educational tool and offers the electronic dental patient record as the entry point for such investigations as well as the repository for all student findings and treatment decisions.

In summary, movement toward an informatics-mediated curriculum in dentistry can be best accomplished by a) the development of an electronic curriculum which supports thorough knowledge base navigation, b) the creation of access routes from that local electronic environment to other literature and databases, c) the availability of computer-based patient simulations, and d) the availability of electronic patient records and clinical databases for the analysis and recording of individual patient care as well as the analysis of both treatment needs and outcomes for larger population groups.

The Problem-Based, Informatics-Mediated Dental Curriculum: Navigation Among Disciplines, Diseases, and Cases

The concept of a completely electronic curriculum for dentistry was first put forward in 1988[28] when it became clear that microcomputing technology would allow the mass storage and instant retrieval of a very large amount of text, images, and sounds in a non-linear (point and click) hypermedia format. At that time, and in a subsequent paper by this author,[29] the focus of the concept was on the ability of a student to move from the factual study of anatomy to the application of those studies in removable prosthodontics, oral surgery, or any other aspect of dentistry. Similarly, it was assumed that in the midst of studying any of the clinical disciplines, a student could return to the underlying basic science concepts of those disciplines with the click of a button. Therefore, what human teachers had generally failed to do in the sixty-five years since the Geis report, could perhaps be accomplished inside the computer: to establish relevance, to suggest conceptual linkages, to offer both logical and visual examples, to reaffirm graphically, and to challenge with realistic patient problems, the integration between the basic and clinical dental sciences.

For the student, it was simply envisioned that each one would be issued a color microcomputer, with appropriate storage capabilities, at the time of acceptance to dental school. The content of all current courses and/or disciplines would be converted to a hypermedia format such that images would be digitized and accompanying text organized, along with a glossary and references, in a way that students could use the materials as their primary source of study material, much as notes and handouts are now used.

When moving from the idea stage to initial prototypes, several challenges became immediately apparent:

1) the need to create an organizational framework for the content of the disciplines taught in the undergraduate curriculum,

2) the need to consider the value and appropriateness of the developing interest among dental educators in the application of problem-based learning to the dental curriculum,

3) the need to apply an appropriate mix of learning theory to the design of the student interface, and

4) the need for a navigational metaphor which students and faculty could both easily use as they moved around what would amount to a small library of information contained in the dental knowledge base that would eventually be created.

Each of these challenges is addressed below.

An Organizational Framework for Content

When the question of organization was first raised, one suggestion was to simply move the current course structure straight into the computer. After all, the traditional problem with any lock-step course structure, that of sequencing, would be overcome immediately as the computer interface would allow the student to find any of the content of any course in the curriculum at any time, and to be able to move to a second course in pursuit of any concept which traversed their common boundaries. As this approach was considered, the weaknesses of such an approach became apparent. First, there was no need to break up the content of any discipline into first, second, third, and fourth year packages as each discipline could be addressed as a whole and repackaged in a fashion which would offer the learner the best overview and overall approach to the discipline. Second, as the discipline-based approach to the curriculum was, in itself, part of the organizational problem, perhaps there should be a search for a more integrative framework for the dental and basic science knowledge base. As we began to explore such frameworks it was apparent that the medical world was awash in several such frameworks which were the products of a branch of science called nosology, defined as the study of the organization of diseases. We also discovered that one such nosology, SNOMED, had already been invoked by the World Health Organization in the preparation of an international index for dentistry, the Oral Status and Intervention (OSI) index, to be used in the description of oral health status.[30]

Another chapter in this volume describes, in considerable detail, the state of medical nosologies, and the efforts of Monteith (see Chapter 8)[31], a coinvestigator in the electronic curriculum project, to apply these nosologies to dentistry. Our current organizational framework, has been drawn initially from the work of Gabrieli.[32] The six additive levels of his nosology include structure, function, diagnostic studies (meaning the conditions of health), clinical medicine (or patterns of disease), etiology, and finally, treatment. Chapter 8 describes the overlay of dentistry to this nosology as the identification of a hierarchy of nodes which lay out the current organizational framework of the discipline. These nodes are of two varieties, containing either knowledge or skill elements. Once the layout of these knowledge and skill nodes has been determined, the process of "filling" each empty node with content, images, references and glossary definitions can begin. Parallel to this, faculty authors can begin to specify which nodes in other disciplines, as well as their own, should be linked to the node they are currently preparing. In time, all nodes in all disciplines will be ready to be dynamically connected into a large knowledge base or knowledge web through which the user can freely navigate.

This model of biomedical knowledge has been adapted to the electronic curriculum project and the applicability of other "non-medical" models grounded in health psychology and community health literature is also being explored. It is our intent to offer the learner more than one reference point with which they can "zoom out" during their study of a particular isolated fact or procedure, thus enabling them to see where this piece of information fits in the larger picture of dental or medical science.

While the nosological approach appears to satisfy the organization of discipline-based information, we have felt that there needs to be a similar approach to the organization of dental, oral, and related systemic diseases. Along this line, it is our intent to organize these diseases so that the learner can follow a given disease from its sub-clinical beginnings through its complete course, showing how, at any stage, the patient and health care team can recognize relevant signs and symptoms or engage in prevention and treatment.

Thus, with an organizational framework for the basic and clinical disciplines, and a second framework for dental and related diseases, we now have in place a two-dimensional learning environment through which a student could navigate. The nodes on each of the discipline and disease axes will be accessible, one from the other, so that when studying a particular aspect of periodontal disease, for example, the student would be able to move smoothly through these two dimensions as described below:

1. beginning from the "clinical" level of the discipline axis (or the "signs and symptoms" aspect of the periodontal disease node on the disease axis) where the symptoms were first detailed, one could link to...

2. the "function" level of the discipline axis in order to explore in depth those physiologic conditions which are operational in a healthy gingival sulcus or the conditions under which microbial activity increases and the periodontal disease process is encouraged, then move on to...

3. the "structure" level of the discipline axis in order to learn more about the anatomy of the gingival sulcus, then on to...

4. the "etiology" level of the discipline axis (or the etiology aspect of the periodontal disease node on the disease axis) to explore which of the possible etiological factors are implicated for this patient, and finally one could link to...

5. the "treatment" level of the discipline axis (or the "treatment" aspect of the periodontal disease node on the disease axis) to explore various treatment options which are available, along with a discussion of those factors which contribute to their success.

Such movement is not possible without some underlying structure for the content, even if all "pieces" of information (data elements) are simply tagged with appropriate labels and retrieved when the correct combination of labels is requested by the learner. This latter "open architecture" model or "semantic net" may eventually become the preferred choice of curriculum designers and informaticians, but for now, a more structured approach is under development.

The Application of Problem-Based Learning to the Electronic Curriculum

The University of Missouri - Kansas City is acknowledged to have been the first dental school to seriously consider the adoption of a problem-based format to their undergraduate curriculum.[33] Tedesco, who organized the first AADS symposium on problem-based learning,[34] and who is a coinvestigator on the electronic curriculum project, has been instrumental in expanding the awareness of dental educators to problem-based approaches to learning in dentistry. In following this lead, the scope of the electronic curriculum prototype was similarly expanded to encompass a problem-based approach to learning, through computer-based patient problems or "cases" as the primary focus for learning available to the student. If these cases are arranged on a "case" axis, the resultant three-dimensional configuration of a "discipline" axis, a "disease" axis, and a "case" axis can be depicted as shown in Figure 9.5 on the following page. The addition of this case-based axis offers the necessary guidance to the student when pursuing the resolution of a specific case within the discipline and disease axes. This approach has been investigated at the Harvard Medical School and is referred to as an orthogonal view of curriculum.[35]

The first-year dental student of the future would, after a brief period of orientation, begin a study of the basic sciences, behavioral sciences, dental disciplines and oral diseases through a series of assigned cases. The patient would be presented to the student not through a written handout, but would be embodied within their first electronic dental patient record. This electronic patient would then be approached using three methods of study, including:

1) independent study and,

2) group study using the electronic curriculum materials or any other learning resources which are needed, with both of these student-driven methods of study being supported through,

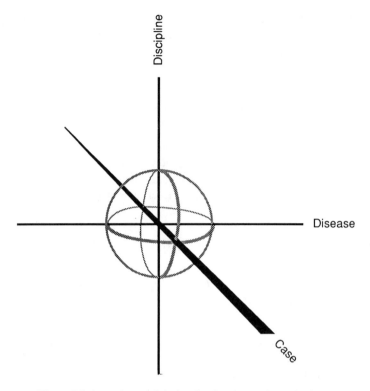

Figure 9.5. An orthogonal design for the electronic curriculum.

3) problem-based tutorials facilitated by basic and clinical science faculty members.

The focus of each case, and therefore of the discussion within the tutorials, would be on the answers to a series of questions along with the reasoning which supports each answer. The questions, with the reasoning displayed in *italics*, are listed below:

1. What are the relevant or potentially relevant findings which this patient has presented with, *and what are the basic science explanations for each of these findings.*

2. What additional questions would you like to ask the patient or what additional diagnostic tests would you wish to order during the examination of this patient, *and why is such information required.*

3. What would you include in the patient's problem list, *why would you include each one, and what is the suspected etiology of each one that you have listed.*

4. When any aspect of the patient's condition is not readily discernible, prepare a differential diagnosis, *provide the reasons for including each disease listed*

in the differential, and describe what additional information will be needed in order to arrive at a final diagnosis.

5. Prepare alternative treatment plans for the patient, including a list of any prescribed medications and/or dental laboratory prescriptions, then identify the plan which is technically preferred and the plan which is best suited to this particular patient, and finally, *articulate the hypotheses on which these selections are based and present the rationale for each of these two selections, with such rationale preferably grounded in arguments within the clinical literature or in available quality assurance data.*

6. Describe the most pertinent complications which may arise during the treatment of the patient, including questions of ethics as well as patient acceptance and/or compliance, *then describe how these complications might best be avoided.*

7. Describe the basis on which the quality of the treatment provided should be assessed in the future, *then provide both a schedule for such assessments and the evidence one would collect in order to determine the continuing quality of the treatment.*

These questions and their supporting arguments should provide a consistent reinforcement for the scientific bases of diagnosis and treatment. They should also encourage, if not demand, an analytical (as opposed to rote) approach to the study of this health care profession.

The Learning Theory Behind the Student/Case Interface

Even with a rather complete organizational framework (the three axes of disciplines, diseases, and cases) and a general notion of what the student is expected to do within that framework (learning dentistry by solving assigned cases), the method of accomplishing this task continues to be under study. What is certain is that we must pay close attention to the learning theory which we prescribe, either consciously or unconsciously, through the design of the user interface. We are consciously trying to follow a body of learning theory literature[36-39] which we believe applies to this field of study. From this work, it is clear that a "worst case" scenario would be a high text, low graphics, page turning design. An equally unappealing analog to this type of electronic book, is that of a wonderfully rich and well-designed environment of text and graphics, through which the student is only expected to *browse.* We are sure that browsing is not learning and, as with an unimaginative electronic textbook, will be devastatingly unsuccessful.

One application of the learning theory to which we have referred is known as methods of inquiry (MOI).[40] We are exploring this avenue since it has shown very successful results with college students and appears to come very close to addressing the conceptual tasks required of health professionals which include analyzing information presented, asking the right questions or generating reasonable hypotheses, collecting the appropriate information, organizing new knowledge and, ultimately, solving subsequent problems. We believe the techniques of MOI can be applied to the electronic environment which we are constructing. To do this successfully we must first take advantage of the potential flexibility of a hyper-media environment to present all information in a pleasing, highly interactive manner, in ways that are not possible with print media, and second, that learners must be required to collect, organize, and display the fruits of their explorations. Our goal is to make the exploration enjoyable, and the collection, organization and display simple. The challenge for the learner should be the intellectual task of assimilating new knowledge and not the idiosyncratic manipulation of software.

At the time of this writing, we are prototyping various interfaces and offering them to in-house students for testing and comment. Our design currently includes the provision of a tool which will allow students to slide text or images from the discipline or disease axes into "case logs" which they must compile for each case. The logs consist of their answers to the seven questions listed above and the rationale which supports each of these answers. Each case starts with the ap-propriate EDPR and empty storage locations (screens) for the answers to each of the seven questions. During the span of time devoted to a given case, each student (working independently and in groups) would be expected to find the relevant answers *and underlying reasoning* from any number of nodes on any of the three axes, then slide them onto a personal "scratch pad". Eventually, when sufficient "chunks" of information have been collected students will be expected to organize all their disjointed information prior to finally transferring their newly acquired solutions into their case logs.

Another form of feedback which has been used in medical[41] and dental[42] simulations involves the availability of an "expert" or "ideal" answer to students who have just completed a case. For beginning students, such information (rein-forcement) is provided after each small step in a case so that they will be more likely to both stay on course for a given case, and learn "model" methods of navigation and exploration within the knowledge base. With our cases, this form of feedback could be provided at the end of each of the seven questions which define a given case. Whether or not this form of guidance will be used has not been decided. As with many learning theories, this might work well for motivated students who would strive to do a good job on each case, but its value to the less well motivated student can be questioned. For those who do not fully explore a case, then prepare hasty and incomplete answers, access to good answers will provide only a quick and superficial review of the case rather than the in-depth retrieval and application we are seeking. There may also be considerable merit in arranging the learning environment so that group study and the tutorials have maximum value, and these might well suffer if any student can "jump" to the correct answers without actually doing the work. Perhaps the use of this feedback method will be used selectively, both for those who are struggling with the problem-based approach to learning and for those outstanding students who are able to move at a much faster pace than their classmates.

We are several years away from even the initial answers to the questions of learning theory. The prototype possibilities described here will undoubtedly evolve further as student trials continue, but the need for some mechanism to enable students to collect and organize the products of their own learning is well supported in the current literature.

Navigation

We envision that learners, when presented with a new case, will first fully explore the EDPR, then immediately start to identify the relevant findings. As they discover findings for which they have no prior understanding or no professional ability to explain (to a patient or colleague, let alone an instructor) they would leave the "case" axis momentarily to explore the "discipline" or "disease" axis. When sufficient information has been found to answer the question at hand, they would return to the "case" axis, record their findings in their case log, then move along to the next question. (We envision that keyboard entry will be minimized, as students will have a software tool which will allow them to capture and drag information from the discipline and disease axes to their case logs, which will remain open on the screen at all times.) At each stage of the case, when new information is needed, the learner would repeat this process until the case log is completed. The discussions with other students, along with more formal discussions within their problem-based tutorials, would provide some assurance regarding the general direction of students' explorations.

In general, when students wish to search for information on a specific topic, disease or related symptom, they would "click" on the icon for the appropriate axis, at which time the root of the nosology for that axis would "pop up" (for example, the discipline axis would present the six choices of structure, function, etc.). If they have a rough idea of where they are heading, they can get there quite easily (as in structure: skeleton: head and neck: mandible: torus). On the other hand, if they know that they are indeed looking for the term torus, they can type the word into a 'FIND __' command and be shown a list of "preferred" locations where the term is discussed in some detail. (To list all the locations in a several hundred megabyte collection of text would be quite time consuming and would yield a number of isolated instances of the term where it was ancillary to another concept. By coding the various parts of each tree with keywords, the searches will be much faster and yield better results.) Such searches can also be partially restricted so that if the skeletal features are indeed being sought, the "structure" level of the nosology could be specified and the search limited to "structural" nodes. Similarly, if one came upon the word "torus" in another branch of the nosology (eg. treatment: oral and maxillofacial surgery: pre-prosthetic surgery: reduction of tori) but did not know what the term referred to, one could invoke the glossary tool, "click" on the word and be shown its definition and at least one, or in this case probably several, photographic images displaying unilateral and bilateral tori, as well as pre- and post-surgical removal photographs. Along with the glossary definition, or any of the images, are displayed the preferred or "key word" locations for information about the term.

Once students have found the location of the topic they are investigating, they would be expected to collect and organize the information presented in a fashion which will be relevant in the support of the case they are researching. For the first few cases, it has been suggested that we guide them through such searches, so they can get the feel of this new method of navigation, however the need for such guidance will need to be tested in the field. Along this line, it has also been suggested that students be provided with a "bookmark" tool which will allow them to mark those nodes in which they have found relevant information for a given case. This will allow them to quickly review the main features of a case by letting them use their bookmarks as a guide to this review.

At least for testing purposes, a corollary to this bookmark concept has also been suggested. Assuming that there will be periodic case tests, whether formative or summative, faculty have often kept a complete log of every (electronic curriculum) location visited so that an analysis can be made of the extent to which a student's navigation was logical and direct, or somewhat questionable. This type of navigational analysis has been done in other software, and has been found to be quite helpful in diagnosing learning deficiencies and providing student counselling.[43] Some systems have been programmed to offer this type of navigational analysis automatically, should the student so request. This methodology is slightly different from the "expert" or "ideal" analysis mentioned earlier in that it does not go into any detail about the case, but simply offers an analysis of where the student has traveled compared to where they might have travelled if all the relevant information had been collected. While helpful for struggling students, a weakness of this feedback mechanism is that it does not account for the prior learning of stronger students into consideration when it suggests that many "collection points" have been overlooked for that particular case.

The illustrated glossary of terms, mentioned above, also includes the correct pronunciation of each word, as well as synonyms, alternate forms of the word and its MeSH (Medical Subject Heading) number(s), should the student wish to move directly into MEDLINE to do a more thorough external search of the literature. (Access to MEDLINE will be provided as a feature of all glossary cards within the electronic curriculum software.) Similarly, students who wish to find images of specific lesions or techniques, will be able to use a look-up feature in the image database to do so. In addition to this access to definitions and images, each knowledge node will include a list of references both used in its development or recommended for further study of individual topics.

Finally, students will have several varieties of "scratch pads" available to them where they can collect information which they know to be important, but are not yet sure how to organize. These "scratch pads" will offer question-answer, information mapping, tree-building, reference gathering and other tools designed with both ease of use and supportive learning theory in mind. All of these navigational tools, the icons, axis hierarchies, glossary, imagebase, case log, bookmarks, and scratch pads, have been designed to assist the students' need to find and organize the information they are seeking, as rapidly and as thoroughly as may be required.

The Need for Prototyping

The electronic curriculum project described in this chapter is now completing the first prototype of the student learning environment which has been described. Initial work has been completed on each of the three axes (discipline, disease, and case) and their respective navigational tools. Cases are now being loaded into the prototypes so that students will have an opportunity to test them while still in a relatively flexible stage. The recent emergence of fast prototyping tools such as HyperCard™, Supercard™, and ToolBook™, have made the design phase of such large projects far more manageable and realistic. It is assumed that several successively improved prototypes will be developed, each time being tested more widely, prior to final coding in a application language such a Pascal or C. Any attempts to develop educational software, particularly of the complex, interdisciplinary variety expected in the health professions, will require extensive prototyping.

The Collection of Electronic Materials for the Informatics-Mediated Curriculum

While the wisdom of prototyping is self-evident, it will take far more effort to overcome the long-standing NIH (Not Invented Here) syndrome which is apparently endemic among academicians. The first major hardship which this syndrome inflicts includes the prospect of individual faculty in many schools working in isolated parallelism as opposed to concentrated synergism. This translates into much duplication of effort and little collaboration in a period of very scarce resources. Secondly, the NIH syndrome easily leads to a number of products that are just slightly different from one another, either in design, software, or hardware, so as to make it impossible to share them at a later stage in their development. Therefore, isolationism at the beginning leads to an absence of accepted standards, which would be desirable at least at the hardware and software levels even if not at the design level.

It is critical that sufficient communication be facilitated among the leaders in dental informatics to insure that as many standards are developed and followed as is possible. One way standards can be promoted and resources shared, is through the development of consortia. The 1990s need to emerge as the decade of consortia within dental and other health professions education. With a small expenditure of funds, and a medium expenditure of time and effort, large projects can be accomplished and many institutions can share in the software or educational materials which are developed. Through collaboration in standards and design, and if such consortia follow the principle that all products which are developed must be end-user modifiable, these collaborations should be very successful.

However, such consortia will not come to fruition if leaders from the ADA, AADS, AADR, and the specialty academies do not see the value of such collaboration. The annual sessions of these organizations must be allowed to take on a more "project-oriented" direction in which collaboration is fostered. This is beginning to happen and will hopefully continue through the decade. Perhaps the most significant collaboration currently underway is demonstrated by the joining of forces by all regional boards, the Texas state board, the AADS, AADE, and the Joint Commission on National Dental Examinations in the development of a computer-based board examination focusing on patient simulations. A non-profit corporation named DISC (Dental Interactive Simulation Corporation) was formed in 1990 to begin work on the design and fund-raising for such a venture. More examples of this nature and magnitude will be needed if dental education is to keep pace with the computerization of the health professions.

Preparing Faculty and Students for their Future Roles in Computer-Based Education and Practice

While the previous section spoke to the politics of standards, inter-institutional collaboration and national leadership, we must not overlook the fact that many of today's faculty remain computer illiterate. Similarly, dental students do not yet perceive dentistry as a profession in which computer skills are essential to their successful practice. It is very likely that by the turn of the century neither of these observations will hold. Leaders within each institution must now take the time to examine their own commitment to faculty development in dental informatics as well as to the preparation of their students for computer-assisted professional life. Planned, incremental change within each institution, designed to gradually improve student and faculty comfort and range within the computer environment is essential.

Informatics-mediated dental practice will evolve and an informatics-mediated dental curriculum will be developed, it is just a question of when and how.

References

1. Rulhman, D.C. and Lowe, J.R. Computer use in a dental clinic, Journal of Dental Education, Vol. 32, No. 2: June 1968; p. 204-214.
2. Bennet, C.G. Dental school applicants record-keeping system, Journal of Dental Education, Vol. 53, No. 2: February 1989; p. 152.
3. Finkelstein, M.W., Johnson, L.A., and Lilly, G.E., Interactive videodisc patient simulations of oral disease, Journal of Dental Education, Vol. 52, No. 4: April 1988; p. 217-220.
4. White, S. ORAD, Journal of Dental Education, Vol. 53, No. 12: October 1989; p. 599-600.
5. Lefebvre, C.A., Richardson, G.B., and Taylor, R.L., Computer-assisted removable partial denture design, Journal of Dental Education, Vol. 54, No. 1: January, 1990; p. 46.
6. Micromedx, Nutriplan professional, Journal of Dental Education, Vol. 52, No. 4: December 1989; p. 738-739.

7. Spohn, E. and Hardison, J. D., Consortium on multi-media information technology to enrich dentistry-COMMITTED, Journal of Dental Education, Vol. 54, No. 10: October, 1990; p. 597-598.

8. Eisner, J., The developing electronic curriculum consortium, Journal of Dental Education, Vol. 54: October 1990; p. 598-599.

9. Buckenham S., Sellers, E.M., and Rothman, A.I., An application of computers to curriculum review and planning, Journal of Medical Education, Vol. 61, No. 1: January, 1986; p. 41-45.

10. Dimge, S.S. and O'Connell, M.T., Cataloging a medical curriculum using MeSH keywords, Proceedings of the 12th Symposium on Computer Applications in Medical Care, 1988; p. 332-336.

11. Personal correspondence from the curriculum coordinators at Emory, Loma Linda, UCLA, and West Virginia dental schools confirm the development of rudimentary curriculum databases in the mid 1980s.

12. Physicians for the twenty-first century, Report of the Project Panel on the General Professional Education of the Physician and College Preparation for Medicine, Association of American Medical Colleges, printed as a supplement to the Journal of Medical Education, November 1984; Part 2, p. 155-159.

13. Association of American Medical Colleges. (1986). Medical Education in the Information Age. Proceedings of the Symposium on Medical Informatics.

14. Salley, J.J., et al, Dental informatics: Strategic issues for the dental profession, in Vol. 39, Lecture Notes in Medical Informatics, Springer-Verlag, Berlin, p. 105.

15. Jaffe, C.C., Lynch, P.J. (1989). Hypermedia for education in the life sciences. Academic Computing; 10-13, 52-57, 73.

16. Shortliffe, E.H. and Perreault, L.E., Medical informatics: Computer applications in health care, Addison-Wesley Publishing Company, Reading, Mass., 1990; 715.

17. Flexner, A., Medical Education in the United States and Canada: A Report to the Carnegie Foundation for the Advancement of Teaching. Bulletin No. 4. Boston, Massachusetts: Updyke, 1910.

18. Gies, W.J. (1926). Dental education in the United States and Canada: A report to the Carnegie Foundation for the Advancement of Teaching. New York: the Carnegie Foundation, Bulletin No. 19.

19. The University of Florida adopted a modular curriculum design in the early 70's, while the University of Texas, at both Houston and San Antonio, adopted a more individualized, media-driven approach to curricula in the late 70's.

20. Neufeld, V.R. and Barrows, H.S., The "McMaster Philosophy": An Approach to medical education. Journal of Medical Education, Vol. 49:1040-1050.

21. Tosteson, D.C., New pathways in general medical education. New England Journal of Medicine, 332, 4, (1990) 234-238.

22. SimpleSoft™ produced by Avanti Systems, Cherry Hill, N.J. and Zanny™, produced by UDAC, Uppsala, Sweden.

23. This symposium was held on April 20/21, 1990 in Alexandria, Virginia and sponsored jointly by the University at Buffalo School of Dental Medicine and the American Association of Dental Schools. A number of papers from the Symposium have been published and can be found in the April, 1991 issue of the Journal of Dental Education.

24. Not integrated with or connected to the dentist's practice management software.

25. A combination of the patient chart, photographs, models, and specialist reports collected for easy review by a student who must prepare a treatment plan or solve an immediate or emergency problem. This can now be accomplished quite successfully using a computer.

26. The use of "trained" patients who simulate all the symptoms and characteristics of a specific disease, in a reliable fashion, so that a series of students can sequentially examine and interview them with the assurance that consistent responses will be provided.

27. Hypertext refers to the non-linear organization of text information characterized by multiple layers and linkages within and between isolated text. Hypermedia escalates this definition of hypertext to include on-screen access to still images, motion video, animation and sound, usually through a "point and click" interface. The "electronic curriculum" described in this paper is a hypermedia application.

28. Eisner, J.E., The future of dental education in an age of information technology, Journal of Dental Research, Vol. 67 (Special Issue, 1988), p. 103.

29. Eisner, J.E., Dental bridges: Electronic and curricular, Minds in Motion, A Publication of York University Press and Apple Canada, Inc., Spring 1989, p. 15-18.

30. World Health Organization, Prevention Methods and Programmes for Oral Diseases, WHO TRS 713 (1984) & Alternate Systems of Oral Care Delivery, WHO TRS 750 (1987).

31. Monteith, B.D., Nosology: A critical link between computers and dental education, practice, and research, in this volume, Chapter 8.

32. Gabrieli, E.R., A new electronic medical nomenclature, Journal of Medical Systems, Vol. 13, No. 6: 1989; p. 355-373.

33. Reed, M.J., A view from the field: Substantial curriculum reform, Journal of Dental Education, Vol. 54, No. 9: September 1990; p. 560-563.

34. Tedesco, L.A., Responding to educational challenges with problem-based learning and information technology, Journal of Dental Education, Vol. 54, No. 9: September 1990; p. 544-547.

35. Dichter, M.S., Greenes, R.A., and Bergeron, B.P. The clinical problem-solving exercise: An orthogonal approach to organizing medical knowledge, Proceedings of the 14th Symposium on Computer Applications in Medical Care, 1990, p. 473-477.

36. Parwat, R.S. (1989). Promoting access to knowledge. Review of Educational Research, 59, 1-42.
37. Glaser, R. (1990). The re-emergence of learning theory within instructional research. American Psychologist, 45; 29-39.
38. Norman, G.R. (1988). Problem-solving skills, solving problems and problem-based learning. Medical Education, 22; 279-286.
39. Waterman, R.E., Duban, S.L., Mennin, S.P., & Kaufman, A. (1988). Clinical problem-based learning. Albuquerque: University of New Mexico Press.
40. Heiman, M. & Slomianko, J. (1988). Methods of inquiry. Cambridge, MA: Learning to Learn, Inc.
41. Patient Simulator II, medical simulations developed and marketed by Knowledge House, Halifax, Nova Scotia, Canada.
42. Finkelstein, M.W., Johnson, L.A., and Lilly, G.E., Interactive videodisc patient simulations of oral disease, Journal of Dental Education, Vol. 52, No. 4: April 1988; p. 217-220.
43. Stevens, R.H., Kwak, A.R., and McCoy, J.M., Mapping student search paths through immunology problems by computer-based testing, Proceedings of the 14thSymposium on Computer Applications in Medical Care, 1990; p. 488-492.

10
Model for Informatics Knowledge and Informatics in the Dental Curriculum

John L. Zimmerman and Marion J. Ball

As we have seen in previous chapters in this book, informatics is a new and evolving field of study and research. Often people ask, "What is informatics?" and "Why do we need to teach informatics to dental students?" This chapter will address the question "What is informatics?" in an educational or academic perspective.

The report, *Physicians for the Twenty-First Century*, recommends that students sharpen and enhance independent learning and problem- solving skills through the study of medical informatics. This model is specific to medical education, but comparisons are easily made with dental education. Opportunities from the study of informatics which benefit the students of the health sciences include:

- managing the information base to treat patients
- treating patients more efficiently and cost effectively by reference to a broad range of experiences documented in national data bases
- providing more time for health care workers to spend on the important personal aspects of patient care through delegation of some information handling and processing tasks to computers
- improving the educational process through the incorporation of information technology and decision-making science and through the utilization of computer-mediated instruction
- broadening and rationalizing the clinical experience in medical education.[1]

Providing health care services to a patient is a rewarding activity. The one-to-one interface of the patient and the health care provider is the foundation of the health care field. Often this fact is overlooked and the more administrative aspects of health care delivery (such as lab testing, billing, patient records) are thrust to the forefront. Also, the health care provider demands the best and most up-to-date information in the course of treating the patient. As malpractice cases become more and more prevalent, the need for current information becomes more critical. In an attempt to clarify and define the field of dental informatics, this chapter will describe various models for informatics knowledge and model curriculum and degree programs that have been established throughout the world. It is our hope that this information will be used by dental educators to design their own innovative curricula in technology and information literacy.

Models for Informatics Knowledge

In addition to working to produce a concise and universally accepted definition for informatics, academicians have also proposed several models for informatics knowledge. These models are an attempt to formalize the numerous informatics applications and basic knowledge into categories. Their intent is to create a more orderly understanding of the scope of informatics which can better serve as a basis for educational programs. There are many taxonomies that can be used and have appeared in the literature. We have, however, chosen to discuss the following five that fit well into the use of computer concepts as applied to health. The five models described below are in use throughout the world. Some models are very similar while others are quite unique and are suited for specialized purposes or views.

Model 1

The model developed by Jan van Bemmel brings order to the myriad of medical computer/information applications being developed. Although most of the information/computer applications now in use are on the first three levels, the majority of the research projects can be classified in the higher levels. Information systems in the professions are used for clinical care, research, education, and administration. This model moves from least to most complex with some overlap.

- systems for communication and recording
  examples: networking, workstations, data representation
- data storage and retrieval, data base management systems
  examples: institutional or departmental information systems, Picture Archiving and Communications System, Medline
- computing and automation
  examples: laboratory automation, imaging, crown fabrication, signal analysis, statistics
- decision support systems, pattern recognition
  examples: expert systems, cell and tissue classification
- therapeutic support systems
  examples: radiotherapy, planning, pharmaco-therapy
- systems and methods for education, research, and development
  examples: simulation and modelling, new methods and systems.[2,3,4]

Model 2

Increasingly students entering graduate and professional programs are computer literate. The challenge for academic health science centers is to expose students to the use of computers and information seeking and management skills in areas within their discipline. The minimum competencies identified by the Association of American Medical Colleges are:

- ability to use bibliographic retrieval systems
- knowledge of computer storage technologies for clinical and research data
- exposure to clinical data bases and decision support
- competency in problem-solving and decision-making techniques.[5]

Model 3

The National League for Nursing has published nursing informatics competencies for nurses in the roles of practitioner, teacher, researcher, and administrator. These competencies are divided into three levels, but the NLN is quick to point out that these competencies assigned to each level should be modified as the general knowledge level increases through time. The NLN has individualized the informatics competencies for each of the nursing roles. These competencies are very expensive and can be obtained from the NLN. The three levels of informatics competencies can be summarized as:

1. User - has awareness, knows, understands, uses, and interacts

2. Modifier- analyzes, manages, critiques, modifies, evaluates

3. Innovator- develops, designs.

The competencies for the practicing nurse reflect their major role functions, such as documenting nursing practice, accessing information, using data and information systems, and coordinating information flow. The nurse administrator's competencies are directing the organization of information, accessing information, using data and information, communicating and networking inside and outside the organization, and assuring ethical standards and data protection. The informatics competencies for the nurse teachers include communication, text processing, data base management, data analysis, and computer-assisted learning. The nurse researcher's competencies are using bibliographic retrieval systems, electronic communication (networking), data management and manipulation, and text processing and graphics applications.[6]

Model 4

The model for informatics knowledge devised by Donald A. B. Lindberg, Director of the National Library of Medicine, consists of seven levels of increasing complexity.

- be computer literate
- use a computer as an independent learning tool
- develop minimal personal skills such as using word processing, data base, and spread sheet applications

- be a knowledgeable consumer: possess sufficient knowledge of technologies and their related issues to enable one to acquire an information system to meet one's needs
- see new applications
- build a system for one's own application using existing technologies and tools
- build new tools.[7]

Dr. Lindberg proposed this model to address the question of what knowledge and understanding should be taught to students at the various levels of undergraduate, graduate, and postgraduate education.

Model 5

In 1988, an Informatics Task Force for the University of Maryland at Baltimore (UMAB), chaired by Marion J. Ball, condensed Lindberg's seven levels taxonomy of understanding into three levels of competency. These levels are summarized below.

Level One a suggested minimum or core computer literacy for the entire campus

Level Two school or discipline-specific knowledge for students in their profession

Level Three an intensive and advanced understanding for the informatics specialist and researcher

UMAB's goal is to make various paths and educational opportunities available to students that will allow them to obtain the competency level appropriate to their own needs, interests, and abilities. For a detailed description of the UMAB Competencies see Table 10.1. UMAB described Level One, campuswide minimum competencies, with the greatest detail of the three levels. Performance at this level, or demonstration of what might be described as basic computer and information literacy, was expected of all students prior to graduation, and included the following skills:

- describe and discuss the basic components and functions of a computer system
- use software applications at a basic level including word processing, spread sheet, data base, statistical and numerical analysis, and educational software
- access electronic data bases and retrieve information relevant to their profession
- utilize data communications equipment to access a remote computing site
- identify and discuss the impact of computers on their profession
- demonstrate beginning computer skills by completing an assignment to organize and report data using a microcomputer
- discuss major social, ethical, legal, and organizational issues involved in computerized information systems.

Table 10.1

Lindberg Taxonomy	UMAB Taxonomy
	I. Campuswide Minimum Competencies
— Computer Literacy	— Use basic informantion handling tools for daily activities such as wordprocessing, electronic mail, library access, statistical analysis. Understand purposes and limitations of computers for clinical tasks.
— Independent Learning	— Understand basic computing and information management sufficiently to read literature in the field. Select and use information systems for learning and professional tasks.
— Minimal Personal Skills	— use computer systems, access databases. Evaluate existing systems, use online bibliographic databases, and understand major hardware and softwsre concepts.
	II. School or Profession Specific Competencies
— Knowledgeable Consumer	— Use specialized systems and databases. Evaluate and make informed decisions about such institutional and personal investments as patient care automation/computerized systems particular to the individual's field.
	III. Informatics Specialist/Researcher Competencies
— See New Applications	— Identify information needs in work environment and select appropriate solutions provided by off-the-shelf technological solutions reguiring only minor modifications.
— Build a System for One's Application	— Identify need. perform system analysis and build information system.
— Tool Building	— Identify research in field, establish scientific method for testing and evaluating solution and system design, publish results in refereed publications.

The second level, profession-specific competencies, was defined with less specificity. The task force concurred that responsibility for defining this level of competencies rested with the schools. This decision resulted in part from the fact that the various schools on campus were then (and remain as of this writing) at very different phases and levels of sophistication in the development of informatics programs and have not published competencies for Level Two. In addition to the minimum competencies, Level One, listed above, dental students should also obtain proficiency in the following areas specific to dentistry.

- demonstrate a working knowledge of the technology and the basic principles of practice management that are used in computerized dental office information systems
- develop a request for proposal for an computerized practice management system and evaluate and rate vendor responses
- understand the strengths and weaknesses of the coding schemes presently used in dentistry, such as ADA procedure codes, ICD-9 diagnostic codes, MeSH terms
- discuss the impact and relevance of large patient information databases that can be used to address issues of quality assurance, mercury levels in patients, the etiology of periodontal disease, and other practice-based research studies
- discuss the future uses of technology in the dental practice, such as automated periodontal probing, computer assisted design of dental restorations, computerized digital radiography and imaging, and computer assisted decision making.

Many dental schools have begun to integrate some of the above Level One and Two competencies into existing curricula. Often these are introduced into already existing courses (horizontal curriculum) rather than offered as new, dedicated courses on informatics (vertical curriculum). The horizontal approach has many benefits, the primary being the readily identifiable relevancy of the newly learned informatics competencies to the practice of dentistry. This approach is also a more effective means to introduce new fields of knowledge into an already crowded curriculum. And in many cases the course developer can minimize the impact of the curriculum committee bureaucracy.

The task force defined the third level, informatics specialist/researcher competencies, with the least specificity. Activities at this level were felt to be the responsibility of the schools and departments within the schools. A good example of Level Three is the UMAB School of Nursing masters program in Nursing Informatics.

Upon completion of this program, the nursing students have obtained competencies in the following areas.

- analyze nursing information requirements for clinical and management information systems
- analyze information needs and technologic issues related to productivity and quality assurance programs in nursing
- develop strategies to manage technological and organizational change and innovation
- apply management and nursing theories and information science to the planning, development, implementation, and administration of nursing information systems
- evaluate the effectiveness of nursing information systems in patient care delivery

- define methodologies related to technology and engineering planning for information systems in health care and nursing
- apply concepts of budget, staffing, and financial management to the design of management information systems in patient care delivery
- apply concepts of nursing theory to the design of health care and clinical information systems
- develop and implement user training programs to support the utilization of clinical and management information systems
- analyze the contribution of information technology to nursing education, administration, clinical practice, and research
- examine the political, social, ethical, and influential forces in health care as they relate to the use of information technology and management
- evaluate hardware, software, and vendor support for technologies that underpin clinical and management decisions in nursing
- examine data base management principles in relation to nursing information system file structures
- apply concepts of programming logic to the analysis of a simple computer program.[8]

A national dental organization, such as the American Association of Dental Schools, should take on a project such as the Nursing Informatics Recommendation put forth by the National League of Nurses. The dental informatics competency recommendations put forth by this group could set the direction for curriculum changes and faculty development as well as continuing education for dental practitioners, researchers, educators, and administrators.

International Educational Health Informatics Programs

Health informatics programs first appeared in European universities in the early 1970s. Today these specialized educational programs are found throughout the world, but the most extensively developed programs remain those in Europe, where the term "informatics" was coined. Existing programs can serve as valuable guides for educators from information science and the health sciences backgrounds. Some dental schools have begun to integrate informatics competencies into their curricula, even fewer schools offer electives in a general informatics topic, but no dental schools have yet offered concentrations or minors in an informatics field.

This is not necessarily a bad turn of events. There are many programs in health informatics, not within dental schools, that can serve the dental community very well. These existing programs can often be modified and tailored to suit the specific needs and interests of the student. This is particularly true of the more advanced degree programs. Due to this lack of informatics programs within dentistry, we shall look at some examples from the health sciences as well as the computer/information sciences. (For additional information an extensive listing of worldwide informatics programs can be found in the May/June 1990 issue of *M.D. Computing*,

Vol. 7, No. 3, p. 172-175. titled "Informatics Programs in the United States and Abroad.") Available in mid-summer 1991, the University of Maryland at Baltimore, in cooperation with the International Medical Informatics Association's Education Working Group 1, will make available via computer network an online database of informatics programs from around the world.

Curriculum Models

Curriculum models may be categorized according to several schemata. One scheme arranges models according to the level at which the graduates of the proposed program will work. Anderson, Gremy, and Pages[9] identified three levels and the International Medical Informatics Association[10] added a fourth level to the list:

- those working or preparing to work in a health field and requiring enough knowledge to use the technologies available
- those acquiring specific knowledge and doing research and developmental work in the field while remaining there
- those acquiring in-depth knowledge in informatics and dedicating full time efforts to the application of informatics in medicine, both in clinical work and research
- those doing advanced research in the field of medical informatics as such.

The utility of this scheme is limited by its focus upon the future activities of the graduates of the informatics programs rather than the content of the informatics programs themselves.

A second scheme differentiates between informatics programs according to the level of study, either undergraduate or graduate. This distinction is blurred by the differences between the higher education systems in Europe and the United States. Thus, its utility is again limited for international comparisons.

From an international perspective, the most useful scheme may be the one which formally recognizes the dualistic nature of health informatics, which is the study of health sciences and information/computer sciences (See Figure 10.1). This scheme acknowledges the fact that health informatics curricula tend to evolve from a base in either the health sciences or information/computer sciences. Such programs tend to be marked by an emphasis in one of the two areas; courses in the other area are then added to the core. Informatics degrees granted may be either academic (B.A., M.A., Ph.D.) or professional (D.D.S., M.D., M.S.N.). Most programs in medical and nursing informatics have been conceived and implemented within an existing health science program such as a medical or nursing school. The other major contributors to the development of health informatics educational programs are the computer and information sciences programs found in the arts and sciences colleges and sometimes within schools of business.

Beside the two traditional contributors to health informatics programs there is the true hybrid, information/computer science and health sciences as distinct fields which have cross-fertilized and produced, as a hybrid of sorts, specialized programs in the various branches of health informatics. These health informatics

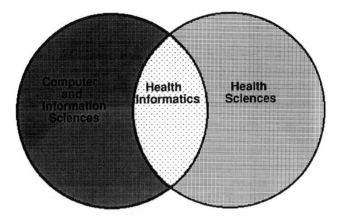

Figure 10.1. The dualistic nature of health informatics.

programs do not start from an established base in either the health sciences or computer/information sciences. A good example of this type of program can be seen in the Health Information Science program at the University of Victoria in British Columbia, Canada.

In summary, the major categories of health informatics educational programs as classified by their curricular origins are:

- informatics programs with an emphasis on information and computer sciences: operations analysis, information science, or computer science degree with a minor or concentration in health
- informatics programs based in the health sciences: health degree with minor in informatics or a concentration in informatics
- specialized informatics programs: hybrid health informatics.

Informatics Programs with an Emphasis on Information and Computer Sciences

This first category of programs is based in computing and information sciences. In Germany, these programs are structured so that coursework in the health sciences account for around 25% of the total (the German differentiation between major and minor fields of study).

There also are excellent programs within the United States that can serve as models. The University of Maryland, Baltimore County, Department of Information Systems Management, offers both a M.S. and a Ph.D. in which the students may specialize in one of six applications areas. Health sciences information is one of the specializations; others include business and law.

Informatics Programs Based in the Health Sciences

In the United States, due in large part to the leadership of the Association of American Medical Colleges and the National Library of Medicine, medical schools have progressed faster than other health science schools in incorporating informatics into their curricula. Although few medical schools have required informatics courses, many are now offering elective courses and establishing base competencies. A much smaller number of nursing, pharmacy, dental, and allied health schools have informatics courses in their curricula.

Very few health degree programs in nursing, dentistry, pharmacy, or medicine allow students to minor in health informatics. One such program in nursing was started in 1988 at the University of Maryland at Baltimore, School of Nursing. The master's program in Nursing Administration gives the opportunity for students to enroll in a health informatics track. This curriculum contains courses in information systems theory, operations analysis, and modeling and simulations — courses offered by the information and computer science departments at its sister campus and required also of their majors.

Specialized Informatics Programs

In the attempt to address the needs of the new and growing field of health informatics, specialized academic programs have been developed by leading informaticians and health educators both in the United States and abroad. These innovative programs are structured to create a balance between study in the fields of health sciences and computer/information sciences, discussed above. An interdisciplinary approach is manifest in these programs. On the graduate level, these programs are often further differentiated by the type of degrees granted. For example, a medical school may offer a Ph.D. in health informatics.

One of the few undergraduate programs is the Bachelor of Science degree program in Health Information Science at the University of Victoria in British Columbia, Canada. Four years of study include a thirteen week cooperative education experience in the third year. Concentrations are offered in administration, computing science, biomedical principles and statistics, and economics. Health care delivery courses replace the business courses under the structure proposed by the Association for Computing Machinery's Curriculum Recommendations for Graduate and Undergraduate Programs in Information Systems.[11]

Stanford University School of Medicine offers a master's degree in Medical Information Sciences. This is an interdepartmental program under the direction of Edward H. Shortliffe and Lawrence M. Fagan. The master's program is two years in length. Most of the core courses are taught in the first year; a major project is completed during the second year. The core curriculum consists of courses in medicine, computer science, decision making, medical computer science, and health policy/social issues with a minimum of 44 units of course work.

Doctoral Programs

In the United States and abroad, the majority of students applying to these programs hold an M.D. degree or are actively seeking one. Curricula tend to follow the standard set by the Association of Computing Machinery, with courses organized in four groups; computer science, health science, integrative studies, and contributing studies. Doctoral degrees in informatics are offered at a growing number of institutions.

In the United States, the National Library of Medicine has supported the development of such programs. Table 10.2 gives a listing of the NLM-supported training programs in the United States. Under its NLM medical informatics research training program, Harvard offers a master's and doctoral program in Applied Biomedical Computing and in Health Decision Sciences at the Harvard School of Public Health. Its postdoctoral program involves apprenticeship in a medical informatics research laboratory at either Brigham and Women's Hospital or Massachusetts General Hospital. Postdoctoral work involves independent research and the acquisition of project experience in such areas as knowledge management, educational applications, simulations, expert systems, and workstation interface design for clinical and educational problem-solving.

Stanford University offers a doctoral program designed to prepare individuals as independent researchers in medical informatics. In addition to completing the core courses and oral examination for the master's program, the students take additional advanced courses, prepare a thesis, complete a teaching assistant service in management information systems courses, and complete a dissertation.

Table 10.2 NLM training grants.

Actrive Training Grants, Fiscal Year 1988
Medical training Research Taining

University of California, San Francisco, California
    John A. Starkweather, M.D.
Harvard School of Public Health, Boston, Massachusetts
    Robert A. Greenes, M.D., Ph.D.
New England Medical Center Hospital, Boston, Massachusetts
    Stephen G. Pauker, M.D.
University of Minnesota Medical School, Minneapolis, Minnesota
    Lael C. Gatewood, Ph.D.
University of Pittsburgh School of Medicine, Pittsburgh, Pennsylvania
    Randolph A. Miller, M.D.
Stanford University School of Medicine, Stanford, California
    Edward Shortliffe, M.D., Ph.D.
Washington University, St. Louis, Missouri
    Charles E. Molnar, Sc.D.
Yale University School of Medicine, New Haven, Connecticut
    Perry L. Miller, M.D., Ph.D.

Sponsored by the National Library of Medicine, Extramural Programs

International Collaboration on Informatics Program Development

Health informatics and particularly dental informatics stand to gain enormously from an international perspective. The Europeans can offer their experience as acknowledged leaders in the development of health science-based and specialized informatics programs for physicians. The United States, where programs in medicine are now being initiated, can share their growing expertise in extending that concept to the other health professions, notably nursing and dentistry. The taxonomies for defining health informatics knowledge and skills highlight issues in program development. Programs in place can provide valuable information for professionals planning and evaluating curricula; these pioneering programs will also help in determining how much impact health informatics can have on the practice of health care. As the University of Maryland Informatics Task Force found, informaticians worldwide are willing to share their experiences and to benefit from those of others. Health informatics holds great promise — promise which these emerging programs are beginning to realize. In the United States, in late 1988, the National Library of Medicine called together a committee chaired by Michael DeBakey to look at its outreach activities as follow-up to its long range plan published in 1986.[12] One of the threads woven into the fabric of this committee's deliberations is the need to integrate the fundamentals of medical informatics into the curriculum and to use the regional medical libraries as well as the National Library of Medicine to foster and encourage this initiative. As the National Library of Medicine begins to look at the information needs of the dentist, the dental profession should extend to the Library a well thought-out plan for the information needs of the dental community. As these efforts are matched across the globe, there is no doubt that health informatics will help to bring the best possible health care to the people of the world.

References

1. Panel on the General Professional Education on the Physician and College Preparation for Medicine. Physicians for the 21 st century, GPEP report. Washington, DC: Association of American Medical Colleges, 1984.
2. Van Bemmel JH. The structure of medical informatics. Medical Informatics. 1984;3: 175-1 80.
3. Van Bemmel JH, Hasman A, Sollet PCGM, et al. Training in medical informatics. Computers and Biomedical Research. 1983;16:414-432.
4. Van Bemmel JH. A comprehensive model for medical information processing. Methods of Information in Medicine. 1983;22:124-130.
5. Panel on the General Professional Education on the Physician and College Preparation for Medicine, 1984.
6. Peterson HE, Gerdin-Jelger U, eds. Preparing nurses for using information systems: recommended informatics competencies. New York: National League for Nursing, 1988: p. 117-138 .

7. Lindberg DAB. The evolution of medical informatics. Medical education in the information age: proceedings of the symposium on medical informatics. Washington, DC: Association of American Medical Colleges, 1986: p. 92-94.

8. Heller BR, Romano CA, Damrosch SP, et al. The need for an educational program in nursing informatics. In: Ball MJ, Hannah KJ, Gerdin Jelger U, et al, eds. Nursing informatics: where caring and technology meet. New York:Springer-Verlag, 1988: p. 339-340.

9. Anderson J, Gremy F, Pages J. Education in informatics of health personnel. Amsterdam: North-Holland Press, 1974.

10. Duncan KA. Educational prerequisites for medical informatics. In: Perez-deTalens AF, Molinoravetto E, Shires DB, eds. Proceedings of the world congress on medical informatics and developing countries. Amsterdam: NorthHolland Press, 1982: p. 163.

11. Duncan KA, Austin RH, Katz S, et al. A model curriculum for doctoral-level programs in health computing careers. New York: Association for Computing Machinery, 1981.

12. National Library of Medicine. Report of panel 4 long range plan: medical informatics. Bethesda: National Institutes of Health, 1986.

11
The Technology Assisted Learning Environment

James F. Craig and Ernest F. Moreland

A technology assisted learning (TAL) center has several functions. The TAL center:

1) emphasizes the use of computer technology

2) is designed to function as a teaching, learning, and support facility

3) may be used for a wide variety of purposes including computer literacy training for students, faculty, staff and administrators, independent learning, information retrieval or on-line literature searching, small or large group instruction, and hardware or software instruction and demonstrations

4) may be created to provide all of the above for an individual department, school or an entire campus.

Role of the TAL Center

In order to facilitate the planning process, the role of technology assisted learning and the TAL center must be established early in the planning process because many of the decisions to be made will be influenced by the role technology assisted learning will play in the curriculum, school or on the campus.

Depending upon a given situation or institution, technology assisted learning may serve as both a primary and a supplementary source of instruction through a single TAL center facility. In this instance, both types of instruction are available on the same hardware and the use is determined by both the faculty and the user. For example, a menu may offer a student a variety of options ranging from assigned dental case simulations for a course in oral diagnosis in which the student's performance will be scored and saved for grading purposes (primary source); to an introduction to wordprocessing; or the use of a dental drug information database which the student elects to use to augment his instruction (supplementary source).

In general, when technology assisted learning is integrated into the curriculum and is used as the primary source of instruction, learners use the technology as a means of instruction and discover other uses of this technology that they may not otherwise have discovered. If the use of technology assisted learning plays a supplementary role in the curriculum, it may not be used at all.

Objectives

Whether the TAL center is campuswide or school specific, the following are some general objectives to be achieved through its use:

1. To assist faculty members in improving their instruction, and, at the same time, to keep the unit cost of instruction reasonable and constant.

2. To involve the faculty in educational research projects, including the application of new technology in instruction.

3. To assist the administration in maximizing the use of their instructional and human resources through the use of technology.

4. To increase the sharing of TAL facilities, hardware, software and personnel among departments, schools, other campuses of the university and other institutions in the area.

5. To develop more precise methods for the measurement of innovative approaches in the solution of instructional problems.

6. To maintain and encourage innovative applications of technology assisted learning by faculty within various disciplines.

7. To provide adequate facilities which are easily accessible for technology assisted learning for students and faculty.

Planning

When considering the creation of a TAL center, serious attention must be given to various aspects of the project: **planning, design, utilization** and **evaluation**. What follows are some basic considerations regarding each of these facets of the project. It is suggested that a committee or resource group be created to coordinate these project activities, and that representatives from various components of the institution be involved in the process. This may include individuals representing the academic, clinical, research and administrative components of the school or campus. It may be useful early in the planning process for this committee to address the **who, what, where, when, how, how much, how many,** and **how evaluated** regarding technology assisted learning and the TAL center. In this regard, following each of these areas are several questions which may be helpful in gathering information to facilitate decision making. The committee may add its own questions in order to address the unique characteristics of each institution.

Who

- Who will use the center—students, faculty and staff? Will the users be from a single department, school or from an entire campus?
- Who will fund or support the center—a department, school, campus, private funds or a combination?
- Who will make the final decision(s) concerning the implementation of the project?
- Who will staff the TAL center and provide guidance and direction for the technology assisted learning program?

What

- What type of interest and administrative support is available or needed for initiating a technology assisted learning program and TAL center in terms of meeting academic or administrative needs and objectives, constructing a facility, equipping a facility, obtaining budgetary support for the ongoing operation of a center, and hiring personnel?
- What type of staff will be needed for the center and what are the job requirements for the staff?
- What type of information, expertise or resources are currently available and will these resources be used to meet the existing needs and objectives for the technology assisted learning environment? If resources are not available, what type of information, expertise or resources are necessary in the area of technology assisted learning that may add guidance or direction to the planning process? In this regard, it is important from the outset to determine the level of administrative and faculty support for technology assisted learning through an assessment of the end-users needs, desires and expectations. This information will facilitate the formulation of the objectives for the project. Several examples include: develop computer literacy skills; develop computer-based educational programs; do data analysis for research projects; conduct online literature searches; and teach students, faculty and staff how to use a dental clinic management system. Keep in mind that many individuals will not be aware of the functions provided through a TAL center. In order to gain support for technology assisted learning, students, faculty, staff and administrators need to know what this technology can do to address their needs. It may be desirable to promote this technology in order to introduce potential users to the ways this technology may meet their needs, such as:
  - Reviewing pertinent literature on TAL facilities and programs which are meeting needs similar to those stated in the objectives for their school.
  - Visiting existing facilities which provide a range of services both similar and dissimilar to those contemplated in their school.

- Developing a file for relevant sources of information, such as hardware, software, furniture manufacturers, architects or facility designers with experience in the area of TAL centers, and professional people willing to serve as consultants.
- Seeking advice from experienced educational and technical personnel relative to problems and solutions involved in developing and operating a TAL center, and encouraging them to share their experience with the appropriate groups or individuals within the school.
- Continually reviewing the needs and objectives to be achieved through technology assisted learning and sharing this information within the school in order to maintain a focus on the critical elements of the project.
- Considering what the space requirements for the TAL center will be and whether such space is available and usable or whether space will have to be acquired or constructed. Space allocation can be a sensitive issue, and involving the appropriate individuals responsible for such decisions early on in the planning process can save time and facilitate the planning process.
- Considering the number and type of personnel that will be required to operate the center and the nature of the services provided by the staff.

Where

- Where will the center be located, that is, within an individual department or school or centrally located on campus and who will make this decision?

When

- When will the plan for the TAL center be available and presented for support and implementation?
- When will the project begin and end, that is, what is the schedule of events that must take place and in what order should they follow?
- When will the facility be available for use? What are the anticipated hours of operation, and will it be available for scheduling classes, demonstrations or other special events?

How

- How will the TAL center be supported? Will the funding come from departmental, school or campus funding, or collaborative arrangements involving support from various sources, including corporate or private funding? Can providing support funding be exchanged for the use of the facilities at pre-arranged times?

- How will the facility be utilized: as a classroom for instruction, for independent study, or both?
- How will the facility be staffed, organized, and equipped?
- How will the level of support and services be evaluated?
- How will the policies and procedures governing the operation of the facility be developed? How will the facility, equipment and holdings be maintained and up-dated?

How Much?

- How much will the facility cost to renovate, construct, equip, operate, staff, maintain and support?
- How much use will be made of the facility and under what arrangements?
- How much will it cost to use the facility, that is, will there be a charge to individuals, departments, schools or programs for access to the facility or for education or training? Will there be a charge for users indirectly or not affiliated with the institution?

How Many?

- How many TAL centers are needed?
- How many users will the facility(ies) accommodate?
- How many pieces of hardware and software are needed to provide support for the user population? How many users will have access to the center?
- How many staff members are required to operate the center?

How Evaluated?

- How will the overall program involving technology assisted learning be evaluated?
- How will the information gathered from the evaluation be used and/or what purpose will the evaluation serve?

Gathering information concerning the **who, what, where, when, how, how much, how many**, and **how evaluated** should provide a basic framework for creating a technology assisted learning environment plan. What follows is more specific information relating to the design, utilization and evaluation of technology assisted learning and a TAL center that must also be incorporated into the planning process in greater detail.

Designing the Technology Assisted Learning Environment

The well designed and properly equipped TAL environment must serve the needs of the user population in order for the TAL center to be successful. For example, the design of the TAL center must be conducive to learning. Additionally, the color selection used in the facility, its location, lighting, acoustics, space, ventilation, and furnishings must complement the learning environment or else they will serve as distractors and make the user feel uncomfortable, depressed or discouraged and may actually dampen the user's enthusiasm toward learning. All of the physical and environmental factors are common problems facing the designer when planning and implementing a technology assisted learning environment.

The information that follows assumes:

- an enrollment of approximately 600 students
- that the facility will be used half time for independent study and the remainder for scheduled classes
- that the facility will be available for use approximately ninety hours a week including evenings and week-ends
- that one full time person will be hired to serve as a TAL center coordinator and report to the appropriate academic administrator
- that student assistants will be hired to provide TAL center coverage evenings and week-ends

Location of the TAL Center

The location of the TAL center is critical if students, faculty and staff are expected to utilize the facility. The location of the center should be on the same floor and within the same building where student activities routinely occur, and ideally, in or adjacent to an area where other types of relevant information or learning resource material is kept. A location of this type facilitates the use of a broader range of instructional materials; makes better use of the users time by having a variety of resources immediately available; and assists in the management and maintenance of the facility.

Space Allocation

Variations exist among schools in the design and arrangement of learning resource or TAL centers. In some schools, a single center will effectively serve the needs of students, faculty, staff and administrators and house a variety of learning resource material ranging from slide tape programs, videocassettes, computer-based education and a broad range of print material. In other schools, individual centers may be used for different purposes where conventional media, technology assisted learning and library materials reside in separate facilities. Ideally, it is desirable to have all resources readily available in a single location, however, differing philosophies, objectives, logistics or overall space requirements may make this impractical or impossible. The recommendations that follow will need to consider such variations within each institution and take these into consideration when deciding whether a single facility or multiple facilities are required.

Study Facilities and Furnishings

The use of the TAL center must be considered in planning for study facilities and furnishings. It may be desirable to select a design that allows for both independent study and formal classes. Several items to consider include:

- If a large number of carrels or desks are to be used, arrange them so they do not have a fenced or regimented appearance. (Figure 11.1). If the facility is to be used for classroom instruction, a more traditional configuration will be required (Figure 11.2). In this case, special consideration should be given to providing an instructor's station equipped with the ability to control the light and audio levels in the room as well as the use of video or projection equipment. A projection screen, adequate storage space, and a chalk or "white board" should also be available.

- In addition to the central TAL center it may be necessary for satellite centers or equipment to be located throughout the building so that the utilization is accessible. Individual study carrels should be considered when satellite locations are used. This allocation of equipment necessitates considering user support, maintenance, and security.

- Furniture used in equipping a TAL center is available in a wide variety of shapes and sizes. In some instances, it may be desirable to enclose or partially-enclose certain areas within the TAL center to restrict use or traffic. Once the decision has been made regarding how the center will be used, the appropriate size and shape of the furnishings can be determined. If the furniture is to be used as a teaching environment, special consideration should be given to providing students with an unobstructed view toward the front of the classroom.

- If projection equipment is to be used, space for this equipment, distance from the projection screen, and light control/dimming need to be considered.

Electrical Considerations

In a TAL center, sufficient electrical power is mandatory and must adhere to local building codes and load requirements. Every carrel or desk should have a minimum of two 110/120 volt electrical outlets. These outlets should be on circuits independent of the room lighting, fused for 20 amperes each with master fusing and circuits planned to prevent overloading. It is also suggested that consideration be given to installing these outlets using flexible cabling, especially if a computer raised floor is used, so that the outlets may be moved if necessary to accommodate changes in the configuration of the room furnishings or computer systems (Figure 11.3). Additionally, special consideration should be given to the installation of

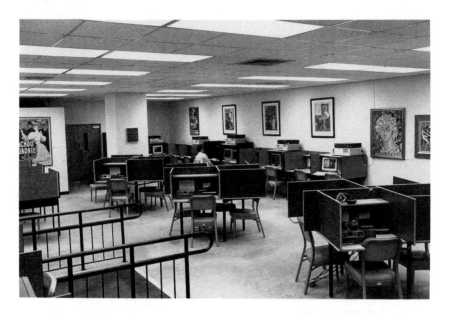

Figure 11.1. Carrel configuration avoiding linear appearance.

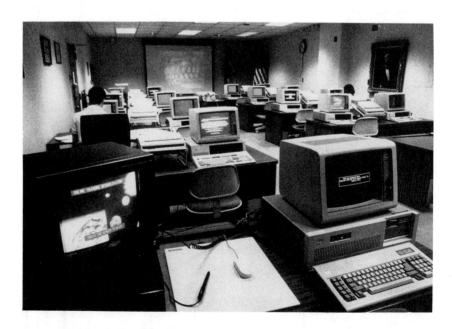

Figure 11.2. Student workstation configuration for classroom instruction.

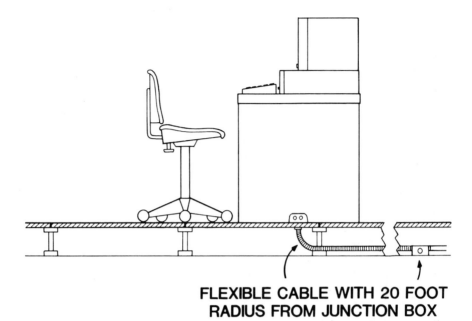

**FLEXIBLE CABLE WITH 20 FOOT
RADIUS FROM JUNCTION BOX**

Figure 11.3. Outlets on flexible cables beneath computer-raised floors.

surge suppressors or a surge suppression system to avoid problems caused by the sudden loss of power or inconsistent supply of power to computer equipment.

Lighting Considerations

Lighting for the TAL center should be designed to meet the specific instructional needs for which the facility will be used. For example, the light controls should be located adjacent to the teaching station so that the instructor may select the optimum light level to accommodate a variety of needs such as use of a large screen television projection system, overhead or slide projector, or note taking during projection. The light should be diffused to eliminate "hot spots" or glare to make viewing information on the computer screen more comfortable for the user.

Ventilation

Instructional environments, including a TAL center, frequently present a cooling rather than a heating problem due to the heat generated from the technology coupled with the body heat generated by large groups of users. This is particularly true when the environment is used for prolonged periods of time. Since conditions vary greatly from one instructional environment to another, and may also vary from floor to floor, or different sides of a building, the ventilation system for the TAL center should be controlled independently in the TAL center. Regardless of the type of ventilation system used, being able to change from a heating situation to a cooling situation at any time in order to maintain a comfortable instructional environment is extremely important. Acoustical Considerations

The TAL center should be equipped with an acoustically treated ceiling and appropriate acoustical separation or treatment of walls and floors. This insures minimum interference from adjacent classrooms, lounges, offices and other areas.

Audio Visual Utilization

The utilization of all instructional equipment is an important consideration in the design of the TAL center. Ideally, the teaching station should be equipped for remote control of a slide projector, videocassette player, videodisc player and large screen television/RGB projection system. It may be desirable to install an audio system for the center for use with audio visual equipment or to accommodate a microphone for the instructor. A wireless microphone is desirable because it enables the instructor to move freely about the classroom providing assistance and yet still be heard by the students. Other considerations may include an overhead projector (with or without a liquid crystal display for use with a computer) and white or chalk board.

Storage Facilities and Security

An active TAL center requires adequate space for storage and security of hardware and software. This space needs to be incorporated into or immediately adjacent to the TAL center. This space is critical and most often overlooked and underestimated when designing a TAL facility. Additional provisions should also be made to secure the hardware in the center and there are a variety of means available commercially for this purpose, varying from the use of cables and/or brackets with locks to hoods that completely enclose and lock-up the equipment when it is not being used. The use of a barcoding system should be considered when planning security for the center to facilitate the circulation of the center holdings. Such a system will maintain an accurate inventory of materials and provide information on utilization, user characteristics, or user preferences, all of which may play an important role in the evaluation of the center.

Floor

It is important to anticipate and plan for future needs and developments in selecting a floor for a TAL center. For example, will the electrical wiring, television coaxial cables or network cables be installed in the floor, walls or ceiling? Wiring should be placed in the least visible location possible and allow for the greatest flexibility in order to permit reconfiguration of existing equipment and furniture or the addition and servicing of new equipment, wiring or cabling. It may be advisable to install computer raised flooring or "false flooring" to provide flexibility. This flooring usually is 6" or more above the actual floor and comes in sections to facilitate access to the space below. Electrical outlets or cable connections can be installed in these flooring sections and can be moved should the room configuration need to be changed. Carpeting provides acoustical dampening for the TAL center and provides a nice aesthetic touch to any study area. It is important that low static carpet be used since static electric discharges are annoying to users and may seriously damage computer hardware and disks. Carpet squares are well suited for installation over computer-raised-flooring since this flooring frequently comes covered with a tile surface. The use of carpet squares, in addition to the acoustical treatment and aesthetic appearance, also provide the advantage of being able to remove stained, damaged or heavily worn sections without having to replace the entire carpet. This is particularly important in areas receiving heavy use.

Utilization of the Technology Assisted Learning Environment

Users should feel the TAL center is there to assist them and to serve as an impetus to learning. The TAL center should provide an environment that is conducive to learning and be operated efficiently and effectively in terms of meeting the needs of the user population.

Whether programs housed in the center are developed "in house" or acquired "off the shelf" the most important single factor leading to the success of a TAL center is how the instructional programs are utilized within the curriculum. The two basic approaches for the use of instructional programs discussed earlier were either a primary or supplementary source of instruction. As the primary source, technology assisted learning is integrated into the curriculum and becomes the source of instruction. As a supplementary source of instruction, technology assisted learning serves as an adjunct to instruction that students may or may not elect to use.

Whether the instructional materials contained in the TAL center are locally developed, off the shelf acquisitions, used as an integral part of the curriculum or a supplementary aid to instruction, every effort should be made to insure the following are taken into consideration.

The programs should:

- be "user friendly" so that software can be used without the constant presence of the instructor or TAL center staff.
- focus on specific objectives, learnable ideas, skills, and techniques directly related to the curriculum or program objectives.
- minimize the amount of effort involved in making changes or modifications.
- provide a high degree of individualization so that each user may progress through the program at his or her own rate.

Guidelines for Selecting Software

While the general considerations listed above should be taken into account when developing or acquiring instructional materials, certain basic guidelines for selecting and purchasing commercially available software need to be established. The following are several items that need to be taken into consideration in this regard:

- The TAL center should establish a selection policy which is endorsed by the school administration and department heads.
- Software should meet the objectives of the various curricular areas and provide for the diverse learning skills and abilities of students.
- The selection of instructional materials should involve the TAL center director or coordinator and selected faculty members or administrators representing the various disciplines or administrative programs within the institution. For example, representatives may include individuals from the school or campus computing center, fiscal or personnel office, the clinical and basic science areas, academic affairs, and faculty development. Only those programs which meet technical and subject matter standards should be acquired. It is suggested that a simple and succinct standardized form be developed for this process.
- Final selection of the software should be the responsibility of a single individual such as the director of the center.
- Sufficient copies of the programs should be acquired and made available to meet the needs of the users. The number of copies will vary depending on whether it is used as a primary or supplementary form of instruction. Other considerations in this regard include:

  a) the cost of the software and the conditions for its use (copyright and/or licensing agreements).

  b) hardware and software requirements and the number of systems available suited for the software specifications.

  c) the number of programs expected to be used at a particular time. For example, is the program an integral part of the curriculum where heavy use is anticipated or supplementary where students may or may not use the program?

  d) Can the program be used by more than one student, or is it designed for a single user?

Encouraging the Use of the TAL Center

The following are suggestions for facilitating the use of the TAL center:

- There should be sufficient, competent, empathetic, and resourceful center staff available to the user population. Use of the center will vary in direct proportion to the quality of staff.
- Hardware and software must be available in sufficient quantities to assure maximum accessibility and utilization.

- The design of the learning or teaching environment must support the purpose for which it was developed.
- The center must be open at all times of the school day and be convenient and comfortable. Before and after school hours, vacations, and weekends must be considered.
- There may be a need to establish satellite learning centers in order to meet special needs and conditions. These satellite centers may be temporary or permanent, but the circulation of hardware or software to meet special needs outside the TAL center must be taken into consideration.
- Loan of hardware or software outside the building may present logistical and security problems, but may have to be addressed. In general, loan of hardware should be avoided. The loan of software is easier to accommodate providing a policy and procedure is established to provide guidance for such a loan policy. The use and loan of all software must comply with legal stipulations such as copyright and/or site agreement.

Staffing

At least one full time person will be required to operate a TAL center. This person will report directly to the appropriate academic administrator and will provide daily service to students, faculty and staff during hours when it is difficult to obtain student assistance because of class schedules and daily requirements. Additionally, this is the time when the center would be under the greatest demand by students and would require constant support. During the evenings and week-ends, the demand can easily be achieved by trained student assistants who would be under the direct supervision of the full time staff person. In general, the TAL staff should:

- Facilitate the application of information technology through a broadbased training and educational program in computer literacy for students, faculty and staff. This program would present various forms of information technology and examine the potential that exists for its application in the areas of administration, education, research, and clinic operations.
- Facilitate the integration of office automation and business applications (in both a dental and non-dental context) on a school wide and departmental basis. This includes word processing, database management, telecommunications, inventory control, electronic mail, fiscal, personnel and project management.
- Facilitate educational applications of information technology including CAD/CAM, computer assisted and computer managed instruction, computer assisted testing, test development and generation, image storage, enhancement and retrieval, computer graphics, computer simulations and games, curriculum and professional development, and didactic and clinical performance evaluation. Facilitate research applications including research design and statistical analyses, tests and measurements, literature searches,

and the use, design and development of dental databases and measures of human performance.

- Encourage collaborative arrangements with other departments, schools, institutions or corporate relationships in order to facilitate the installation of state of the art information networks in the school and on campus.

The committee may want to expand or reduce the role of the TAL center to staff beyond the scope of the items listed above. Carefully defining the role of technology assisted learning in the curriculum will help refine the focus the TAL center and its staff serve.

Software Organization and Cataloging

The organization and cataloging of software is imperative. Users need to know what is available, where it is located, and what they need to do in order to use a program. An on-line database of the TAL center holdings may provide a useful tool to the users in this regard or this information needs to be available in a printed form for circulation to departments as a reference in planning their instructional programs. In some cases, it may be desirable to make this information available for a modest fee. Each school or TAL facility may have a different approach for cataloging their holdings, but it is advisable to have the holdings cataloged. It may be desirable to include information regarding TAL center policies and procedures within the catalog. This would help clarify hours of operation, loan policies, available hardware, course offerings, instructional support services and the names and phone numbers of support staff if assistance is needed.

Hardware

The kind and amount of hardware obtained and the way it is made available is a matter of great importance to the success of the TAL center. Unfortunately, hardware may often be purchased without serious consideration being given to the role that this technology will play in the curriculum, the software available for use within the curriculum and its required hardware support configuration, or the level of reliability or performance of the hardware or its manufacturer. An important factor in determining the type of hardware to be purchased is whether there is a sufficient amount of locally produced or off-the-shelf compatible software available.

In making hardware decisions one should attempt to standardize equipment by purchasing from a single manufacturer whenever possible. Some of the advantages of standardization include:

- It is easier to teach users to properly operate one type of delivery system.
- It is easier to stock spare parts and train a technician to make repairs on a single type of delivery system.
- A standard type of equipment may provide savings through discounts realized through ordering a greater number of a single system rather than a fewer number of a variety of systems.

- There is less clerical and technical work involved in maintaining an inventory of spare parts for a single type of hardware.
- There will be fewer operational failures because users will not be confronted with a wide variety hardware configurations and types.

When considering the purchase of hardware, obtain information about the system being considered from a reputable source such as a colleague or systems analyst. Additionally, request a demonstration of the desired hardware in the environment in which it will be used, and test it for a period of time to see if it performs the functions for which it is intended. The following items should be considered when ordering hardware:

1. Functionally meets technical specifications

2. Reputation of the manufacturer

3. Reputation of the vendor

4. Quality and reliability of performance

5. Cost to maintain and repair

6. Cost to purchase

7. Can it be up-graded and/or networked

8. Local service available

9. Ease of operation

10. Portability

11. Attractiveness of design

The order of the items implies relative importance in the decision-making process, however, each situation may require a variation in this order according to user requirements.

Maintenance

The hardware utilized in the TAL center is useless unless it is properly maintained and serviced regularly. Staff and user motivation will be lost quickly if they are constantly confronted with hardware problems resulting from inadequate maintenance. Furthermore, students will lose precious learning time and patience if they are constantly confronted with malfunctioning technology.

In order to service and maintain hardware properly in the TAL center, it is recommended that a service policy be negotiated at the time the equipment is purchased unless technical support is available in house. It is usually advantageous to employ a full time technician for preventive maintenance and to solve technical problems "in house." Various types of test equipment and an ample supply of parts for hardware repair will be required in the latter case.

If a technician is employed for maintenance and repair, records should be kept in order to monitor hardware performance and provide guidance in maintaining a sufficient supply of spare parts.

Integrating the Use of Technology Assisted Learning into the Dental Curriculum

In order to integrate the use of technology assisted learning into the dental curriculum, it is of utmost importance that the programs to be developed or purchased for use in the center be an integral part of the curriculum. That is, to remove these programs from student use would, in fact, remove a portion of the curriculum itself. The ultimate challenge, however, is to develop a positive attitude toward the use of computers on behalf of the user population.

What follows is a list of initiatives that took place at the University of Maryland Dental School and led to the gradual acceptance and integration of technology assisted learning in the curriculum. This list of actions is not a recipe for success. It is shared with others with the intent that several of the events may be helpful in initiating a similar program in other institutions.

In the events that follow, a concerted effort was made in each instance to (1) satisfy an individual need or need within the curriculum; (2) provide an opportunity for gaining recognition for the individual, department, school or institution; or (3) provide a means of obtaining credit for promotion, tenure or merit increment. It seemed that the greater the number of these items that were associated with a given activity, the greater the opportunity there was of achieving the desired result and vice-versa.

1. **Introduced faculty to the use of computer-generated graphics through the acquisition of a computer for this purpose in order to enable faculty to produce their own slides for instruction and formal presentations.**
The purchase of this system was in response to faculty members who expressed a constant need for professionally produced graphic slides for their lectures and presentations. This new system was introduced to the departments through a memo sent encouraging each department chairman to ask one of their faculty members to design a logo slide for their department to see how easy the system was to use. Of course, this service was "free," and faculty were encouraged to use their departmental logo slide in their lectures and professional presentations. Once the faculty saw the graphics capability of the new system, the requests for these slides soared. This provided faculty with high quality graphic slides which added a "professional touch" to their lectures and professional presentations, and in many cases offered them the opportunity to gain hands-on experience. Another benefit for the faculty using these slides occurred frequently when someone from their audience would complement them on the quality of their presentation slides. The use of this system "soft-sold" the technology, and eventually, requests for these slides and the opportunity to see and use the system were coming in from the entire campus.

2. Used a microcomputer system to develop and demonstrate a program called BORDEXAM in order to meet the expressed need of the Dean for improving student performance on the National Board Exams.

It was anticipated that developing a program designed to meet the specific needs of the school would serve as a direct pathway for adding microcomputers (and ultimately, interactive videodisc technology) to the school's academic program. The program included a didactic and clinical exam, with the latter requiring students to view images simultaneously as part of the examination process. The overall plan was to gain a commitment for the use of microtechnology for testing in the didactic area, and to gain support for technology assisted learning applications within the curriculum. The results proved favorable, as the faculty and administration grew more receptive toward the use of microcomputers for academic purposes. Students enjoyed and preferred using technology assisted learning in preparing for their exams, and their overall performance on the National Board Exam improved. The program also served as a means of developing computer-literacy skills among students and exposed and encouraged faculty to the use of technology assisted learning for academic applications.[1,2,3,4,5]

3. Developed a co-operative joint venture with the Information Resources Management Division (IRMD), the campus-wide computing unit, in order to gain a TAL center.

Space is a valuable commodity on the University of Maryland at Baltimore (UMAB) campus. In this case, IRMD needed space for the installation of a center for teaching computer literacy skills and the Dental School needed microcomputers for students to use to prepare for their board examinations. Working co-operatively, a portion of the school's Independent Learning Center, used for viewing independent learning programs, such as slide-tape and videocassette programs, was modified to include a microcomputer lab or TAL center. In exchange for the space allocated for this facility within the Dental School, the center was to be available to all students and faculty on campus for "walkin" use when it was not formally scheduled for use; be scheduled for use by anyone on campus up to fifty-percent of the time for formal classroom instruction through prior arrangement; and to include a Level III interactive videodisc authoring system in order to introduce this technology and demonstrate its potential for educational purposes to administrators, faculty, students and interested visitors. The ultimate goal for initiating this joint venture was to obtain additional equipment and support for introducing technology assisted learning and computer literacy training into the dental curriculum and to gain access to a Level III interactive videodisc system while offering a broad range of individuals the opportunity to gain "hands-on experience" with technology assisted learning. IRMD also gained attention and recognition for their well-equipped TAL center which attracted the attention of health science professionals from around the world. Additionally, the demonstration of technology assisted learning became a routine part of a visitors tour. The Dental School also took advantage of the center and demonstrated various applications of technology assisted learning when recruiting new students and faculty members to the school.

4. Developed a "Generic Dental Disc" in order to expose dental students, faculty and staff to the emerging developments in the use of videodisc technology and to encourage its use in dental education.

This project was realized through the co-operative joint venture initiated between the campus IRMD and the dental school.[6] The production of the disc would be used for several purposes. It would create discipline-specific courseware in the dental curriculum and show the potential for the use of this technology as an integral part of a curriculum. The "Generic Dental Disk" would also focus attention on the emerging field of "dental informatics" on the campus. It would gain attention and publicity for the development of the "Generic Dental Disc" and the use of this technology which would benefit IRMD, the Dental School, the campus and the university in general, and be used to encourage the development and use of other "generic" image bases in the health sciences by demonstrating how this disc could be interfaced with microtechnology and become a powerful and innovative instructional tool.

5. Publicized and demonstrated the use of technology assisted learning and the TAL center at every opportunity in an endeavor to gain as much national and international attention as possible for the individual authors and their departments, the school and campus administration, and the institution.

The ultimate goal was to encourage the use of technology assisted learning and the TAL center by demonstrating its utility in an academic discipline and simultaneously, "soft-sell" it as an educational tool to students, faculty, administrators and a broad range of health professionals. This gained recognition for a broad range of individuals, and generally, made the "decision-makers" more comfortable with the expanded use and acquisition of technology assisted learning and the use of a TAL center.

6. Created an administrative unit within the school to focus attention on the use of information technology in dentistry, in this case, the Division of Dental Informatics.

Through the creation of this Division, it provided an administrative unit within the school for coordinating all computer related activities. Ultimately, this resulted in obtaining grant support from the Pew Foundation, a part of which was devoted to developing a strategic plan for information resources and dental simulations. This effort continued to gain national and international recognition for the school, campus and university and provided funds for hiring personnel, purchasing hardware and software and providing release time for faculty to create computer-based educational programs and simulations.

7. Encouraged faculty to publish information regarding technology assisted learning applications in order to share this information with other dental schools and to gain recognition for faculty for promotion and tenure purposes.

Through the "Software Review" section in the **Journal of Dental Education**, faculty had a means of publishing information on software they developed or were currently using for technology assisted learning. Additionally, faculty were encouraged to publish the results of their research regarding the use of technology assisted learning and to present their findings at national or international meetings as an additional mechanism for gaining recognition for promotion and tenure purposes. This point is particularly important to the overall success of a technology assisted learning program in an academic institution.

8. Integrated computer literacy skills into the dental curriculum and the Schools' faculty development program.

Through the assistance of various administrators, computer literacy skills were integrated into the dental curriculum and the faculty professional development program. Examples in the curriculum included a basic introduction on how to use the microcomputer followed by how to use spreadsheets, develop financial projections, do wordprocessing, prepare a resume, prepare a business plan,[7] and conduct on-line literature searches.[8] In the area of professional development, courses and their presenters included:

- Introduction to Computers
- Word Processing and Graphics
- On-line Literature Searching
- Decision Support Systems in Oral Pathology and Diagnosis
- Patient Simulations in Oral Diagnosis and Oral Medicine
- AUTOCHART- An Automated Dental Charting System for Clinical Practice
- Informatics for the Dental Practitioner
- Strategies and Design Principles for Effective Dental Simulations
- Evaluation of Dental and Skeletal Development: A Multimedia Presentation

In order to encourage faculty participation in these faculty development courses, the courses were offered at different times and on different days to accommodate faculty schedules. Participation in faculty development courses was recorded through the Office of Professional Development to document individual efforts toward professional growth and development. The goal was to have 100% of the faculty receive computer literacy training within a single year. The results achieved from the efforts above have been very positive and technology assisted learning and the use of the TAL center continues as a high priority within the school. Again, the key elements for encouraging the use of technology assisted learning in the curriculum were:

1. Satisfying an individual need or a need within the curriculum

2. Providing an opportunity for gaining recognition for the individual, department, school or institution

3. Providing a means of obtaining credit for promotion, tenure or merit increment.

Evaluation of the Technology Assisted Learning Environment

The systematic and frequent evaluation of technology assisted learning will certainly be worth the time and effort, and the results should provide valuable guidance and direction for both operating the TAL center and improving the effectiveness of the technology assisted learning program. Several areas to consider in the evaluation include:

- the performance of the center director and/or staff
- environmental conditions such as study facilities, user comfort and whether users are satisfied with the services being provided by the center and/or center staff
- whether the needs and objectives of the user population, department, school or campus are being achieved
- whether student performance is being enhanced or improved through the use of technology assisted learning
- whether hardware and software are meeting performance standards
- whether there is adherence to or the need for modification or change of operational policies and procedures governing the use of the facilities, software, and hardware
- whether there is a change in the level of acceptance toward technology assisted learning as a means of instruction
- whether users are satisfied with the performance of the hardware and software
- whether the TAL center has had a positive influence on establishing hardware and software standards for the user population, the school, or campus
- whether technology assisted learning has encouraged or influenced the establishment of new program directions or the expansion of support services
- whether there has been a change in attitude or the level of usage toward technology assisted learning or the TAL center involving the academic, clinical, administrative, clerical or research activities and programs
- whether there has been a positive change in the level of administrative support and the allocation of funding toward technology assisted learning and/or the TAL center

Collecting information or data on the above items will provide a more accurate perspective regarding the operation and direction of the TAL center and insight as to whether the initial needs and objectives for the center are being met or achieved.

Summary

Although numerous topics addressing technology assisted learning and the planning, design, utilization, and evaluation of a TAL center have been presented, **it is important to emphasize that the role of technology assisted learning and the TAL center must be clearly defined before any other activities actually take place**. Additionally, planning will be facilitated if a committee is established to guide the planning process and to address the who, what, where, when, how, how much, how many, and how evaluated questions of technology assisted learning and the TAL center. While the approach to each project may differ among institutions, at a minimum, a plan should include:

- the needs to be addressed and/or objectives to be achieved through technology assisted learning and the establishment of a TAL center
- the identification of existing and required resources, including hardware, software, personnel, and cost estimates
- the proposed time schedule and list of activities to be coordinated
- line staff organizational charts and job descriptions for the TAL center staff
- the services to be provided along with the anticipated policies and procedures for the center
- the means of providing technical support, maintenance and service for the center
- construction and/or renovation plans
- the level of budgetary support required initially for "start up" and annually for "on going" support
- a plan for evaluating the many facets of the technology assisted learning program and the TAL center and a schedule indicating the frequency for conducting these evaluations along with an action plan for using this information once it is obtained.

This list is not intended to be exhaustive; however, many aspects must be considered and planned before initiating a technology assisted learning program and TAL center. Once this information is available and organized into a comprehensive plan, it should be presented to the appropriate decision makers for support and/or revisions. Following this review and approval the committee is on the way to creating a technology assisted learning environment. As the plan is implemented, constant day-to-day changes will occur. These changes may require a review, revision or delay in achieving the original plan and objectives. The important thing to remember is to work closely and carefully together when such situations arise in order to avoid making decisions hastily or that may compromise the overall goals for the TAL center. Additionally, planning for the use of information technology may be very frustrating because of the rapid changes that continually take place in the development of new technologies. While this may present the planners with a certain level of frustration, it cannot be avoided. In this day and age, there are few things that do not change by the moment.

References

1. Park, Jon K. and Craig, James F. Comprehensive Radiographic Interpretation Utilizing Interactive Videodisc Technology: Introduction to the Intraoral Survey. New Educational Programs paper, Journal of Dental Education, Volume 53, Number 1, pp. 47, January, 1990.

2. Siegel, Steven M., Davidson, William M., Christ, Diane and Craig, James F. Orthodontic Diagnosis and Treatment Planning Using Interactive Patient Simulations. New Educational Programs paper, Journal of Dental Education, Volume 53, Number 1, pp. 47, January, 1990.

3. Siegel, Michael S. and Craig, James F. Evaluation of Oral Diagnostic and Management Skills Using Interactive Patient Simulations. New Educational Programs paper, Journal of Dental Education, Volume 53, Number 1, pp. 49, January, 1990.

4. Craig, James F., Plotkin, Jeffrey I. and Ball, Marion J. Integrating the Use of Interactive Videodisc Technology into the Dental Curriculum, Proceedings of the Symposium on Computer Applications in Medical Care, Washington, DC, November, 1990.

5. Craig, James F. and Barry, Sue C. Interactive Videodisc Applications in Dental Education: A Case Study in Oral Histology. In MEDINFO 89, Proceedings of the Sixth Conference on Medical Informatics, Part I, edited by Barber, Barry; Cao, Dexian; Quin, Dulie; and Wagner, Gustav, published by Elsevier Science Publishing Company, Inc. New York, N.Y., October, p.722-724, 1989.

6. Craig, James F. The Potential For Computer and Optical Videodisc Technology in Dental Education (book chapter). In Computer Applications in Dentistry, Dental Clinics of North America (Zimmerman, John L., editor) Volume 30, Number 4, October, p. 713-720, 1986.

7. Craig, James F. and Manski, Richard Reducing the Costs of Computer-Literacy Through Resource Sharing. Journal of Dental Education, Vol. 53, No.8, p. 498-500, August, 1989.

8. Grace, Edward G., Craig, James F., and Cohen, Leonard A. Maryland Introduces Dental Informatics Into Curriculum. National Library of Medicine News, published by the Department of Health and Human Services, Public Health Service, National Institutes of Health, Vol. 45, No. 5-6, May-June, p. 3, 1990.

12
Instructional Design and Informatics

Jane Terpstra

You may have heard the old phrase, "Look before you leap." Whatever the source of this sage advice, it is the message of this chapter. It takes assessment, planning, understanding, creativity, and integration to bring technology and education together in an effective manner.

The investment in this process is well worth the effort. It can prevent two possible tragedies: 1) education without technology and 2) technology without education. Education without technology is a tragedy because students are not given all possible opportunities to learn. However, merely installing instructional technology does not ensure learning. The messages transmitted via technology must be instructionally effective or the technology soon becomes an expensive exhibit, extinct before its time.

The purpose of this chapter is to describe the process by which to look and ponder before leaping into instructional technology.

Needs Assessment

One way to determine changes needed in an educational program is with a needs assessment. Burton and Merrill define an educational needs assessment as the process of determining goals, measuring the discrepancy between what ought to be and what actually is, and establishing priorities for action.[1] Applying this definition to informatics, goals for instructional technology are determined and a comparison of the current system is made with the ideal delivery system needed to meet these goals. Resource limitations often require that changes take place over time, thus requiring prioritization of necessary changes.

There are several strategies for conducting a needs assessment: interviews, surveys, and program comparisons. In combination, these provide a complete overview of needs. However, implementing even one can yield valid information for decision making.

By interview and survey, needs assessments provide an internal perspective of needs. For interview needs assessments a questionnaire is designed, often by a committee, to standardize information gathering. See Table 12.1 for an example

Table 12.1.Needs Assessment: Internal Perspective

1) What are your standards for preparing successful dental professionals? (Examples: dental board exam scores, percent of students completing dental school, percentage of graduates successfully practicing in dental professions, and contributions of graduates to the field)
2) How have dental students at your institution performed in meeting these standards? What are the specific areas in which dental students at your institution need to improve?
3) What are the goals and objectives for the dental courses at your institution?
4) Using course examination scores or other measures of student achievement of course goals and objectives, list specific areas in which dental students at your institution need to improve.
5) Based on the above comparisons, list and prioritize changes needed in the dental program at your institution.

of internal needs assessment items. Interviews are conducted either by a consultant or a small committee. Dental education administrators, faculty, staff, students, and alumni should be included to gain a broad spectrum of information. Results are then compiled into a narrative report and distributed to participants and decision makers. Survey needs assessments are similar to the interview strategy, except standardized items and possible responses take less time to implement and results are easier to compile. The tradeoff for this time savings is less diversity of information gathered. Also, more time and effort must be spent in designing survey items to ensure a complete overview of needs as reported in the statistical summary of survey results.

Program comparison needs assessments offer an external perspective of needs. A dental education committee reviews other dental education programs' curricula, course syllabi, print and nonprint instructional media, and facilities. Refer to Table 12.2 for examples of external needs assessment items. Information may be obtained via phone interviews, print materials obtained from the dental schools, and on-site visits. Results are summarized into a narrative report for participants and decision makers.

Using the data from one or several of these needs assessment strategies, instructional technology needs can be listed and prioritized by dental education decision makers. The dynamic nature of educational institutions necessitates

Table 12.2.Needs Assessment: External Perspective

1) Comparing the dental curriculum at your institution with peer institutions, list differences in courses offered.
2) Comparing the course syllabi used at your institution with peer institutions, list differences in goals and objectives.
3) List differences in print and non-print instructional media used in the dental curriculum at your institution compared with peer institutions.
4) In what ways do your classroom, laboratory, and learning resource facilities differ from peer institutions?
5) Based on these comparisons with peer institutions, list and prioritize changes needed in the dental program at your institution.

ongoing, periodic reviews of specified needs and priority lists in order to progress toward the ideal dental instructional delivery system.

Matching Needs with Educational Technology

Once educational needs have been identified, a plan of action and timeline for meeting each identified need is developed. How do you match the needs with available technology to create a plan of action? Again, look and ponder before you leap. In this case, several analyses help lead to effective decisions. These include analyses of 1) the educational goals and objectives, 2) the advantages, disadvantages, and requirements of technologies, and 3) the human and financial resources available.

First, educational goals and objectives should be analyzed. Many goals and objectives may already be met with existing technologies in the dental education program, while others may require a change to be effectively met. Compare past student achievement with educational goals and objectives to determine those requiring an alternate approach.

Every technology has characteristic advantages and disadvantages as well as requirements when applied to education. Media selection models can be applied to assist in determining these characteristics.[2,3,4] See Table 12.3 for a summary of relevant aspects of these media selection models as applied to informatics.

As an example, a need may be identified for increased interaction between lecturers and learners to teach diagnosis skills effectively. In this case the technology being considered is a set of computer simulations presented during large group lectures via a projection system.

According to the media selection models, computer simulation is an appropriate media to teach integrated skills to learners. Is it the best choice? Should alternate technologies be considered? To answer these questions, consider the advantages, disadvantages, and requirements of the technology under consideration. See Table 12.4 for a review of the computer simulations criteria. A decision regarding use of this technology to meet the increased interaction need must be made by the dental school based on an analysis of these criteria.

Finally, human and financial resources should be considered. Leadership, acceptance, adaptability, and motivation are critical human factors among administrators, faculty, staff, and students. When considering a specific technology or several possible technologies, discuss the options with individuals who will be directly involved. Include their reactions, both positive and negative, in your analysis. Financial resources shape technology decisions and are integrally linked to the human factors of leadership, acceptance, adaptability, and motivation. A financial analysis should include an account of the finances currently available as well as an investigation of other possible funding sources.

Technology selection for dental education is the determination of a balance point between technology needs and results of the analyses. Reaching perfect balance is improbable. However, one plan of action or several alternate plans must

Table 12.3. Appropriate Technologies for Instructional Goals

Instructional Goal	Appropriate Technologies
Verbal Information Skills: * ** *** - identifying	- Computer-Based Instruction (CBI)
- naming - distinguishing	- Compact Disc-Read Only (CD-ROM)
- classifying	- Interactive Videodisc Instruction (IVI)
Information Processing Skills: ** ***	- Interactive TV (broadcast or closed circuit)
- problem solving - analysis	- Interactive Videodisc Instruction (IVI)
- synthesis	- CD-ROM
- evaluation	- Compter-Based Instruction (CBI)
	- Expert Systems
Motor or Perceptual Skills: * ** ***	- Interactive TV (broadcast or closed circuit)
	- Computer-Based Instruction (CBI)
	- Interactive Videodisc Instruction (IVI)
	- Simulator Practice

* Adapted from Selecting Media for Instruction by Robert Reiser and Robert Gagne, Copyright 1983 by Educational Technology Publications.
** Adapted from The Selection and Use of Instructional Media by A. J. Romiszowski, Copyright 1974 by John Wiley & Sons, Inc.
*** Adapted from Media Selection Handbook by Mary Robinson Sive, Copyright 1983 by Libraries Unlimited, Inc.
Used by permission of the publishers.

be determined and weighed by representatives from all levels of involvement before a final plan is chosen.

Evaluating and Selecting Versus Creating Instructional Software

Developing instructional technology programs often takes a tremendous commitment of human and financial resources. The effort is worth the investment if no suitable existing programs can be found for dental curriculum needs. However, before beginning development, seek and evaluate existing programs.

Begin by searching through catalogs listing educational technology programs as well as dental journals, newsletters, and conference exhibits. Next, contact vendors and authors to obtain demonstrations or complete programs to evaluate.

Table 12.4.Example of Analyzing a Technology for a Specified Need

Need:
Increased interaction between lecturers and learners to teach diagnosis skills

Technology Under Consideration:
Computer simulations presented during large group lectures via a projection system

Advantages:
- Highly interactive
- Stimulate discussion
- Present case complexity in a manner that can be reviewed visually
- Allow almost instantaneous views of aspects of the case for reinforcement
  and review during lecture

Disadvantages:
- Projection equipment is necessary for large group viewing

- Realistic visuals from photographs or video motion are limited without adding laser
  or compact discs
- Computer technology requires pre-lecture setup and equipment checks
- Lecturers must become familiar with the technology to use it effectively in lectures

Requirements:
- Computer, keyboard, and monitor
- Projection system for large group presentations
- Simulation software that meets curriculum objectives

Develop an evaluation form to standardize the evaluation process for all reviewers and programs. There are numerous evaluation models to assist in this process.[5,6,7] Categories included in most models are content and goals, design and technical quality, instructional management, learner guidance, support materials, cost analysis, and motivation. Suggested criteria for each category are listed in Table 12.5.

When an evaluation form is prepared, invite relevant faculty and learners to review the program and support materials. Encourage repeated viewings of the program for a complete and accurate assessment. Interactive TV programs can be videotaped to accomplish this.

Once the standardized evaluation forms are completed by all reviewers, compile the results into a summary report for decision makers and participants. Compare the results to arrive at a decision of whether the instructional technology programs can be recommended to meet the current needs of the dental curriculum.

Creating Instructional Technology Programs

For needs which cannot be addressed with existing programs, consider developing instructional technology programs. However, before starting such projects, carefully consider the answers to these questions: First, is there faculty interest in program development; is at least one appropriate faculty member willing to serve

Table 12.5. Criteria for Evaluating Instructional Technology

Contents and Goals:
- Goals and objectives match curriculum needs.
- The content matches curriculum needs.
- The content is accurate.
- The content is complete.
- Emphasis and sequence of content is appropriate for learners.

Design and Technical Quality:
- Displays are uncluttered.
- Text is readable.
- Display format is consistent throughout the program.
- Graphics and animation accurately illustrate content.
- Display banners provide orientation information.
- Color is effectively used for instructional emphasis.
- Color-coding is effectively used for orientation.
- Sound effects/music match program goals and objectives.

Instructional Management:
- Learner control is provided.
- Feedback is accurate and instructional.
- Achievement mastery is defined.
- Learner response data and records are accurately kept.
- Data and records are accessible to the instructor.
- Summary statistics are available.
- Printout of learner data and records is possible.
- The option to correct and update content is provided
- The option to correct and update content is provided to the instructor.

Learner Guidance:
- Instructions are accessible.
- Instructions are helpful.
- Options are clear.
- The method of responding is understandable.
- It is possible to exit and later resume interactivity with the program.

Support Materials:
- Start-up instructions are clear.
- Program goals and objectives are clearly stated.
- The appropriate audience for the program is specified.
- The content provided is accurate.
- Learner worksheets, test items, or other support materials contain accurate content.
- Information and references to promote further learning are provided.

Cost Analysis:
- Instructional effectiveness justifies the cost.
- Long-term use justifies the initial investment.
- Evaluative data from pilot testing and reviews provide support for purchase.
- *Written/verbal contracts include continued vendor/author support.*
- *Program updates will be available for minimal fees.*

Table 12.5. (continued)

Motivation:
- Learners attend to the program.
- The program is interactive rather than passive.
- Groups of learners discuss program content.
- Learners seek further content after completing the program.
- The program provides a challenge to all learners.
- Feedback prevents learner confusion and failure.

Adapted from Computer-Based Instruction: Methods and Development by Stephen Alessi and Stanley Trollip, Copyright 1985 by Allyn & Bacon; Evaluating Educational Software by Carol Doll, Copyright 1987 by American Library Association; and Instructional Software: Principles and Perspectives for Design and Use by Decker F. Walker and Robert D. Hess, Copyright 1984 by Wadsworth, Inc. Used by permission of the publishers.

as the content expert? Second, are there funding sources for a pilot project or complete program development? Third, are there rewards for development members, the dental school, and the institution? The development team may include content experts, an instructional designer, a computer graphic artist, a computer programmer, a photographer, TV production personnel, and a project evaluator. Possible rewards are the potential for improved instructional effectiveness, tenure credit, program publication and marketing, conference presentations, and recognition of instructional innovation and professional awards. Finally, is there administrative leadership and support for developing instructional technology programs? If the answers to these questions are "Yes", such projects will likely succeed. If the answers are "No", it is wise to postpone development until changes in resources and motivation can be obtained.

The process of developing instructional technology programs is complex. Many steps are completed in several months to several years, depending on the complexity and scope of the project. Several authors have developed descriptions of the sequential development process.[5,8,9,10] For an overview of essential steps in creating instructional technology programs, see Table 12.6.

Principles of Instructional Technology Design

Learning is an active process progressing from perception to transfer to memory and, finally, to mental manipulation of available information. Certain learning principles seem to apply to all effective instruction.[11] Perception principles are guidelines for the early stage in cognition in which information is gathered from the environment through the senses. Memory principles provide guidelines for effective mental acquisition and processing to transfer perceived information into memory. Concept formation and problem-solving principles apply to mental methods of consolidating, categorizing, analyzing, and synthesizing information stored in memory.

Table 12.6.Essential steps in Developing Instructional Technology Programs

Sequential Steps	Instructional Technologies			
	CBI	IVI	CD-ROM	ITV
Develop Program Goals and Objectives	X	X	X	X
Research and Script Program Content	X	X	X	X
Develop Performance Measures	X	X		X
Flowchart Program	X	X	X	
Write Script and Storyboard Visuals	X	X	X	X
Design Screen Display Format	X	X	X	
Review Script & Storyboard for Accuracy, Completeness, and Style	X	X	X	X
Prepare Final Script and Storyboard	X	X	X	X
Design Computer Program	X	X	X	
Produce Photographs Needed		X	X	X
Produce Graphic Art/Animation Needed	X	X	X	X
Produce and Edit Motion Video Segments		X		X
Review Produced Visuals	X	X	X	X
Revise Produced Visuals, if Needed	X	X	X	X
Arrange Interaction via Telecommunications				X
Produce and Transmit Live Program				X
Write Computer Program, Including Textual Content	X	X	X	
Review Computer Program	X	X	X	
Revise Computer Program	X	X	X	
Design Support Materials	X	X	X	X
Proof Support Materials for Accuracy	X	X	X	X
Print Support Materials	X	X	X	X
Obtain Check Disc		X		
Pilot Test Program	X	X	X	X
Revise Program as Needed	X	X	X	X
Obtain Master Disc		X	X	
Implement Program and Evaluate Effectiveness and Motivation	X	X	X	X
Periodically Review and Update Program	X	X	X	X

Adapted from Computer-Based Instruction: Methods and Development by Stephen Alessi and Stanley Trollip, Copyright 1985 by Allyn & Bacon; The Videodisc Book: A Guide and Directory by Rod Daynes and Beverly Butler, Copyright 1984 by John Wiley & Sons, Inc.; Author's Guide: Design, Development, Style, Packaging Review by Harold Peters and James Johnson, Copyright 1978 by CONDUIT; and Reaching New Students Through New Technologies by Leslie Purdy, Copyright 1983 by Kendall/Hunt Publishing Company. Used by permission of the publishers.

During instructional technology development, perception, memory, and concept formation/problem-solving principles need to be incorporated. See Table 12.7 for a listing of relevant principles.

Table 12.7.Learning Principles Relevant to Instructional Technology[a]

Perception Principles:
- Make the organization of the message apparent.
- Divide difficult concepts and skills into small parts or steps.
- Relate new concepts and skills to those already known.
- Balance novelty with familiarity, complexity with simplicity, and uncertainty with certainty.
- Ensure that text colors are visible to all learners, including those with color-blindness.
- Allow time for visual, aural, and verbal information to be encoded.
- Organize information to increase the amount that can be perceived at a time.
- Use highlighting techniques to accentuate critical information.

Memory Principles:
- Design content that is organized and meaningful to the learners to promote long-term memory retention.
- Group similar concepts and skills in the program.
- Design interaction to include repetition and questioning with feedback to promote short-term memory retention.
- Feedback should be interesting, useful, informative and rewarding to promote retention.
- Present content using more than one sensory mode for effective retention.
- Highlight critical cues for initial learning; reduce or eliminate these cues for advanced learners.
- During interaction, add cues as necessary until the learner can respond correctly.
- Repeating questions incorrectly answered or responses incorrectly made to facilitate retention.
- Practice spaced over time is more effective than massed practice.
- Provide step-by-step demonstration and practice for effective skills acquisition.
- Match the sensory modes of testing with the sensory modes used in instruction.

Concept Formation/Problem Solving:
- Include a wide variety of examples and non-examples of concepts and skills during instruction.
- Present concrete before abstract content.
- Present simplified visuals before realistic visuals.
- Allow the learner time to study content and skills presented and to study corrective feedback.
- Provide a means of recording, testing, and changing alternatives to teach problem solving skills.

[a]   Adapted from Instructional Message Design by Malcolm Fleming and W. Howard Levie, Copyright 1978 by Educational Technology Publications. Used by permission of the publisher.

Strategies for Integrating Instructional Technology into a Non-Technology Based Curriculum

Change is a difficult process. Although routine is comforting and secure, there can be no progress without change. Simply identifying instructional technology needs through needs assessment will not ensure that these needs will be met. This takes a commitment to change, acquisition of resources to institute change, and development of a technology adoption process.[12]

Commitment to change is expressed as a reciprocal relationship of leadership and trust among dental administrators, faculty, staff and students. When leaders emerge, their first role is to develop a funding strategy to support needed instructional technology. This entails an investigation of possible funding sources, a determination of the most relevant sources, the design of a plan to implement the technology, a written proposal requesting project funding, and lobbying efforts to gather support for the plan.

At times when fewer grants are available, creative funding strategies may be needed. Consortium projects involving several institutions, project support from technology equipment vendors, foundation support, alumni and dental student fundraising, and other strategies may offer alternative funding sources. Where there is a will, there is almost always a way.

Once funding is secured for any change from a pilot project to large-scale implementation, a technology adoption program can begin. Leaders in adoption are often administrators, faculty, and staff members who have become interested in the instructional technology. They develop methods to promote awareness of the new technology, provide information about the technology, train users, test the technology in the curriculum beginning on a small scale, and help others in the dental school to adopt, adapt, and integrate the instructional technology into the curriculum.

Evaluation of Instructional Technologies

Evaluation is an essential step during pilot projects and implementation of new technologies. Several models are applicable to the evaluation of instructional technologies.[13,14,15,16] Such models include three major areas of analysis: 1) faculty and student reactions to the new technologies, 2) an objective analysis of student achievement, and 3) cost-effectiveness.

Faculty and student reactions to new instructional approaches can be gathered through interviews or questionnaires. Questions about the learning environment, reactions to instruction via new technologies, and their perceived instructional value can be addressed in this evaluation phase. Such issues are critical to the evaluation process as they provide information regarding human issues such as acceptance, teaching and learning preference, and motivation.

Determine student achievement by evaluating post-test scores for items related to pilot program content. The critical issue to determine is whether students are able to demonstrate satisfactory performance following innovative instruction.

Cost-effectiveness can be measured in terms of human resource savings and time and financial resource savings. Measures of human resource savings are the amount of time faculty and students are freed by the use of new instructional technologies. Capital investment and operational costs calculated as a per student cost over time provides a measure of practicality for new technologies.

A balanced review of all of these evaluation measures provides valuable information to determine which new technologies, if any, to expand from the pilot phase to large-scale implementation in the dental curriculum.

Table 12.8. Storage Capacities of Emerging and Current Technologies

Technology	Storage Capacity

CD-I:
(specially designed compact disc
and joystick used in conjunction
with a standard television)
	- 7,000 still images
	- 72 minutes of partial
	  screen motion video
	- 2-19 hours of digital audio, depending on
	    the desired fidelity
	- 300,000 pages of text
	- a combination of the above

CD-ROM:
(compact disc player used in
conjunction with a computer)
	- 4,500 still images
	- 60 minutes of full
	  screen motion segments
	- 8 to 32 hours of digital audio,
	    depending upon the desired fidelity
	- 200,000 pages of text
	- a combination of the above

DVI: (DVI technology board and CD-ROM used in conjunction with a computer screen	- 40,000 still images - 72 minutes of full screen motion segments - up to 44 hours of digital audio - a combination of the above
IVI: (videodisc player used in conjunction with a computer)	- 54,000 still images per side - 30-60 minutes of full video per side - 1-4 hours of audio per side - a combination of the above

Emerging Technologies with Possible Dental Education Applications

Although the future of instructional technology is difficult to predict, there are several emerging technologies that warrent continued investigation: Compact Disc Interactive (CD-I), Digital Video Interactive (DVI), expert systems, and expanded two-way communications for interactive TV.

Compact Disc Interactive (CD-I) is a self-contained multimedia system under development. CD-I combines digital audio with still images, partial screen motion segments, text, and computer data stored on a standard-sized compact disc. Programs will run on a specially designed compact disc player and standard television; no computer is necessary. Learners will interact with the programs using a joystick device developed for the system. With current capabilities, a single CD-I disc can hold up to 650 megabytes of information. The capability to store digitized motion video as well as other information is made possible by a specially engineered digital compression and decompression system. For a comparison of current CD-I storage capacity with other technologies, see Table 12.6. As this technology develops, storage capacity may increase. Digital Video Interactive

(DVI) is an emerging technology that combines digitized audio, still images, full screen motion segments, and text to create interactive instruction. See Table 12.8 for a comparison of current DVI storage capacity with other technologies. Programs are stored on compact discs and delivered via computer with a CD-ROM player and with a specially engineered DVI Technology interface board and software installed. Increased compact disc storage capacity is possible with DVI's system for compressing and decompressing digital information. As this technology develops, an even larger storage capacity may be possible.

Expert systems, precursors of artificial intelligence, are large databases containing a knowledge base in a defined content area and heuristics or rules enabling simple to complex learner queries to gather information. Although expert systems cannot yet mimic complex mental skills nor converse with the learner, such systems can serve as valuable reference guides and decision-making aids. Expert systems are often stored on large capacity disk drives or compact discs and are delivered via computer with a hard drive or CD-ROM player added. Future development may enable even larger knowledge bases, simultaneous interaction between knowledge bases linked electronically, and communication methods approaching natural conversation between learners and expert systems.

Combining two-way visual and audio communication with televised instruction will offer even more interactivity for distant learners. There are two emerging technologies that make this possible: PC Networking and fiber optic delivery. PC Networking enables simultaneous voice and full color images to be sent via a single modem. By adding a Voice-Too modem, a standard MS-DOS computer becomes a two-way audio and visual communication site for telecourses, teleconferences, and expert consultations. Images such as photographs, slides, and radiographs can be simultaneously displayed on learners' computer monitors and discussed. Adding optional writing tablets, Telewriters, to the system allows handwritten notes and drawings to be transmitted between the origination site and distant sites. By adding a digitizing camera system at distant sites, learners can appear on computer monitors at the origination site and other sites to ask questions or discuss content. Also, learners can see and interact with each other using this system.

Fiber optic delivery of interactive TV enables digitized transmission of televised instruction along with images and computer data via fiber optic telephone lines to a standard television. A specially engineered converter is added to the incoming line to decode the digitized information for screen presentation. With a digitizing camera system, two-way visual and audio communications will be possible for telecourses, teleconferences, and expert consultations. Although fiber optic delivery has not received approval from the Federal Communications Commission at this time, its development warrents continued investigation.

Summary

This chapter provided a look to preceed your leap into instructional technology. Needs assessment shapes decisions for change in the dental curriculum. Matching these educational needs and objectives with current and emerging technologies requires an analysis of their advantages, disadvantages, and requirements compared with possible resources. When making an instructional technology decision, consider whether programs delivered via the technology under consideration can be selected or developed to meet the educational objectives. Follow proven sequential steps and design principles to develop effective instructional technology programs. Plan the integration of instructional technology into the dental education curriculum and its adoption by individuals involved at all levels. Finally, begin the process over again as different curriculum needs and instructional technologies emerge.

References

1. Briggs, L. (Ed.). Instructional Design: Principles and Applications. Englewood Cliffs, NJ: Educational Technology Publications, Inc., 1977.
2. Reiser, R. and Gagne, R. Selecting Media for Instruction. Englewood Cliffs, NJ: Educational Technology Publications, 1983.
3. Romiszowski, A.J. The Selection and Use of Instructional Media. New York, NY: John Wiley & Sons, Inc., 1974.
4. Sive, M.R. Media Selection Handbook. Littleton, CO: Libraries Unlimited, Inc., 1983.
5. Alessi, S. and Trollip, S. Computer-Based Instruction: Methods and Development. Englewood Cliff, NJ: Prentice-Hall, Inc., 1985.
6. Walker, D. and Hess, R. (Eds.) Instructional Software: Principles and Perspectives for Design and Use. Belmont, CA: Wadsworth Publishing Company, 1984.
7. Daynes, R. and Butler, B. The Videodisc Book: A Guide and Directory. New York, NY: John Wiley & Sons, Inc., 1984.
8. Peters, H. and Johnson, J. Author's Guide: Design, Development, Style, Packaging Review. Iowa City, IA: CONDUIT, 1978.
9. Purdy, L. (Ed.). Reaching New Students Through New Technologies. Dubuque, IA: Kendall/Hunt Publishing Company, 1983.
10. Fleming, M. and Levie, H. Instructional Message Design. Englewood Cliffs, NJ: Educational Technology Publications, 1978.
11. Havelock, R. G. The Change Agent's Guide to Innovation in Education. Englewood Cliffs, NJ: Educational Technology Publications, 1973.
12. Gagne, R. M. and Briggs, L. J. Principles of Instructional Design. New York, NY: Holt, Rinehart, and Winston, 1974.
13. Romiszowski, A.J. Designing Instructional Systems. New York, NY: Nichols Publishing Company, 1981.
14. Scriven, M. Evaluation in Education: Current Applications. Berkeley, CA: McCutchan Publishing Company, 1974.
15. Stufflebeam, D.L. The Relevance of the CIPP Evaluation Model for Educational Accountablility. Journal of Educational Research and Development, 5 (1), 1971.

Select Bibliography

American Interactive Media: Compact Disc Interactive. Los Angeles, CA: Philips/PolyGram Corporation, 1988.

Burgess, J. Wire War: Putting America on Line. The Washington Post, October 22, 1989.

DVI Technology: The Multimedia Solution. Santa Clara, CA: Intel Corporation, 1990.

DVI Technology. Santa Clara, CA: Intel Corporation, 1990.

The Future of Fiber. Washington, DC: Opt In America.

Gayeski, D. and Williams, D. Interactive Media. Englewood Cliffs, NJ: Prentice-Hall, Inc., 1985.

Heines, J. M. Screen Design Strategies for Computer-Assisted Instruction. Bedford, MA: Digital Press, 1984.

Hilton, J. and Jacobi, P. Straight Talk About Videoconferencing. New York, NY: Prentice Hall Press, 1986.

Introducing PC Networking. New York, NY: Optel Communications, Inc.

Luskin, B. J. CD-I: A Call for Professional Design and an Ubiquitous Format. The Journal, 18(1), 58-59.

13
Tools for Technology Assisted Learning: Teaching Problem-Solving Skills with Patient Simulations

Lynn A. Johnson

Introduction

This chapter discusses the need to teach problem-solving skills to dental students and describes the development, formative evaluation, implementation, and planned summative evaluation of the Dental Diagnosis and Treatment (DDx&Tx) System, a series of patient simulations designed to teach these problem-solving skills. A separate discussion summarizes the role of evaluation in guiding the development process of all instructional technology products, with examples provided from our experiences with the Dental Diagnosis and Treatment (DDx&Tx) System.

Teaching Problem-Solving Skills

A survey of the literature reveals that dental educators generally recognize the need to develop problem-solving skills as preparation for the practice of dentistry. Early research suggested that persons who choose a career in dentistry may tend to be somewhat inflexible and more interested in the application of knowledge than in theory.[1] More recent work indicates that dental education in its present form may reinforce those inclinations.[2] An analysis of test instruments at one dental education institution found all test instruments used in one academic year were classified according to Blooms' Taxonomy at levels one and two—Knowledge and Comprehension; none were classified at any of the other four levels—Application, Analysis, Synthesis, or Evaluation.[3]

Research employing the Myers-Briggs Type Indicator indicates that dental students are more likely to fall toward the "feeling/sensing" poles rather than the "intuitive/thinking" direction characteristic of the decision maker.[4,5,6] These findings suggest a need for teaching strategies that will strengthen problem-solving skills.

Among a wide range of methodologies that have been described for teaching problem-solving skills to health care providers,[7,8,9,10,11] many researchers consider patient simulations one of the most effective.[12,13,14,15]

Documented use of medical simulations demonstrates that they can be a powerful tool for the instruction of health care skills.[16,17] Videodisc and other computer-based instructional technologies have received attention from dental educators at the annual meeting of the American Association of Dental Schools and other health care meetings.

In the clinical teaching setting, it is often difficult to match the skill level of the student with the unique problems of special patients such as the geriatric or disabled patient. Patient simulations offer a supplementary learning experience which can be sequenced and tailored to the particular educational needs of the individual student. Each student may progress from simple to complex patient encounters at his or her own rate. Patient simulations permit students to master required skills in less time and with fewer "live" patient encounters.[18,19] Research has shown that interactive videodisc patient simulations shorten the time required for learning and that the skills learned are retained longer.[20]

Research has also demonstrated that to acquire the problem-solving skills necessary to diagnose and treat a complex patient, students and practitioners require properly sequenced experiences with numerous and varied patients.[14,16,21] Interactive videodisc simulations effectively implement a learning system that presents a properly sequenced series of experiences tailored to the skill level of each student user.

The Dental Diagnosis and Treatment System

In response to the need to teach problem-solving skills, the University of Iowa College of Dentistry developed the Dental Diagnosis and Treatment (DDx&Tx) System. The DDx&Tx System currently consists of a series of interactive videodisc patient simulations, and a management system. An authoring tool is planned for the future. This section describes the components of the DDx&Tx System (see Figure 13.1), the history behind the project, and how it is being integrated into the curriculum.

DDx&Tx System Components

DDx&Tx patient simulations use a laser reflective videodisc controlled by a computer. As illustrated in Figure 13.2, the student views two television screens and communicates with the simulation via a microcomputer keyboard. One screen displays videodisc images while the other screen displays computer text. The microcomputer allows the student to gather textual information on the patient's disease, to give a differential diagnosis, and to prescribe and sequence treatment. The microcomputer is also used to provide feedback about the problem-solving process. The videodisc presents high-resolution visuals of the clinical, radiographic, and histologic features of the patient's disease.

The management system uses a local area network to connect all the students to a central microcomputer. The patient simulations, the management system, and student demographic and performance information reside on this central

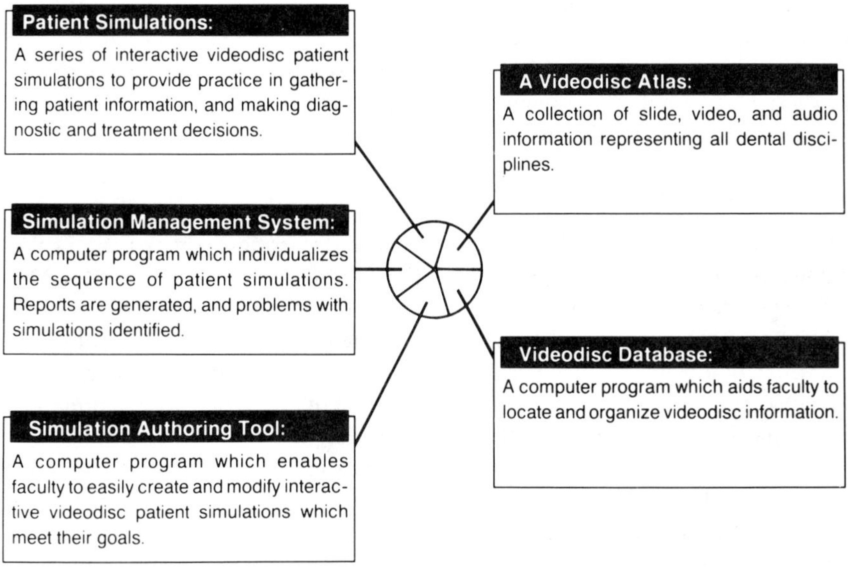

Patient Simulations:

A series of interactive videodisc patient simulations to provide practice in gathering patient information, and making diagnostic and treatment decisions.

A Videodisc Atlas:

A collection of slide, video, and audio information representing all dental disciplines.

Simulation Management System:

A computer program which individualizes the sequence of patient simulations. Reports are generated, and problems with simulations identified.

Videodisc Database:

A computer program which aids faculty to locate and organize videodisc information.

Simulation Authoring Tool:

A computer program which enables faculty to easily create and modify interactive videodisc patient simulations which meet their goals.

Figure 13.1. The DDx&Tx System components.

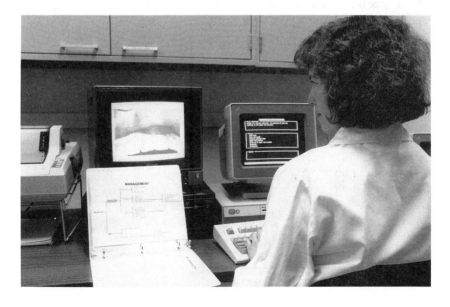

Figure 13.2. A student using the DDx&Tx System.

microcomputer. The management system software assigns patient simulations, tracks student progress, and generates reports.

The authoring tool will enable faculty to write a patient simulation easily. Authors will be able to concentrate on presenting a patient, not on creating an operationally correct patient simulation.

Patient Simulations

Three software components combine to form one patient simulation: 1) the simulation driver program, 2) five model files, 3) and individual patient files. The driver program presents information from the model and patient files, permits movement within the program, scores the student's work, and controls the sequence of computer and videodisc material. The model files contain the information that is common to all patients, while each patient file contains the information that is specific to the individual patient simulation.

Each individual simulation contains five major sections and a varying number of minor sections (see Figure 13.3). The patient profile section presents the patient's chief complaint and the videodisc images. The investigation section enables the student to gather information about the patient's chief complaint, medical, dental and social history, and physical findings. The student selects a question and receives the patient's response. The student may ask all questions or choose only those questions that appear appropriate. Menus permit questions common to most patients to be grouped into categories; this encourages students to learn a systematic approach to information gathering.[22] A student can ask additional questions by selecting from a series of fill-in-the-blank questions. Because natural language interviews are not necessarily superior to other methods,[23] the prepared list of questions can be used for the more practical purposes of speed and accuracy.

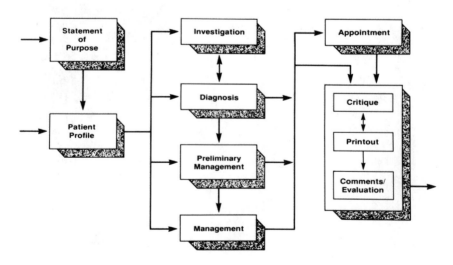

Figure 13.3. DDx&Tx Patient Simulation Map.

The diagnosis section uses a decision tree, similar to one in Figure 13.4, to encourage students to make a series of deductive decisions, rather than a single diagnostic judgement. At the end of Diagnosis, the student has prepared a list specifying the patient's problems.

The student may advance to the management section only after entering a problem. This emphasizes that a clinical diagnosis precedes patient management. Management also uses a decision tree to encourage systematic problem-solving. For beginning dental students, patient management consists of a series of treatment decisions for each problem in the diagnosis list. This results in a treatment plan which does not account for social, psychological, or financial factors. Advanced students must account for this additional patient information.

The critique section contain the student's scores, the correct diagnosis and management, follow-up information and visuals, and detailed feedback for each simulation section. The critique for Investigation describes the information that is vital to the correct diagnosis and management of the disease. The critique of Diagnosis and Management reports the optimal decision path, accompanied by an expert's rational for each decision. The Follow-up describes the treatment outcomes and presents clinical and microscopic visuals of the disease. A printout reinforces the critique and repeats the student's diagnosis and management decisions. This lets the student immediately compare his or her problem-solving with that of an expert.

Management System

The patient simulations solved one instructional problem and created three other problems. First, it became evident that the sequence in which students complete simulations is critical. Each student needs to be presented with an individualized sequence of simulations that ensures mastery of clinical problem-solving skills. Random assignment of patient simulations does not guarantee this mastery. Second, recording completed simulations and student performance on each simulation is time-consuming. Third, to maintain our high standard of quality, we continually evaluate and revise simulations. Our recordkeeping and evaluation/revision process needed to be streamlined.

Our solution to the problems of mastery, record keeping, and evaluation/revision consists of a management system and database operating on a local area network. The management system sequences the patient simulation for each student. The database holds student demographic and performance information. The local area network links all the student workstations to a central microcomputer. This single microcomputer contains all of the patient simulations, the management system, and the database with its associated information.

The management system organizes the patient simulations into a series of patient simulation models. Each model differs in content, difficulty, and instructional techniques. Using a model and its associated patient simulations, the management system assigns a simulation to a student. If the student passes the simulation, it counts toward fulfilling a mastery requirement for the model. If the

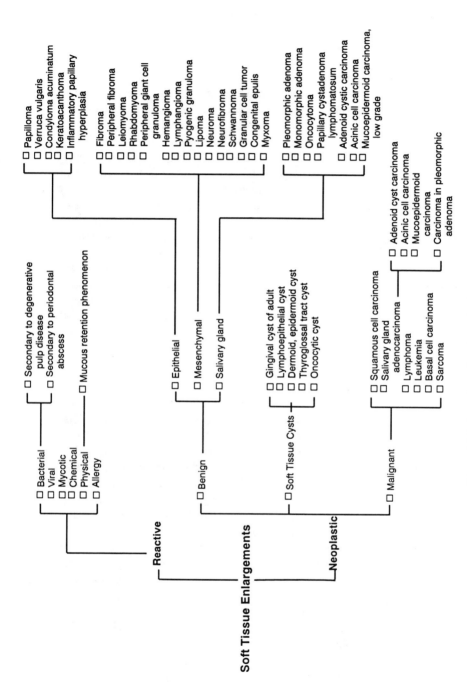

Figure 13.4. A portion of an Oral Diagnosis decision tree.

student fails this and similar simulations, he or she receives an easier simulation or an equivalent simulation with instructional prompts.

The primary objective of the management system is to ensure that each student masters diagnosis and treatment planning. A student must complete the mastery requirement of each model before advancing. The management system helps to guarantee mastery by individualizing the sequence of simulations for each student. A student who quickly masters diagnosis and treatment planning completes fewer simulations than other students.

The database associated with the management system stores student demographic and performance information. The database uses this information to generate reports about an individual student, or about a group of students.

At the end of each simulation, students may comment on the simulation's strengths and weaknesses. At regular intervals, students complete an evaluation form summarizing a patient simulation. The management system stores these comments and evaluations. When requested, an evaluation report about a specific simulation or model is printed. These evaluation reports act as a quality control mechanism for the patient simulations and the simulation models.

Authoring Tool

In order to write hundreds of high quality patient simulations with ease, faculty need to concentrate on a simulation's content; authors should not be distracted by the mechanics of writing operationally correct patient simulations.

Our solution to the authoring problem is an authoring tool. The authoring tool will prompt the author for the information required by a simulation. This includes the patient's record, clinical photos and radiographs, the patient's response to questions, the correct diagnosis and treatment plan, and feedback. The author will need only to "fill-in-the-box" in order to complete a patient simulation that operates correctly.

The authoring tool will include prompts that help maintain instructional consistency among the many simulations. These prompts will also help ensure a high level of quality for all the patient simulations. Revision to the simulations will be made using the same authoring tool.

Imagebase: Videodisc and Database

A large number of patient simulations require a large quantity of visual and audio material that is easily and quickly accessed. A single-sided videodisc can hold 54,000 still images, 30 minutes of motion, or some combination of the two. It can also hold up to one hour of audio. The first edition of the videodisc that accompanies the DDx&Tx System, the Videodisc Atlas, contains 33,000 slides, eleven minutes of video, and two minutes of audio information representing all oral health care disciplines. Endodontics, Operative Dentistry, Oral Diagnosis, Oral Medicine, Oral Pathology, Oral and Maxillofacial Surgery, Orthodontics, Pediatric Dentistry, Periodontics, Prosthodontics, and Preventive Dentistry are all represented by still images. The related disciplines of Dental History, Radiology, Histopathology, and Dermatology also have slide collections on this videodisc. Prosthodontics, Operative Dentistry, and Dental Hygiene provided video information from an intraoral camera. Temporomandibular joint sounds represent the dental audio content; the remainder of the audio on the videodisc is original music.

For the videodisc to be useful, faculty need to easily find the audio and video information they require for a patient simulation. To assist faculty in this search, a computer database has been constructed describing all of the Atlas information. Using American Dental Association (ADA) treatment codes and International Classification of Diseases (ICD) diagnostic codes, faculty can easily find the required audiovisual information for a patient simulation.

The History and Development Process

The DDx&Tx System has been developed over five years through a cooperative arrangement between three University of Iowa departments—the College of Dentistry, the University Video Center, and the Weeg Computing Center. The project started in 1985 when the School of Art and Art History at the University of Iowa placed 36,000 images on a videodisc that could hold 54,000. The College of Dentistry placed 900 slides on that videodisc, 600 of which came from the Department of Oral Pathology/Radiology and Medicine. Once the videodisc was completed, work on the Oral Disease Simulations for Diagnosis and Management (ODSDM) began. (This boost into videodisc technology by the School of Art and Art History may be the only time art has launched a major innovation in dental education.)

The DDx&Tx System has developed in six phases:

Phase 1 - Prototype Patient Simulations

Phase 2 - Formative Evaluation and Implementation of Prototype

Phase 3 - Management System and Videodisc Atlas Development

Phase 4 - DDx&Tx Patient Simulation Development

Phase 5 - Formative Evaluation of the DDx&Tx System - Patient Simulations and Management System

Phase 6 - Summative Evaluation of the DDx&Tx System - Patient Simulations and Management System

Phase 1 - Prototype Patient Simulations: When the School of Art and Art History videodisc was completed, Weeg Computing Center agreed to support the design and programming of the prototype ODSDM patient simulation project. An instructional designer and programmer worked with two faculty members to design a patient simulation program that would teach the clinical problem-solving skills of diagnosis and treatment of oral diseases. The work started in Fall, 1985 and finished approximately one year later.

Phase 2 - Formative Evaluation and Implementation of Prototype: An extensive formative evaluation of the ODSDM project was conducted in the Fall, 1986 to the Winter, 1987.[24] Twenty-one third year oral diagnosis students completed six to eight simulations for a total of 188 completed patient simulations. Observations, questionnaires, and interviews were used to gather data. The goals of the formative evaluation were to find design flaws in the conceptual design of the ODSDM patient simulation software and in each individual patient simulation. The results of this formative evaluation aided the design of the DDx&Tx patient simulations and indicated revisions required by the individual patient simulations. Subsequently, the simulations were then integrated into the third year oral diagnosis curriculum and the second year oral pathology curriculum. Based on the strong positive results, it was decided to expand the scope of the ODSDM project. This new project is known as the DDx&Tx System.

Phase 3 - Management System and Videodisc Atlas Development: The management system was designed in the Winter and Spring of 1987 and programmed in the following Fall. The first version was implemented with the ODSDM patient simulations in the Winter of 1988. Two computer programmers, an instructional designer, and two dental faculty were involved its design.

The DDx&Tx Videodisc Atlas was designed and produced in approximately one year (January, 1987 through February, 1988). Available faculty and graduate student slide collections along with new simulation-specific material were transferred to one-inch videotape. Motion and audio demonstrating disease symptoms were also obtained when ever possible. Multiple photographers, faculty from all departments, video production personnel, and an instructional designer made up the large team of persons required to produce this videodisc.

A videodisc combined with a computer database catalog is an imagebase. The database allows faculty to find the required images easily. A database programmer, multiple faculty members, an instructional designer, and many data entry clerks are required to complete the database portion of the imagebase.

Phase 4 - DDx&Tx Patient Simulation Development: Based on the results of the ODSDM formative evaluation, the DDx&Tx patient simulations were designed and programmed. New features of the simulations include computer graphics that present dental charts, and expanded video functions that provide intra-oral clinical visuals and motion as answers to student inquiries. In addition a treatment planning component was added. Students can categorize, select, and sequence the treatments required of prosthodontic patients. Additional functions include automated questionnaires and comments for ongoing evaluation. The design of the new functions involved six faculty, an instructional designer, and two programmers. It started in Spring, 1987 and was completed in Fall, 1990.

Phase 5 - Formative Evaluation of the DDx&Tx System: A formative evaluation of the DDx&Tx System is currently underway. It examines the DDx&Tx patient simulations and the DDx&Tx management system. The patient simulation portion of the formative evaluation examines the instructional design of the patient simulations and six individual patient simulations. The management system formative evaluation examines sequencing, implementation, recordkeeping, and ongoing evaluation issues associated with patient simulations.

Phase 6 - Summative Evaluation of the DDx&Tx System: A summative evaluation to measure the effectiveness of the DDx&Tx System is planned for the

Fall, 1991. It will consist of five parts. A detailed description of each part is contained in the Summative Evaluation portion of this chapter.

Authoring Patient Simulations

Authoring and writing patient simulations are not equivalent terms. Authoring entails the design, writing, and pilot-testing of a series of patient simulations; writing is the creation of a single simulation.

Authoring a series of patient simulations is a multi-step process with three major parts: 1) design the model for a series of patient simulations, 2) write the individual patient simulations, and 3) pilot-test the patient simulations with students.

Designing the simulation model is the most critical, intellectually stimulating, and time consuming task of the authoring process. The author needs to define the audience and goals. Who will use this series of patient simulations? Will the simulations emphasize diagnosis, treatment, or both? The decisions concerning audience and goals will impact the rest of the authoring process. The audience and goals determine which components to include in the simulation. Starting with decision trees, each component will be built, one at a time. The last component to be built is the investigation section. Once an author has built all of the components, the simulation model should be submitted to an expert review. Colleagues' input will improve the simulation model. Model components should be reviewed for accuracy and appropriateness of depth and breadth, always keeping in mind the intended audience and goals.

When the simulation model has been reviewed and revised, the author is ready to write the individual patient simulations. The first step is a brief description, or scenario, of each simulated patient. These scenarios include clinical photos, radiographs, study models, histopathology slides, TMJ sounds, and other audio or visual materials required to accurately portray the patient. These scenarios and patient history information are used to create the actual simulations. Each component requires specific information. This may mean responses to critical questions, a correct diagnosis pathway, or a computer graphic to portray the patient's chart. Once all the simulation material has been specified, the Critique is written. The Critique summarizes the vital information for Investigation and includes a rationale for each decision in Diagnosis and Management. The rationales explain why certain diagnoses were excluded and the consequence of incorrect decisions. Once the Critique is completed, someone familiar with the simulation software will make sure the simulation executes properly. The simulation is now ready to be pilot-tested with students.

Authoring is not completed when the simulation is operating. Authors need to gather information on the correctness and effectiveness of the simulation and use this information to refine the simulation. Pilot-testing involves student review. Authors should revise the simulation based on what is learned from the student pilot-test sessions. If the revisions are extreme, the author should conduct another pilot-test. If the revisions are minor, no additional pilot-testing is necessary.

The Integration of Patient Simulations into the Curriculum

The DDx&Tx patient simulations are presently being used in four courses. The third year oral diagnosis course has used patient simulations since Fall, 1986; the second year Oral Pathology and dental hygiene Oral Pathology courses have used patient simulations since Spring, 1987; and the third year dental hygiene Periodontics course has used patient simulations since Spring, 1990. Each of these courses uses simulations that focus on, but are not limited to, clinical diagnosis. Simulations that will also focus on clinical diagnosis are for the third year Periodontics, Pediatric Dentistry, Endodontics, Prosthodontics, fourth year Family Dentistry courses and the fourth year dental hygiene Pediatric Dentistry course. Discussions are underway to vertically integrate comprehensive care patient simulations into numerous courses spread over three years of the dental curriculum. These simulations would focus on the total care, or gestalt, of the simulated patient. They would include treatment planning and take into account psychosocial, financial, and physical characteristics which may limit a patient's oral health care.

Students would be introduced to the concepts involved in the comprehensive care of patients and plan the treatment for a few basic patients during their second year. In the third year,, students would complete a series of discipline-specific patient simulations with increasingly difficult comprehensive care simulations interspersed. During the fourth year students would be expected to care for twenty-five simulated comprehensive care patients. It is anticipated that it will take three to four years to author these simulations and complete the curriculum integration.

Computers assist with the instruction of treatment planning on two levels. The DDx&Tx System provides students with practice and feedback about their diagnosis and treatment problem-solving skills. The College's Dental Information System (DENIS) allows students to enter their treatment plans for clinic patients directly into the collegiate computerized patient management system. Both systems have parallel treatment planning components. During the development of the shared components, the DDx&Tx and DENIS staffs consulted with each other. This cooperative development provides for a merging of instruction and clinic practice. Students practice, via patient simulations, skills taught in the classroom; students apply, via real patients, the skills practiced with simulations.

Where We Are: Where We Are Going

Approximately 30 Oral Diagnosis patient simulations for third year dental students were written for the ODSDM project. Ten more were written for the DDx&Tx System for a total of 40 simulations. Modifications were made to these simulations so that they meet the needs of second year dental students in the Oral Pathology course, and third year dental hygiene students in their Oral Pathology course. Twelve simulations for third year dental hygiene Periodontology have also been authored. Additional patient simulations are currently being written in Prosthodontics, Periodontics, Endodontics, Oral Diagnosis, Oral Pathology, Pediatric Dentistry, and comprehensive care.

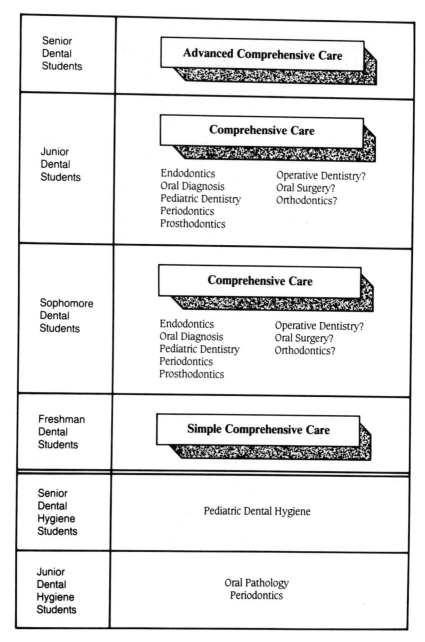

Figure 13.5. A plan for integrating patient simulations into the oral health care curriculum.

Videodisc	Database	
Radiographs:	Image Information:	Contributor:
Panorex	Tray Number *	Name
Bitewings	Slot Number *	Department
Periapicals	Frame Number	Institution
	Image Type	
Clinical Photographs:	Slide Identifier	Patient:
Full Face	General Description	Patient Identifier **
Frontal		Birthdate
Occlusal Maxillary	Diagnosis:	Sex
Occlusal Mandibular	ICD-9 Code	
Relevant pathology or	Diagnosis Comments	Histology:
areas of interest		Diagnosis
	Treatment:	Magnification
Models (optional):	ADA Code	Stain
Pre-operative mounted models	Treatment Comments	
		Radiology:
Motion:	Anatomy:	Radiograph Type
Working right and left	Location	Interpretation
Centric Relation Centric Occlusion	Tooth Number	
Balancing left and right		
Protrusive		
Opening Closing		
Closest speaking space		
Audio:	* Used only for production	
TMJ sounds	** Not available outside the University of Iowa	

Figure 13.6. Description of the videodisc and database contents.

Figure 13.5 contains the design for a vertical integration of comprehensive care patient simulations into the dental curriculum. It also indicates where in the dental and dental hygiene curricula we envision implementing discipline-specific patient simulations.

During 1991, a second edition of the Videodisc Atlas is planned. Poor quality and outdated images from the first edition will be removed. New images representing simple comprehensive care and discipline-specific patients will match a standardized imagebase definition. (See Figure 13.6 for a description of this imagebase.) With the second edition of the Videodisc Atlas, the database will be build as material is submitted.

Related Research

The second edition of the Videodisc Atlas may be the last videodisc imagebase we produce. We are currently exploring the development of a digital imagebase. With support from Apple, Inc., we are developing a prototype radiologic imagebase, using digitized and enhanced radiographs. This prototype digital imagebase is scheduled for completion in Spring, 1991.

A series of research projects involving patient simulations are currently underway. A summative evaluation of the dental hygiene periodontal simulations is scheduled to be completed in January, 1991. Preliminary summative evaluations are being conducted for the third year Oral Diagnosis, and second year Oral

Pathology patient simulations. Both are scheduled to be completed in May, 1991. Based on the results of these preliminary studies, a complete summative evaluation is scheduled for the 1991-1992 school. It is described in more detail later in this chapter.

The Evaluation of Computer-Based Instructional Materials

The Need for Instructional Evaluation

A systematic approach to program development involves the identification of educational needs, specification of program goals, and design of instructional strategies that create effective learning conditions for the targeted students. Evaluation plays changing roles through the phases of program development, but its consistent goal is to maximize the program's potential for success. A systematic approach to curriculum was introduced by Ralph Tyler in Basic Principles of Curriculum and Instruction.[25] Tyler was the first to advocate that all instructional projects should have clearly defined goals, provide learning experiences directed at achieving these goals, and evaluate the strengths and weaknesses of the project in accomplishing these goals. Tyler proposed a cyclical approach to instructional product development that encouraged developers to try out the products, identify weaknesses, and suggest improvements, followed by redevelopment and reappraisal. "In this [cyclical] way we may hope to have an increasingly more effective educational program rather than depending so much upon hit and miss judgement as a basis for curriculum development." (p. 123)

This section describes the three major types of evaluation used in the development of instructional technology products. Examples from the DDx&Tx System illustrate the nature of decisions at each phase and the roles that evaluation plays in facilitating problem-solving.

Needs Assessment: The Initial Evaluation

Introduction—What's the Problem?

A needs assessment is the initial phase of all instructional projects. Its goals are to establish the need for the project and the product's feasibility. The major questions involve the product's audience, content, medium, and setting.

Audience

The DDx&Tx team first focused on the following questions regarding the audience:

- Who needs patient simulations? Dental students? Dental hygiene students? First year? Second Year?...
- Are there sufficient numbers of dental and dental hygiene students to justify the cost of development and implementation?

- Are the needs of dental and dental hygiene students too diverse to be met by a single simulation package?

The goal of the DDx&Tx System is to teach problem-solving to dental and dental hygiene students. For the prototype ODSDM phase, the audience was limited strictly to second year and third year dental students in Oral Diagnosis and Oral Pathology courses. At the completion of a formative evaluation of the ODSDM project, the audience for the second phase, the DDx&Tx System, was expanded to include dental and dental hygiene students of all skill levels. The variability of student expertise required flexible software that would accommodate the varied needs of each group.

Content

At each phase of the simulation project, the design team searched for answers to these content questions:

- What should be the breadth of the content?
- What content justifies the investment, given the resources?
- Do the simulations duplicate content that is already being sufficiently taught in the dental and dental hygiene curriculums?

In the prototype stage the content was limited strictly to Oral Diagnosis and Oral Pathology. While it addressed treatment issues, it focused on the formation of a differential diagnosis. This decision was based on the interest of the faculty and the design team. For the second phase, content experts from all dental disciplines were consulted. The content capabilities of the Diagnosis section were slightly expanded, and the simple ODSDM treatment approach was expanded to include a multiple-phased treatment planning approach.

Medium

While the design team considered audience and content issues, it concurrently examined the variety of media available to present the patient simulations. A few of the questions addressed include:

- What media format stores large amounts of still visuals?
- What media format allows students to quickly receive extensive and immediate feedback regarding their decisions?
- What media format stores large amounts of demographic and performance data?
- What media format allows faculty to author patient simulations in a reasonable amount of time?

A literature review revealed two findings that would help ensure the learning of problem-solving skills. These include student practice in diagnosing and treating numerous and varied patients. Interactive videodisc was the medium selected to present the large number of varied patients. The videodisc can store up to 54,000 still images on a single side; the computer controls the presentation of visuals, text, and graphic information. The computer also permits immediate feedback to students regarding their performance and stores extensive amounts of data.

Summary

The first phase in developing any instructional product, whether technology-based or not, is a needs assessment. The following questions must be answered: What are the goals of the product? Who is the audience? What media should be used? How will the product be used? Is the product even feasible? What people are required to complete the project? What personnel are required to implement the product? Also, many decision makers require designers to project costs for development, evaluation, and implementation. If the product is a technology project, the needs assessment must determine what hardware will be required to develop and deliver the product.

The result of the needs assessment is a predesign document that answers all of the above questions and includes an initial content outline. This document will provide administrators with the information required to decide whether to pursue the project to completion.

Formative Evaluation: The Process Evaluation

Introduction—Why Bother?

Formative evaluation helps the instructional software designer during the early developmental stages, to increase the likelihood that the final product will achieve its stated goals. Information is systematically collected for the purpose of providing design and content information to decision-makers to improve the final product. The term "formative" implies that information is collected during the formation of the instructional product so that revisions might be made at a lower cost.

The formative evaluation is a cyclic process of review, revise, and refine.[26] Two cycles occur during a formative evaluation: the Expert Review and the Pilot-Test. Figure 13.7 illustrates these two cycles. The expert review provides suggestions from content and instructional technology specialists, while the Pilot-Test provides feedback from the client—the student.

Evaluation Questions

The formative evaluation of the ODSDM product addressed two levels of questions. The first level included macro-level issues addressing the conceptual design of the patient simulations; the second level addressed each individual patient simulation:

Macro - Design questions:

- What improvements are required to the design of the simulation model?
- Is the interface easy-to-use? Are students able to concentrate on the simulation instead of operating the computer?

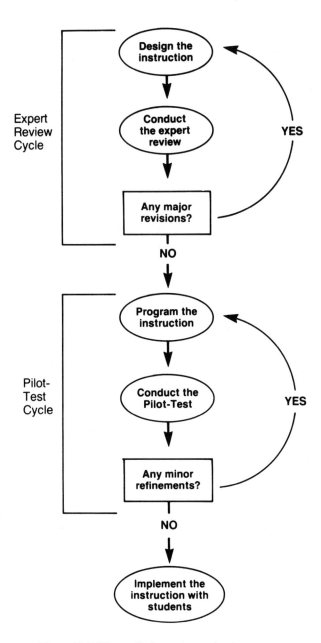

Figure 13.7. The cyclic formative evaluation process.

- Is the use of a decision tree the correct organizational structure for diagnosis and treatment?

- Is information gathering via menus sufficient? Should open-ended questions be available?
- Are the videodisc images of sufficient quality?

Micro - Simulation questions:

- Is the diagnosis and treatment correct?
- Is the information necessary to diagnose and treat the simulated patient provided?
- Does the level of difficulty match the targeted skill of the students?
- What is the average time required to complete a patient simulation?

Strategies

The following strategies, described in detail below, were used in the formative evaluation of the ODSDM project: expert review, pilot-test, interview, and questionnaire.

Expert Review

The expert review should be conducted with two types of specialists—a content specialist and an instructional technology specialist. The content specialist reviews the subject matter for audience appropriateness and content validity;[5] the instructional technology designer checks for sound utilization of instructional principles and appropriate use of the medium. Checklists, informal discussions with the evaluator taking notes, and open-ended questionnaires will provide the information required to improve the instructional product. It is recommended that the expert review team should not be involved with the design of the simulation model.

Lavell[27] performed an extensive formative evaluation of a series of periodontal patient simulations for dental hygiene students. The expert review team included two periodontists, two dental hygienists with extensive periodontal expertise, and an instructional designer. The periodontists and dental hygienists reviewed the content of her simulation model; one periodontist reviewed the content of each individual patient simulation. The instructional designer reviewed the design of the simulation model and of each individual patient simulation.

Pilot-Test

As significant portions of an instructional product are completed, pilot-tests with one to three students from the target population should be conducted.[18] By trying out small but representative portions of a program and making design revisions early, major overhauls may be avoided.

During a pilot-test, a student completes a representative number of patient simulations—usually five to six. An observer present during the pilot-test records student's reactions, questions, and approaches. Prior to the pilot-test, students are instructed to verbalize their thoughts, describe difficult and easy sections, and explain approaches to problems and answers to questions. If observation is not possible, students are instructed to write their thoughts and reactions.

Simulation authors should attend one or more pilot-sessions. Our experiences have shown that the authors gain valuable insights when they witness the students using the system. Authors more clearly understand the need for improvements suggested by students and suggest revisions that might otherwise be overlooked.

Interview

Additional information may be attained if the pilot-test is followed with an informal interview[28,11] or a questionnaire.[5] The interview and questionnaire should focus on the high point and low points of the program, and aim at obtaining a deeper understanding of difficult sections. Asking the student for instructional ideas may provide a fresh perspective for a troublesome simulation. All troublesome simulations should be revised and subsequent pilot-tests conducted until no further modifications are identified.

During interviews, the evaluator asks students about their work, how simulations compare with their previous experiences, and how they perceive the use and value of the patient simulations. Brief structured interviews elicit biographical, demographic, and other standard information. Longer, open-ended interviews uncover discursive information. Whenever possible, each participant should be interviewed. If this is not possible, a random sample plus individuals with a special insight or whose position is particularly noteworthy should be interviewed.[29]

We interviewed every student who was pilot-tested. We started with a standard interview form and added questions as we uncovered new issues, and deleted irrelevant questions. Thus, we continually formatively evaluate our interview form.

Questionnaire

Most evaluations will use observations and interview techniques. However, paper and pencil questionnaires can prove effective in large studies and provide quantitative information in smaller studies. Questionnaires can be used to sustain tentative findings. Fixed questions supply quantitative summary data, while open-ended questions supply supporting and unexpected commentary. Questionnaires should not be used in isolation. Participants should also prepare written comments, or complete checklists.[30]

Originally, our questionnaires were paper and pencil questionnaires consisting of Likert-scale and open-ended questions. We are presently experimenting with placing the same questionnaires on the computer. Currently, we place a required questionnaire at the end of each new patient simulation. Once five students have completed the questionnaire, the data is reviewed. If major revisions are needed, the changes are made and the simulation, with its questionnaire, is completed by five additional students. If revisions are not necessary, the questionnaire is replaced with a comments option. If a student has a question about a simulation, or wishes to suggest changes, the student can leave comments on the computer. These comments are reviewed once a semester. If the comments result in extensive changes, the questionnaire is again turned on; if the changes are minor, the comments option remains.

Considerations of Emerging Technologies

Depending upon the technology product being developed, additional specialists may be required to participate in the expert review. Videodisc, Digital Video Interactive (DVI), and other technologies use motion, audio, or still images. While content experts evaluate the subject matter, audio and video specialists should assess the quality and appropriateness of the audio, motion, and still information. Also the instructional technology designer should review the video and audio control functions. An Instructional Technology Attribute Checklist is included in the Appendix A for this purpose.

Limitations of Formative Evaluation

Formative evaluation is restricted in providing all of the answers about software design. Evaluation assists designers and producers to choose among alternatives, but it is limited in generating these options. The formative evaluation team needs to be receptive to all the ideas, comments, and criticisms generated by the expert reviewers and students, and use this information to improve the product. The primary outcome of a conscientiously applied formative evaluation is a markedly improved product. A secondary outcome is a staff that has developed a broader base of experience about how the user interacts with instructional software.

Summary

The process of formative evaluation involves the identification of deficiencies, and the revising of a product based on feedback from external content specialists and students. Revisions based on this feedback can maximize the instructional product's potential for success.

Summative Evaluation: The Product Evaluation

Introduction—What Results/Outcomes?

The purpose of a summative evaluation is to provide information regarding the merit and worth of an instructional package to decision makers. Decision makers may include administrators considering the cost of the instructional package, instructors examining their content and ease of use, or researchers studying their effectiveness. The summative evaluation of instructional products should provide the information these decision makers may want.

A summative evaluation may consist of one study or a series of studies, each investigating different evaluation questions. A list of questions to be answered should be started during the needs assessment and continue through the formative evaluation. It may be concluded during the implementation of the instruction.

Evaluation Questions

Questions that arose during the needs assessment of the DDx&Tx System that are to be addressed in the Summative Evaluation include:

- Can other institutions successfully use these patient simulations?
- Is the audience appropriate?
- Is the level of difficulty appropriate for the audience?
- Is the use of videodisc appropriate? Is it cost effective?

Questions that arise during the Formative Evaluation that may be addressed in the Summative Evaluation could include:

- Is the interface easy to use?
- Are there sufficient supporting functions, such as help and decision summaries?
- Are the critiques succinct, yet informative?
- Is the breadth of content neither too broad, nor too narrow?
- Do the simulations fulfill the stated goals, in that diagnosis simulations provide diagnosis practice, and treatment planning simulations provide treatment planning practice?
- Are the simulations sufficiently documented? Does the documentation include operation instructions, guidance for authors, implementation suggestions?

In a perfect world, the summative evaluation team should consist of external evaluators and the summative evaluation should be conducted at a site different than the development site. But the cost of such an evaluation frequently prevents this from happening. External consultants can make a summative evaluation more credible. They provide a fresh, unbiased perspective and a perception of credibility that developers cannot bring to an evaluation of their own product.

The first task of the evaluation team is to select questions from the list that was compiled during the needs assessment and formative evaluation. Add the requests of various decision makers. Using that list, design the components of the summative evaluation. Each component should address a separate list of questions.

Strategies

Each component of a summative evaluation will answer a certain set of questions. The strategy used to answer these questions may be the quantitative result of a controlled psychometric technique or it may be a qualitative summary of opinions based on facts, surveys, or interviews. The summative evaluation for the DDx&Tx System is contained in Figure 13.8. It contains both quantitative and qualitative components. The history and theory behind each of the components is discussed, accompanied by examples from the DDx&Tx System evaluation. It should be noted that the summative evaluation is just beginning as this chapter is being written. We expect that it will undergo its own formative evaluation and that its final shape, while answering the same questions, may be altered.

Learning Validation

Ralph W. Tyler[25] took a behavioral objective approach to evaluation. He summarized his theories (p.69) as follows:

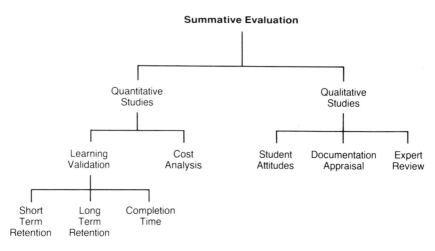

Figure 13.8. The summative evaluation of the DDx&Tx System.

The process of evaluation is essentially the process of determining to what extent the educational objectives are actually being realized by the program of curriculum and instruction. However, since educational objectives are essentially changes in human beings, that is, the objectives aimed at are to produce certain desirable changes in the behavior patterns of the student, then evaluation is the process for determining the degree to which these changes in behavior are actually taking place. (Used with permission from The Basic Principles of Curriculum and Instruction by Ralph W. Tyler. ©c 1950 by the University of Chicago. All rights reserved. Published January 1950. Third impression 1951.)

Many of the techniques used to determine learning effectiveness are based on Tyler's work. Learning validation measures the degree to which an instructional product's stated objectives satisfy the needs of the defined audience. Ultimately the learning validation should measure the degree to which the instruction transfers to the world outside the dental school. However, in practice this seldom occurs. For example, Smith[31] evaluated an interactive videodisc package intended to teach interview skills to social workers. Instead of observing students in actual interviews with clients, Smith used a written post-test. Although this method may have measured formal learning, it provided no information about whether the learning contributed to the students' actual interview skills.

The use of pre- and post-tests can provide useful information.[11,18] The difference between these test scores quantifies learning. Post-tests given immediately after instruction measure short term retention, whereas follow-up tests, given from six weeks to six months after instruction, measure long term retention.[5] An effective learning validation should also report the amount of time needed to complete each part of the instructional package.[11] Administrators are always interested in reducing teaching time. Furthermore, computer-assisted instruction can accurately record the time spent learning computerized information, as long as students know how to stop and restart the timing for breaks.

A learning validation should always use as many randomly selected students as possible. Sample sizes less than 30 jeopardize the validity and reliability of the evaluation.[32] Any evaluation performed with less than 30 students should describe sample behavior and not attempt to generalize beyond those students.

The learning validation of the DDx&Tx System will measure short and long term retention, and the average amount of time required to complete a patient simulation. The primary goal of the DDx&Tx System is to teach the clinical problem-solving skills of diagnosis and treatment planning. A Randomized Solomon Design will measure the learning effectiveness of the patient simulations with dental and dental hygiene students. Case studies will be used to measure problem-solving skills. Each case study will consist of appropriate clinical photographs of the patient, written responses to questions, and clinical findings. Ten different case studies representing the range of dental problems will comprise each test.

Students will be randomly assigned to two groups—a control group and an experimental group. The control group will maintain the normal clinic schedule. The experimental group will complete simulated patients in lieu of real patients. The computer will record the elapsed time required for a student to complete each simulation.

A total of three open-book tests will be given: one pre-test, an immediate post-test, and a deferred post-test. To control for learning caused by the pre-test, one-half of each treatment group will complete the pre-test; all students will complete both post-tests. The deferred post-test will occur eight weeks after the immediate post-test. Students will be allowed two hours for each test.

Cost Analysis

A cost analysis answers the question "How much does it cost?" Administrators need to know hardware and software costs, update costs, costs for support personnel, and initial and recurring costs. A cost analysis should provide itemized and totaled costs with a summary that is easy to understand. A suggested Cost Analysis Worksheet is included in the Appendix. It includes hardware, software, documentation and administrative costs. Hardware and software costs are broken into three categories:

Hardware	Costs Software Costs
1. Off the shelf	1. Operating system (on hand) (text editor, compiler)
2. Standardized	2. Programming tools (able to buy) (development utilities)
3. Unique	3. Instructional technology (need to build) packages

The Cost Analysis Worksheet has two columns for each category. Investment costs include acquisition, installation and start-up costs. Recurring costs cover maintenance, operation, and modification expenses. Because the information technology industry constantly changes, projections can only accurately be made for one to two years. Projections beyond that should contain a qualification that changes are likely to occur.

This Cost Analysis breakdown works well for most instructional technology packages. However, the DDx&Tx System has certain unique features. The DDx&Tx System is designed to allow faculty to author patient simulations and to modify patient simulations authored by other faculty. To accommodate these authoring and modification capabilities, we include the time that authors spend to write or modify the simulation content, and the time support personnel spend to operationalize these patient simulations. Our experience shows that after a simulations model has been designed, the author takes an average of two days to write a single patient simulation; the computer support person takes one to two days to make the simulation work.

Learner Attitudes

Surveys can provide important information about student attitudes toward the instruction. Other sources of information such as open-ended comments, checklists, learner notes, observations, and personal interviews should supplement survey information.[29]

Alessi and Trollip[18] report the importance of gathering qualitative information. A statistics professor at the University of Illinois wanted to compare the impact of a computer-based instruction package to traditional statistics instruction. The class was divided into a control group which received the traditional series of lectures and laboratory sessions and an experimental group which received most of its instruction from the computer. Both groups received the same semester exam and the experimental group did better. However, the following semester not a single student from the experimental group took a follow-up statistics course, while a number of students from the control group did. The computer-based training achieved its instructional objective of teaching statistics, but failed in the affective goal of fostering an interest in statistics. If a qualitative follow-up study had not been conducted, this important information would have been overlooked.

In the summative evaluation for the DDx&Tx System, learner attitudes will be measured by a survey which students will complete after they have completed their patient simulations. A similar follow-up survey will be given six months later. In each survey students will be asked for their perception of how the simulations helped them to diagnose and/or treat their patients. In the follow-up survey, they will be asked to give specific examples whenever possible.

Documentation Appraisal

Instructional software documentation is written for the instructor, the learner, administrator, or other user. Check the instructor's manual for implementation procedures for the hardware and software, such as how to use a test generator, a detailed project description, specific goals and objectives, prerequisite skills, possible pre- and post-tests, instructional suggestions and strategies, field-testing results, and supplemental worksheets or activities.

Check the administrator's manual for a succinct summary of identifying characteristics. Included should be a list of hardware components and purchasing information for unique peripherals such as CD-ROM or videodisc players.

Evaluators should also check for descriptions of potential hardware problems and their remedies. A suggested Documentation Checklist is contained in the Appendix C.

The Documentation Appraisal for the DDx&Tx System will involve four reviewers. The documentation consists of an Author's Guide, a System Guide, and a User's Guide. Two authors will examine the Author's Guide for completeness, accuracy and ease of guidance through the authoring process. Their examination will be conducted while they are authoring a series of patient simulations. Two computer support persons will review the System Guide. They will examine it for hardware and software information, set-up support, and accuracy and clarity of making the simulations execute properly and implementing them with students. Their review will be conducted while they are actually providing support for a simulation author.

Expert Review

Although expert review was addressed during the formative evaluation, it is recommended that additional content experts review the implementation version of a product.[33] Correlating the subject matter with major texts and other media is important, especially if the instruction is part of a curriculum. Questions to address in the summative evaluation are: Is the age level appropriate? Is the scope and sequence appropriate? Are the concepts and facts accurate? Is the content free of racial, social, ethnic, and sexual bias?

The expert review of the DDx&Tx System will have the usual content validation; however, it will have another characteristic that is unique to the nature of the DDx&Tx System. The DDx&Tx patient simulations have been designed to be modified by other institutions to meet the unique requirements of that institution. When experts review these patient simulations, they will also note changes needed for the simulations to fit the requirements of that institution.

Considerations for Emerging Technologies

Videodisc and other instructional technologies are expensive to implement into a curriculum. Dental educators should insist upon a careful evaluation of each product. In the case of videodisc and other visual media the following questions arise: Does it depict a problem or situation that cannot be better depicted by another medium? Is the video information central to the concepts being taught or supplementary? Is it the best medium for the content? Does the video demonstrate rather than explain? Does the video present multiple examples of a topic, rather than just one? Are the still frames developed using proven design principles? Are video control options available to the learner? Could a less expensive form of technology have accomplished the same instructional task? Just as a content expert evaluates instruction for content validity, an instructional technology expert should evaluate the instructional product for its use of the technology.

Summary

The summative evaluator has a diverse set of measurement tools available to investigate the learner's skill acquisition and attitude. Additional tools are available to determine the ease with which an instructional package can be implemented, and the support that is provided. Because each tool has differing strengths and weaknesses, most evaluators use a combination of tests, observations, surveys, and checklists in order to provide a complete and accurate picture of the effectiveness of an instructional product.

Acknowledgements

I wish to express my sincere appreciation to Gilbert E. Lilly, Head, Department of Oral Pathology, Radiology and Medicine, the University of Iowa. His vision, trust, and commitment of energies and resources encouraged the growth of instructional technology at the University of Iowa College of Dentistry. My deepest thanks also goes to the faculty and staff at the College of Dentistry for their contributions in supporting the authoring of patient simulations. I thank the University Video Center for their videodisc production support and the Weeg Computing Center for their software design and programming support. I also thank Kristin Eveson for her help in preparing this manuscript.

References

1. Kirk BA, Cummings RW, Hackett HR. Personal and Vocational Characteristics of Dental Schools. Pers Guid J. 1963;41(6):522-527.
2. Hendricson WD, Berlocher WC, Herbert RJ. A Four-Year Longitudinal Study of Dental Student Learning Styles. J Dent Educ. 1987;51:175-181.
3. Rinchuse DJ, Zullo T. The Cognitive Level Demands of a Dental School's Predoctoral, Didactic Examinations. J Dent Educ. 1986;50(3):167-171.
4. Erskine CG, Westerman GH, Grandy G. Personality Styles of First-Year Dental Students. J Dent Educ. 1986;50(4):221-224.
5. Reeves TC, Lent RM. Levels of Evaluation for Computer-Based Instruction. In: DF Walker and RD Hess, eds. Instructional Software: Principles and Perspectives for Design and Use. Belmont, CA: Wadsworth Publishing Co, 1984: p. 188-203.
6. Silberman SL, Cain MJ, Mahan JM. Dental Students' Personality: A Jungian Perspective. J Dent Educ. 1982;46(11):646-651.
7. Elstein AS, Shulman LS, Sprafka SA. Medical Problem-Solving: An Analysis of Clinical Reasoning. Cambridge, MA: Harvard University Press, 1978.
8. Russell IJ, Hendricson WD, Lawlor RW. A Prospectively-Designed Assessment of the Condition Diagramming Method for Teaching Diagnostic Reasoning. Proceedings of the Twenty-Fourth Annual Research in Medical Education Conference. Washington, D.C., 1985.

9. Lau J, Parker SG. Casual Reasoning in Medicine: Analysis of a Protocol. Cognit Sci. 1984;8:363-385.

10. Berner ES. Paradigms and Problem-Solving: A Literature Review. J Med Educ. 1984;59(8):625-633.

11. Steinberg ER. Teach Computers to Teach. Hillsdale, NJ: Lawrence Erlbaum Associates, 1984.

12. Frederiksen N. Implication of Cognitive Theory for Instruction in Problem-Solving. Rev Educ Res. 1984;54(3):363-407.

13. McGuire C. Medical Problem-Solving: A Critique of the Literature. Proceedings of the 23rd Annual Conference in Research in Medical Education. (p.13). Washington, D.C.: Association of American Medical Colleges, 1985.

14. Blancher MC. A Role for Clinical Case Simulations in Basic Medical Science Education. Physiologist. 1985;28(5):422-424.

15. Barnett 0. Computer-Based Simulations and Clinical Problem-Solving. Med Inf. 1984;9(3/4):277-279.

16. McGuire C. Simulation Techniques in the Teaching and Testing of Problem-Solving Skills. J Res Sci Teach. 1976;13(2):89-100.

17. Woodbury PA. Computer Assisted Evaluation of Problem-Solving Skills of Primary Health Care Providers. J Contin Educ Nurs. 1984;15(5),174-177.

18. Alessi SM, Trollip SR. Computer-Based Instruction: Methods and Development. Englewood Cliffs, NJ: Prentice-Hall, 1985.

19. Finkelstein MW, Johnson LA, Lilly GE. Interactive Videodisc Patient Simulations of Oral Diseases. J Dent Educ. 1988;52(4):217-220.

20. Alessi SM. Fidelity in the Design of Instructional Simulations. J Comput Based Instruct. 1988;15(2):40-47.

21. Lilly GE. Educational Program Emphasizing Problem-Solving and Decision-Making. Unpublished Manuscript, 1984.

22. Ausbel DP. Educational Psychology: A Cognitive View. New York, NY: Holt, Rinehart, and Winston, 1968.

23. Small DS, Weldon LJ. An Experimental Comparison of Natural and Structured Query Languages. Hum Factors. 1981;25(3):253-263.

24. Finkelstein MW. A Formative Evaluation of Oral Disease Simulations for Diagnosis and Management. A paper submitted for publication.

25. Tyler RW. Basic Principles of Curriculum and Instruction. Chicago: University of Chicago Press, 1950.

26. Flagg BN. Formative Evaluation for Educational Technologies. Hillsdale, NJ: Lawrence Erlbaum Associates, 1990.

27. Lavell NC. Interactive Videodisc Periodontal Patient Simulations: A Formative Evaluation. Unpublished master's thesis, University of Iowa, Iowa City, IA, 1990.

28. Call-Himwich E, Steinberg E. Myth and Reality: Essential Decisions in Computer-Based Instruction Design. (Report No. MTC-R-18).

Washington, DC: Advance Research Projects Agency (DOD), 1977. (ERIC Document Reproduction Service NO. ED 152 239)

29. Stufflebeam DL, Shinkfield AJ. Systematic Evaluation: A Self-Instructional Guide to Theory and Practice. Boston, MA: Kluwer-Nijhoff Publishing, 1985.

30. Parlett MR, Hamilton D. Evaluation in Illumination: A New Approach to the Study of Innovative Programmes. In: D. Hamilton et al., eds. Beyond the Numbers Game. London: MacMillan Education, 1977.

31. Smith RC. Full-Scale Pilot-Testing of Florida's Videodisc Training Project. Paper presented at the Fifth Annual Nebraska Videodisc Symposium, Lincoln, NE, 1984.

32. Isaac S, Michael WB. Handbook in Research and Evaluation. San Diego, CA: EdITS Publishers, 1982.

33. Otte RB. Courseware for the 80's. Tech Horiz Educ J. 1984;12(3):80-91.

Appendix A: Instructional Technology Attribute Checklist

This checklist is intended as a guide only. Check the appropriate column for each technology attribute. Check —

      *Not Applicable if the attribute is not appropriate to the instructional package

      *Included if the attribute is included in the instructional package

      *Excluded if the attribute is appropriate to the instructional package, but not
          included

	Not Applicable	Included	Excluded
SOFTWARE ATTRIBUTES			
Program operates correctly			
Industry standards used			
Access speed is reasonable			
Generates reports			
Audio and visual material indexes			
Modifiable by instructor			
Specialized controls			
Program map			
STOP motion			
Forward one section			
Backward one section			
Slow forward			
Slow reverse			
Fast forward			
Fast reverse			
Browse			
Audio on/off			
Frame display on/off			

	Not Applicable	Included	Excluded
VISUAL ATTRIBUTES			
Reduced jitter			
Sound over still			
Limited "talking head"			
Clear sharp visuals			
Smooth & quick motion			
Accurate representation of colors			
Special effects enhance not distract			
AUDIO ATTRIBUTES			
Narration/music is clear			
Consistent audio levels			
Narration synchronized with visuals			
Multiple audio channels			
SUPPORT ATTRIBUTES			
Hardware requirements listed			
Simple installation instructions			
All peripheral drivers included			
Updates available			
Phone support			

Appendix B: Cost Analysis Worksheet

Cost Analysis Worksheet - Hardware

	Product _____		Product _____	
	Investment Cost	Recurring Cost	Investment Cost	Recurring Cost
Off the shelf hardware (on hand) Computer Equipment Peripherals				
Subtotal				
Standardized hardware (able to buy) Computer equipment Peripherals				
Subtotal				
Unique hardware (need to build) Parts Labor				
Subtotal				
Hardware Total				

Cost Analysis Worksheet - Software

	Product _____		Product _____	
	Investment Cost	Recurring Cost	Investment Cost	Recurring Cost
Operating software Text editors				
Compilers				
Subtotal				
Programming tools Authoring languages				
Design utilities				
Graphics packages				
Subtotal				
Instructional packages				
Subtotal				
Software Total				

Cost Analysis Worksheet - Summary

	Product _____		Product _____	
	Investment Cost	Recurring Cost	Investment Cost	Recurring Cost
Documentation				
Instructor's manual				
Learner's manual				
Technical manual				
Other				
Documentation Total				
Administration				
Maintenance contracts				
Faculty time				
Support personnel				
Facility expenses				
Other				
Administration Total				
Hardware Total				
Software Total				
GRAND TOTAL				

Appendix C: Documentation Checklist

This checklist is intended as a guide only. Check the appropriate column for each documentation characteristic. Check —

Not Included if the characteristic is not a part of the documentation or is not applicable

Included - Poor if the characteristic is poorly written

Included - Adequate if the characteristic is of average quality

Included - Well Done if the characteristic is of above average quality

	Not Included	Included		
		Poor	Adequate	Well Done
Rationale				
Goals & objectives				
Audience				
Prerequisite skills				
User options				
Hardware listing and set-up description				
Software implementation description				
Evaluation summary				
Instructional suggestions & strategies				
Curriculum integration strategies				
Supplemental activities				

14
Informatics and Issues Related to Assessing, Assuring and Improving Quality of Care

James J. Crall

Quality Assessment and Quality Assurance in Health Care

Defining Quality of Care

Numerous frameworks have been proposed to capture the concept of quality in health care. Those concerned with defining quality have emphasized aspects including accessibility, acceptability, effectiveness, efficiency and provider competency.[1] Others interested in developing approaches for characterizing and evaluating quality have depicted health care as a composite of attributes and elements comprising structure, process and outcome dimensions[2] or have subdivided care into technical and interpersonal features.[3] An Institute of Medicine (IOM) committee recently collected and evaluated over 100 definitions of quality of care and subsequently developed the following consensus definition: "quality of care is the degree to which health services for individuals and populations increase the likelihood of desired outcomes and are consistent with current professional knowledge".[4] Desired outcomes in this context include consideration of health status, patient satisfaction and well being, and overall quality of life. Others[5] have expanded upon that definition slightly by stating that in addition to increasing the probability of desired outcomes, quality should be measured in terms of the degree to which care decreases the probability of undesired outcomes.

Quality Assessment and Quality Assurance

Methods and strategies for affecting quality in health care generally are grouped according to three major areas: quality assessment, quality assurance, and quality improvement. Quality assessment denotes measurement of the technical and interpersonal aspects of care and the outcomes of that care.[6] Although quality assessment is considered to be a useful first step for monitoring performance and identifying problems, additional procedures are necessary to prevent or remedy deficiencies and ensure acceptable performance. Historically those procedures have been considered the realm of quality assurance.

Quality assurance generally connotes a cyclic series of formal systematic activities aimed at monitoring performance, identifying problems, designing actions to remedy those problems, and carrying out follow-up evaluations to ensure that corrective actions have been effective and are sustained.[6] With proper implementation and adequate support, traditional quality assurance approaches can positively influence quality of care by:

1) prompting attention to high-priority areas of clinical care,

2) prompting development and use of relevant indicators of care,

3) stimulating analysis of appropriateness and effectiveness,

4) serving as a basis for targeted education and other approaches to improvement and

5) stimulating sorely needed improvements in clinical information systems.[7]

At the same time, traditional quality assurance approaches have been criticized for:

1) lacking an internal focus (being of use to external parties, but not to those involved in the delivery of care),

2) being focused primarily on clinicians and not on processes or systems that influence patient care and its outcomes,

3) focusing on isolated aspects of care and not on episodes of treatment provided to patients over time,

4) not fostering integrated analyses of effectiveness and efficiency,

5) reducing morale by relying on inspections and by failing to support professional instincts for self-assessment and improvement and

6) not providing a basis for answering fundamental questions regarding reasonable expectations for performance under different circumstances.[7,8]

Extensive systems to support quality assurance activities of this nature have been developed and widely applied in hospital facilities. Application of the traditional quality assurance model to ambulatory care settings has been quite limited owing to a number of problems, not the least of which is the lack of efficient methods for collecting and disseminating useful information in a timely manner.[9]

Quality Assessment and Quality Assurance in Dentistry

Quality Assessment

Numerous quality assessment approaches have been used to evaluate dental care.[10] For the most part, those approaches have evolved as by-products of efforts in medicine. For example, retrospective record audits have been used extensively for evaluations of hospital care and have been advocated for use in dentistry. Focused approaches include the use of procedural audits for various tracer conditions[11] and monitoring of retreatment of the same tooth or region.[12] Drawbacks associated with current applications of the techniques cited above, which rely heavily on manual collection and analysis of data, relate to the considerable time and expense necessary to evaluate recurring episodes of care, the typically low yields, and the lack of critical information in most practitioners' records. A more direct approach, patient examinations, has also been criticized as being costly, obtrusive and of questionable reliability.[13] Among less-obtrusive and less-expensive approaches, patient assessments of quality have received considerable attention in the literature[14] but are not commonplace in dentistry. Automated assessments (such as statistical profiles of data on insurance claims submitted by practitioners) can identify unusual practice patterns, but are of limited value in determining appropriateness of treatment due to the absence of critical elements (such as diagnoses) in most dental claims data.

Internal and External Quality Assurance Programs

To a large extent, dentistry involves the delivery of ambulatory, primary care services (services directed toward prevention or early detection and treatment of disease and long-term management of chronic conditions over recurring episodes of care).[9] Unlike their medical counterparts, a large majority of dentists practice in independently owned, solo or two-person private offices and are generalists.[15] Given those attributes, it is not surprising that formal quality assurance programs are not pervasive throughout the dental care delivery system. Organized programs operating within dental care facilities that fit the traditional quality assurance model are found largely in accredited group practices and institutional settings (for example, hospital dental departments). The system in place at the dental care facility for employees of the R. J. Reynolds Company in Winston-Salem, NC exemplifies an extensive, multi-faceted dental quality assurance program.[16]

In addition to internal quality assurance programs, various types of quality assurance activities are mandated in conjunction with some third-party payment arrangements. For example, various office assessment instruments[17,19] have been developed and used by third-party payors and regulatory bodies to evaluate providers who wish to participate in certain alternative delivery and/or financing systems. Although the use of office assessment instruments is becoming more commonplace, evidence of the effectiveness of that approach in terms of modifying provider behaviors or improving outcomes of care is lacking.

Many consider state and regional board examinations, state licensure laws and established educational standards as external quality assurance measures. Board and licensure examinations and educational standards do not constitute quality assurance activities in the traditional sense outlined above since they do not focus directly on the actual delivery of health care services. Rather those mechanisms attempt to provide some degree of protection to the public by ensuring that practitioners possess the necessary knowledge and skills (thus the potential) to provide quality care. Extensions of those original measures (such as re-examination of providers prior to relicensure and/or recertification and periodic reaccreditation of educational institutions) more closely conform to the traditional quality assurance model in that they are cyclic activities and may involve mechanisms for remedying identified deficiencies. However in most cases, direct assessments of patient care and its outcomes have not been incorporated into those activities heretofore. Likewise some consider third-party-payor utilization review programs as being quality assurance activities. In most cases the primary objective of those programs is cost-containment, not quality assurance.

Thus in summary, several approaches for assessing various quality-related aspects of dental care have been devised. However, relatively few organized, ongoing programs are in place to consistently monitor, evaluate and provide information that might be used to improve dental care in those settings where the majority of services are provided.

Barriers to Effective Quality Assurance in Dentistry

Efforts to establish effective quality assurance systems in dentistry face the same barriers that apply virtually throughout the entire ambulatory primary care sector. Problems that must be addressed include the lack of uniform data collection and storage systems (not to mention the lack of consensus on what constitutes appropriate data elements), a paucity of data on which to base criteria and standards of care and difficulty in achieving changes in provider behavior because practitioners are generally isolated and largely insulated from peer pressure.[9] In addition, because of the relatively low unit costs of dental services and the need for quality assessment and assurance procedures to be cost-effective, resources available for monitoring and evaluating dental care typically are quite meager. The above factors argue for the development of efficient data collection and communication methods that minimize human involvement.

Information Systems and Issues Related to Quality of Care

Quality of care embodies many broad issues as outlined in the opening paragraph of this chapter. Specific aspects for which electronic information systems (dental informatics) are likely to be useful for enhancing quality of care include accessibility, preventive care, appropriateness of diagnosis and treatment, continuity of care and adverse outcomes.[20] Three established strategies for monitoring quality of care involve case finding, provider profiles and population-based measures.[20] Examples of potential uses of informatics to enhance the quality of dental care are provided below.

Accessibility

Access to care refers to the ability to obtain needed care in a timely manner. Accessibility is of particular concern for individuals enrolled in prepaid health care programs (such as dental capitation plans) where providers receive a fixed payment for services regardless of whether or how many services are provided for enrollees in the plan. On a broader scale, access may be a problem for individuals whose care is financed through public programs (for example, Medicaid recipients) because of the historically low levels of reimbursement provided under most public financing schemes. Electronically collected data can serve as an efficient means for monitoring access by providing information on visit rates and service utilization patterns across patient populations.[20]

Preventive Care

Dentistry has been a leader among professions in the development and provision of preventive services for large segments of the population. In spite of the benefits obtained from the application of various preventive measures, many individuals in the population remain susceptible to preventable dental diseases.[21,22] For the most part, preventive services have been administered on a population-wide basis (with relatively little consideration for specific risk factors or customization of preventive therapies). As additional findings regarding individual risk factors and constellations of characteristics that signal patients who are at varying levels of risk for different diseases become available, individualized preventive care will become increasingly important. Electronic information systems hold considerable promise as tools for both research and improved patient management in that regard. Again on a broader scale, informatics can facilitate comparisons of patients and providers' use of preventive services (and examine relationships between utilization and outcomes of care), flag patients who require intensive preventive therapy and monitor compliance with recommended preventive guidelines.

Appropriateness of Care

Unlike medicine where quality review criteria have existed for many conditions for some time, criteria and standards for evaluating appropriateness of diagnostic and treatment regimens in dentistry are only beginning to be developed and tested. One exception is the area of diagnostic radiology where guidelines for the use of dental radiographs have been established.[23] Additional activities related to the development of quality review criteria (e.g., indications for various procedures) have been undertaken recently by various dental specialty groups. Beyond that, the American Dental Association has begun the task of developing practice parameters which seek to aid in establishing what types of services constitute appropriate care for particular conditions.[24] Information systems can facilitate evaluations of appropriateness by monitoring compliance with pre-established guidelines and criteria and by signaling tracer conditions or sentinel events (conditions that would not be expected to occur or that have been identified as warranting further review). Automated information systems also can be used to track individuals who have specific conditions or who have received certain services for purposes of monitoring outcomes of care.[20]

Continuity of Care

The general model for providing primary dental care involves the delivery of diagnostic, preventive and if necessary rehabilitative services on a recurring basis over multiple treatment episodes. Because of the chronic, preventable and largely irreversible nature of the two major disease processes that prompt individuals to seek dental services (caries and periodontal disease), continuity of care is considered to be highly related to the maintenance of oral health. Many existing practice management software packages include a provision for identifying patients who are due to return to the practice for maintenance care. Not commonly found in existing systems are information management features that would allow practitioners to identify the characteristics of patients who are more likely to fail to return for follow-up care.[20]

Adverse Outcomes

As part of the process of developing criteria and standards of care, many professional groups have adopted a format which includes explicit listings of expected or desired outcomes along with unexpected or adverse outcomes. Identification of adverse outcomes can be facilitated by applying electronic information systems to the monitoring of various types of sentinel events (for example, preventable disease and disability or need for certain types of treatment or retreatment). Another use of electronic information systems to detect unexpected and potentially adverse outcomes involves the collection of data on patient satisfaction or dissatisfaction with treatment.

Future Uses of Information Technology to Improve Quality

In a recent publication, Barnett and Winickoff[25] stated the following: "There are two major factors which limit extensive quality assurance activities: (i) it is time-consuming and difficult to gather data on clinical practice; and (ii) after the initial measurements have been made, those concerned with implementing quality assurance protocols are often totally exhausted and unwilling to undertake the necessary efforts to re-examine the issue on a regular basis after corrective action has been taken." Although that statement was not intended to reflect directly on quality assurance efforts in dentistry, it certainly would appear to apply. Barnett and Winickoff[25] went on to emphasize the potential for using an automated medical record system to enhance quality assurance activities. Upon further examination, it becomes clear that quality assurance (QA) to those authors is very closely linked to quality improvement (QI), an approach that increasingly is being applied in health care settings.

Quality Improvement

The concept of "quality improvement" (also termed "continuous quality improvement") refers to a set of techniques for continuous study and improvement of processes and outcomes of care to satisfy the needs and expectations of "customers" (internal and external recipients and purchasers of services or products).[1] Quality improvement approaches have been used extensively in industrial settings,[26,27,28] and only recently have been advocated and applied in health care operations.[7,8,29,30] Quality improvement has been characterized as being an information-driven, statistically-based process; however, effective communication is also a major area of emphasis in the application of quality improvement approaches.[29]

The Joint Commission on Accreditation of Healthcare Organizations (JCAHO) has been a prominent activist in the continued development of approaches for assessing and assuring quality, primarily in hospitals but more recently in other types of health care settings.[31] A major emphasis by the JCAHO of late has been the development of indicators that can provide more objective, quantitative measures that can be used to monitor and evaluate patient care.[32] The continued development of indicators, practice guidelines, criteria and standards of care is likely to be a prominent activity throughout health care in the years to come.[33] Through its Agenda for Change, the JCAHO also has begun to incorporate elements of the quality improvement approach into its accreditation activities[34] and to examine the potential for developing an interactive medical management information system to facilitate "continuous flow" of data between the JCAHO and the organizations and facilities it surveys.[32] Similar professional initiatives for primary care facilities that are not routinely accredited (such as dental and medical offices) would appear to hold considerable potential for improving quality of care.

In noting the potential for quality improvement via computer-based record systems, Barnett and Winickoff[25] characterized the use of peer comparison feedback as "a powerful quality assurance intervention", citing evidence of significant improvement in provider performance and patient management. The effectiveness of that approach appears to be related to the degree of personal involvement and engagement which results when providers compare and contrast their individual performance with that of their peers. Linking deviations to particular patients where poor performance is perceived as relevant by the responsible provider and providing feedback in time to allow for corrective actions are also deemed to be of critical importance.[25] As noted earlier, traditional quality assurance programs have not achieved overwhelming success along those lines.

Potential for Informatics to Enhance QA and Facilitate QI

Electronic record systems and workstations would appear to have the capability to enhance quality of care as follows:

1) by facilitating the collection, storage and retrieval of relevant information on patient characteristics, clinical findings and treatments in a timely and efficient manner

2) through standardization of important data elements

3) by providing decision support that can lead to more appropriate and effective services for individual patients

4) by achieving "real-time quality assurance" (influencing patient care in a positive manner at the time of treatment).

Combined with techniques such as peer evaluation feedback and other methods advocated as part of continuous quality improvement, informatics holds the potential to enhance individual provider and collective professional performance by:

1) countering the effects of isolationism inherent in the dental care delivery system

2) providing information that can positively influence patient care in a timely manner

3) linking providers to centralized support facilities and to networks of their peers.

Summary

Regardless of the setting, quality assurance programs are generally conducted for one or more of the following purposes:

1) to identify providers whose care is of such poor quality that immediate actions need to be taken to restrict their ability to practice;

2) to work with providers whose care is determined to be substandard in order to identify problems and corrective actions necessary to return performance to acceptable levels;

3) to improve the average level of quality of care delivered by a community of providers and

4) to motivate and assist providers to achieve high levels of quality.[6]

Traditional quality assurance approaches have not been implemented effectively in ambulatory primary care settings such as those wherein most dental care services are provided. Informatics holds considerable promise for enhancing quality of care by providing practitioners with a basis for peer group comparison and by facilitating the introduction and use of quality improvement approaches that have proven successful in industrial settings and are becoming more popular in health care.

References

1. Palmer RH. Defining quality of care. In Ambulatory health care evaluation: principles and practice. Chicago: American Hospital Publishing Co., 1983: p. 13-16.
2. Donabedian A. Evaluating the quality of medical care. Milbank Mem Fund Q 1966; 44:166-203.
3. Donabedian A. Explorations in quality assessment and monitoring, vol 1: the definition of quality and approaches to its assessment. Ann Arbor, MI: Health Administration Press, 1980.
4. Institute of Medicine, Committee to Design a Strategy for Quality Review and Assurance in Medicare. Health, health care and quality of care. In: Lohr KN, ed. Medicare: a strategy for quality assurance: a report of a study by the committee of the Institute of Medicine, Division of Health Care Services, vol I. Washington, DC: National Academy Press, 1990: p. 19-44.
5. U.S. Congress, Office of Technology Assessment. The quality of medical care: information for consumers. Washington, DC: U.S. Government Printing Office, 1988 (OTA-H-386).
6. Committee to Design a Strategy for Quality Review and Assurance in Medicare. Concepts of assessing, assuring, and improving quality. In: Lohr KN, ed. Medicare: a strategy for quality assurance: a report of a study by the committee of the Institute of Medicine, Division of Health Care Services, vol I. Washington, DC: National Academy Press, 1990: p. 45-68.
7. Roberts JS, Schyve PM. From QA to QI: the views and role of the Joint Commission. In: The quality letter for healthcare leaders. Rockville, MD, Bader Associates, Inc., May 1990.
8. Berwick DM. Continuous improvement as an ideal in health care. N Engl J Med 1989; 320:53-56.
9. Palmer RH. The challenges and prospects for quality assessment and assurance in ambulatory care. Inquiry 1988; 25:119-131.
10. Crall JJ. Informatics futures in dental education and research: quality assurance. J Dent Educ 1991;55:257-261.
11. ADA Office of Quality Assurance. Guidelines for the development of a quality assurance audit system for hospital dental programs. Chicago: American Dental Association, 1983.
12. American Dental Association Quality Assurance Project. Quality assurance in dentistry: executive summary, part 3. J Am Dent Assoc 1979; 98:429-435.
13. Marcus M. Quality assurance systems. In: National round table on dental quality assurance, summary of proceedings. Chicago: W.K. Kellogg Foundation, 1983: p. 5-21.
14. Cleary PD, McNeil BJ. Patient satisfaction as an indicator of quality care. Inquiry 1988; 25:25-36.
15. ADA Bureau of Economic and Behavioral Research. The 1988 survey of dental practice. Chicago: American Dental Association, 1988.

16. Quality assurance program. Winston-Salem Dental Care Plan, Inc., Winston-Salem, NC, August 1989.

17. Schoen MH. A quality assessment system: the search for validity. J Dent Educ 1989; 53:658-661.

18. Morris AL, Bentley JM, Vito AA, et al. Assessment of private dental practice: report of a study. J Am Dent Assoc 1988; 117:153-162.

19. Gotowka TD. Personal communication re: dental office assessment instrument developed by AEtna Healthcare Systems, Inc., 1987.

20. Steinwachs DM, Weiner JP, Shapiro S. Management information systems and quality. In: Goldfield N, Nash DB, eds. Providing quality care: the challenge to clinicians. Philadelphia: American College of Physicians, 1989: p. 160-181.

21. Miller AJ, Brunnell JA, Carlos JP, et al. Oral health of United States adults: national findings. Washington, DC: National Institute of Dental Research, 1987. (DHHS publication no (PHS) 87-2868).

22. National Institute of Dental Research. NIDR releases results of new schoolchildren's survey. Bethesda, MD: NIDR Digest, 1988.

23. Center for Devices and Radiological Health, Department of Health and Human Services. The selection of patients for x-ray examinations: dental radiographic examinations, 1987. (DHHS publication no (FDA) 888273).

24. ADA News. House gives parameters a green light. Chicago: American Dental Association, November 5, 1990: p . 6, 16 .

25. Barnett GO, Winickoff RN. Quality assurance and computer-based patient records. Am J Public Health 1990; 80:527-528.

26. Deming WE. Quality, productivity and competitive position. Cambridge, MA: Massachusetts Institute of Technology, Center for Advanced Engineering, 1982.

27. Juran JM, Gryne FM, Jr. Quality planning and analysis. New York: McGraw-Hill Book Co., 1980.

28. Crosby PB. Quality is free. New York: McGraw-Hill Book Co., 1979.

29. Batalden PB, Buchanan ED. Industrial models of quality improvement. In: Goldfield N, Nash DB, eds. Providing quality care: the challenge to clinicians. Philadelphia: American College of Physicians, 1989: p. 133-159.

30. Laffel G, Blumenthal D. The case for using industrial quality management science in health care organizations. JAMA 1989; 262:2869-2873.

31. Couch JB. The Joint Commission on Accreditation of Healthcare Organizations. In: Goldfield N, Nash DB, eds. Providing quality care: the challenge to clinicians. Philadelphia: American College of Physicians, 1989: p. 201-224.

32. Joint Commission on Accreditation of Healthcare Organizations. Characteristics of clinical indicators. QRB 1990 15: 330-339.

33. Leape LL. Practice guidelines and standards: an overview. QRB 1990: 42-49.

34. Joint Commission on Accreditation of Healthcare Organizations. Agenda for Change. Update 1988; 2:1,5.

15
Research Frontiers

James A. Lipton

Introduction

Dentistry and oral health research will undergo many changes in the coming years. The resulting "new dentistry" will be much broader in scope than at present, characterized by a greater variety of techniques to diagnose and treat a larger number of orofacial conditions, and a more diverse array of approaches to prevent disease and foster positive oral health. Among the key factors responsible for these changes are (1) the tremendous knowledge "explosion" and fundamental advances currently taking place in such fields as molecular and cell biology, the neurosciences, immunology, biomaterials, computer science, and biotechnology; and (2) the increasing application of these advances to clinical practice.

Underlying and facilitating many of these changes are the rapid developments in information science and computer technology. Acquiring, processing, managing, and communicating through automated systems the ever increasing amounts of information pertinent to dentistry will come to dominate many aspects of dental practice and oral health research, as it has started to do already in medicine. Computers already are being used to assist in developing diagnoses and treatment plans, as well as in the actual performance of clinical procedures. These technologies and the biological advances are helping dentistry to become a more research-oriented profession.

This chapter will consider some of the exciting research frontiers in dental informatics, which is the field that applies computer technology and automated information systems to the cognitive, information processing, and communication tasks of oral health research, practice, and education. The chapter is organized as follows:

I. Major Research Issues and Opportunities in Dental Informatics

A. Constructing Computer-Based Resources for Managing and Disseminating Oral Health Research Information

B. Applying Computer Technology to Generating Information in Oral Health Research and Delivery of Clinical Care

The principal foci will be on the application of informatics and computer technology to dental practice and to basic and clinical oral health research. Informatics research in dental education has been addressed elsewhere in this and other books,[1] and will not be discussed here.

I. Major Research Issues and Opportunities in Dental Informatics

A series of recommendations will be proposed and opportunities highlighted for future research in dental informatics in this section. Several basic assumptions have influenced their development. First, the particular research opportunities and recommendations in dental informatics must be relevant to the general aims of oral health research and to the specific information needs of dental practitioners.

Second, the responsibilities of the dental research and practitioner communities in regard to dental informatics should be to: (a) identify the perceived needs in informatics; (b) perform the highest quality research that will provide the clinical, epidemiological, and basic science knowledge to be included in the information systems; (c) test and evaluate the usefulness of the systems that are developed; and (d) utilize the informatics resources in dental research and clinical settings.

Third, the purely technological aspects of informatics, such as development of computer hardware, work stations, and most software, should be supported primarily, if not solely, by organizations outside of dentistry, such as the National Library of Medicine and other components of the U.S. National Institutes of Health (NIH), or private industry.

Fourth, to receive support from the major funding agencies in the United States, such as the National Institute of Dental Research, NIH, particular dental informatics research proposals must be of high scientific quality and fit within the general mission of these agencies.

The mission of the National Institute of Dental Research (NIDR) and goal of oral health research is to improve people's oral health through such approaches as basic science laboratory experiments, clinical investigations, epidemiological surveys, and behavioral and health services studies into the causes, prevention, diagnosis, and treatment of oral diseases and conditions. Ultimately, the research findings must be brought to the dental practice setting and adapted for clinical applicability. This leads to the first major way that dental informatics can contribute to the "new" dentistry.

A) Constructing Computer-Based Resources for Managing and Disseminating Oral Health Research Information

Recommendation # 12: Propose Overall Goals for Research in Dental Informatics

1.1 Develop knowledge bases oriented primarily to the information needs of dental practitioners. These would supplement existing resources that are more suited to the needs and perspectives of the research community and non-dentists. New knowledge bases should be: a) practice-oriented and user friendly, providing advice about what to do in various situations, when to do it, and how to interpret clinical evidence; b) adaptable to different levels of expertise and experience, and able to dispense advice and guidance that will lead the clinician to where he/she should be; and c) able to provide simultaneous user access to large quantities of information that combine such clinically relevant information as image data, graphics, three-dimensional objects, and text.

1.2 Develop prototype projects to investigate the integration of diverse information database systems for dentistry, such as in clinical decision-support research for various clinical oral conditions. Expert systems would serve as the primary component of the linkage mechanism.

1.3 Establish electronic network communications, using automated information systems, through oral health research and dental practitioner communities so that information dissemination and specific collaborations can take place rapidly and conveniently.

1.3.1 Research groups need the ability to transfer and share knowledge bases and problem-solving methodologies, so that they can compare alternative approaches and cooperate on the development of knowledge bases per se.

1.3.2 Practitioner populations, clinical and epidemiological researchers need standardized interfaces with pre-existing clinical and population record systems. Wide dissemination of most systems for decision support will depend on development of a standardized method for interfacing with large information systems, such as those in hospitals, private and public clinics, those from private insurance companies and government insurers, and those kept in national, state and local databases.

1.3.3 Practitioner communities and clinical investigators need an automated system to store and retrieve standardized patient records. Such systems offer large databases of patient information on which to conduct both prospective and retrospective studies, and for use in clinical decision analysis and development of expert systems. However, because these databases represent mostly local collections of information, any studies will be limited until the databases are linked nationally, providing the foundation, for example, for broader scope decision support systems.

The remainder of this part of the chapter will describe how the above recommendation can be realized through an action plan, consisting of several recommendations for research and applied activities to occur over the coming years.

Existing Data Bases and Sources of Information

There is a wealth of existing databases that are relevant to the activities of basic and clinical oral health researchers. However, there are few, if any, that are designed specifically for the practitioner.

Probably the most accessible and economical source of all biomedical information is the National Library of Medicine, whose computer files consist of more than 20 biomedical databases. MEDLINE is the best known, and contains more than 20 years of bibliographic data from over 3,500 major medical biomedical journals. Of these, over 400 are from the dental field. MEDLINE is easily accessed through GRATEFUL MED, a software package designed to simplify the process of searching the NLM's Medical Literature Analysis and Retrieval System (MEDLARS). In addition to MEDLINE, GRATEFUL MED provides access[3] to references on such subjects as Acquired Immunodeficiency Syndrome (AIDS); audiovisual programs in the health sciences; the cancer literature; over 600,000 records for printed books and serials related to the biomedical sciences; more than 15,000 organizations that act as information resource centers; non-clinical aspects of health care delivery (such as administration and planning of health facilities, services and manpower, and health insurance); and various effects of drugs and related chemicals. The National Institute of Dental Research has developed a database, DENTALPROJ, which contains summaries of ongoing dental research projects funded by such organizations as the NIDR, Department of Veterans Affairs, and Department of Defense. DENTALPROJ is part of MEDLARS and can be accessed through GRATEFUL MED.

Recommendation # 2: Improve the Usefulness of Existing Biomedical Databases for Dental Researchers and Clinicians through DENTLINE

2.1 To facilitate the use of NLM databases by dentists, a system should be developed that contains all references in MEDLARS related to oral health and diseases. This would be called DENTLINE, and made available through GRATEFUL MED.

2.1.1 To make DENTLINE most relevant to dentists, it should contain databases with information about such topics as: (a) new dental products, grouped by clinical area or purpose; (b) drugs most relevant for practitioners; and (c) journal articles, books, and audiovisual resources, grouped by particular oral health topics or dental specialty areas.

2.1.2 Alternately, information could be grouped according to clinical issues, such as: prevention, frequency, cause, assessment for risk, diagnosis of oral diseases; and treatment, its outcome, and its cost-effectiveness.

2.2 In preparation for DENTLINE, research has to be conducted as to who needs and uses information among dental practitioners, when, for what purposes, what is the outcome, who benefits, and how satisfied are the users.

2.3 In addition, an assessment should be made before constructing DENTLINE of the adequacy of dental and oral health coverage in MEDLARS, especially MEDLINE, and the usefulness of the current organizational structure, especially the indexing terms employed for oral health topics using the current structure and content of Medical Subject Headings, or MeSH terms.

For those interested in basic science topics that are not included in MEDLARS, several useful private information retrieval sources are available. These include BIOSIS, CAN/SND, DIALOG, and STN International. Other clinical information retrieval services include Embase plus and PaperChase.

Proposed New System of Organizing Oral Health Information Resources

The types of information contained in MEDLARS that will be accessed through DENTLINE are referred to as bibliographic databases; these are "fact locators" which indicate where the information can be found external to the current database. However, future dentists functioning in a research-based practice also will need access to information that will enable them to perform various computer-assisted procedures, such as decision analysis for diagnosis and treatment planning. This will require expert systems to coordinate operations on vast amounts of linked data that were collected by such efforts as: oral epidemiology studies; health services research; biomedical investigations involving molecular and cell biology; registries for particular diseases; and patients' dental and medical records that contain information from oral and physical examinations, laboratory tests, radiographic and magnetic imaging, treatment provided and its outcome, and so forth. These types of information are collected in factual databases, which consist of structured knowledge that is acquired, processed, stored and disseminated through automated electronic systems. Factual database systems are "fact providers."[4] In the future, all of these data sources will have to be easily accessible to the dental researcher and practitioner. To do so, a new system should be developed.

Recommendation #3: Develop a National Automated Information System of Computer-Based Resources for Oral Health

This system that could be accessed by dentists and researchers via personal computer.

3.1 The particular resources in this central system would include information from such sources as: bibliographic databases (such as MEDLINE, DENTLINE); national and local epidemiological surveys; practice-linked data banks (such as clinical patient records, image data, three-dimensional objects, graphics, text); health services research databases (for example, organization, delivery, and financing of dental care); biomedical research data banks (such as biomolecular databases such as GenBank); and biomedical knowledge bases, consultation systems, and expert decision systems.

The National Library of Medicine (NLM) has begun to develop such a central accessing system for medicine. This effort, started in 1986, is called the Unified Medical Language System (UMLS); its purpose is to facilitate the retrieval and integration of information from many machine-readable sources, such as those listed in recommendation #3.1.[5] The final products will be a thesaurus and a set of computer programs that will be able to compensate for differences in the vocabularies or coding systems used in different computer-based information sources.[6] The NLM is providing the technical expertise and coordinating the system design for the project. However, information to be included in the databases and computer-based resources has to be developed, supplied, and financed by public and private health care organizations or agencies. For example, the American Medical Association is assisting the NLM in obtaining and coordinating information input from the private sector. Currently, there is no dental component to the UMLS.[7]

3.2 Over the next 10-15 years, dental informatics researchers should become involved in activities that will lead to an integrated dental component in the UMLS. This component would be located in the National Automated Information System of Computer-Based Resources for Oral Health.

The next step is to determine which types of databases are needed, and proceed with their development. To initiate this activity, several important research topics now will be discussed for which computer-based resources should be established or improved, information collected and transmitted to the centralized National Automated Information System, where it would be organized, maintained, and prepared for dissemination to the research and practitioner communities.

i) Epidemiology of Oral-Facial Diseases

To date, oral epidemiology has relied mostly on original data collected by clinical examinations that were performed by the investigators themselves or specially trained staff. This may be adequate when such common conditions as caries and periodontal diseases are studied. However, the "new" dentistry will be concerned with oral disorders that are far less prevalent in the general population. Dependence solely on original data collection would be far too costly. Therefore, to obtain large databases on relatively infrequent oral conditions, other epidemiological approaches will have to be utilized.

Recommendation # 4: Initiate New Approaches to Collecting Information About Oral Diseases

4.1 As the scope of oral conditions that come under the domain of dentistry broadens in the future and relatively less common oral and craniofacial disorders come to be studied and treated, it will become increasingly important to develop descriptive databases that utilize such existing data sources as national statistical reports, disease registries, hospital records, third-party claims, and medical records. In addition, there will have to be an increased number of epidemiological surveys of purposive samples or special groups to collect an adequate amount of information about specific conditions so that knowledge bases could be developed for purposes of decision analysis.

4.2 The information must be collected using standardized records, organized into an accessible format, maintained and updated by a central source, and made available to both scientists and clinicians in a user-friendly system.

4.3 A directory of these studies in all relevant areas must be developed, kept current, and disseminated to researchers and clinicians so that multiple sources of information can be easily accessed, when needed, through automated systems.

One approach could utilize computer technology to facilitate the development of an efficient national surveillance system[8] of orofacial conditions to provide current data on trends not only in tooth loss, caries, and periodontal diseases, but also such areas as craniofacial anomalies, temporomandibular disorders, orofacial pain, soft tissue disorders, taste and swallowing dysfunction, salivary diseases, and other orofacial conditions which are within the broadened scope of oral health researchers and dentists. Surveillance systems have been developed in the United States for conditions involving but not specific to the oral cavity,[9] for military populations,[10,11] international oral health,[12,13] and particular types of dental practitioners.[14]

The major need is for standardization and transmission of findings on a systematic basis to a national (or international) focal point. The central agency in the United States could be the Centers for Disease Control, National Institute of Dental Research, National Center for Health Statistics, or National Technical Information Service. These organizations could store and publicize the data bases, and coordinate computer networks to make the information readily accessible to researchers. Eventually, records from virtually every orofacial epidemiological study involving original data collection, when initial analysis is completed, could be routinely stored in this computer bank for dissemination. Data from dental insurance groups also could be added to the bank, if this source would be made available.[15]

The existence of such a national database could stimulate cohort (prospective or longitudinal) and case-control (retrospective) analytical epidemiology studies of less common or relatively rare oral conditions, especially exploration of the etiologies of disorders such as temporomandibular disorders, orofacial pain syndromes, and other oral conditions about which relatively little is known regarding causation.

ii) Risk Assessment

These centralized databases would be very helpful in addressing the high priority research topic of risk assessment and the identification of risk factors for various oral disorders. The situation today appears to require the development of new databases for risk assessment studies. This seems especially true for caries, as stated recently: "For purposes of identifying previously unrecognized risk factors, existing publicly available data bases are unlikely to be of much value. With few exceptions, only variables that concern already recognized risk factors will have been included."[16]

Recommendation # 5: Develop Risk Assessment Databases

5.1 In the future, new approaches to collecting data for risk assessment should be tried. These approaches include:[17]

5.1.1 Collecting data periodically from computerized dental records of a selected group of clinicians distributed throughout the country who are trained to maintain complete records and additional information regarding potential risk factors, including host factors, environmental measures, and behavioral variables;

5.1.2 Coordinating additional data collection with other ongoing studies in related fields where other variables associated with general health are being studied;

5.1.3 Developing central registries, similar to those for cancer, to monitor oral conditions; and

5.1.4 Starting a national database clearinghouse to which state, federal, and individual investigators could submit oral health data for compilation and sharing, thereby facilitating the establishment of small, multisite longitudinal studies of potentially high-risk populations from many different geographic regions.

iii) Clinical Dental Care

The research-based dental practice of the future will depend on a number of concepts taken from clinical decision analysis[18,19] to determine the most appropriate diagnostic tests for particular oral disorders. These include sensitivity (or the proportion of people with a disease who have a positive test for the disease), specificity (or the proportion of people without the disease who have a negative test), predictive value (or the probability of disease, given the results of a diagnostic test - positive or negative predictive value), and accuracy (or the proportion of all test results, both positive and negative, that are correct). For both diagnosis and treatment, quantitative decision-making methods can be utilized. In the clinical situation, these most often include decision analysis (which is based on probabilities for particular outcomes of alternate courses of action), and cost-effectiveness analysis, (which determines the monetary costs and effects on quality of life for alternative courses of action to achieve a particular health outcome).[20,21] These concepts have been employed in various areas of dentistry, including caries detection,[22] surgery,[23,24] endodontics,[25,26] pulp capping,[27] medication of special patients,[28] periodontal diseases,[29] dental pain,[30] general dentistry,[31] and dental radiography.[32,33,34,35,36,37] However, information specifically collected for these types of databases is rarely found.[38]

Recommendation # 6: Develop Databases for Decision Analysis

6.1 To provide the data which can be used by practitioners to determine the values and knowledge bases needed for constructing decision analytic models and expert systems, especially in cases of less common oral conditions, it will be necessary to develop a set of standardized clinical recording formats to be used in all studies involving particular conditions. Assuming this standardization can be achieved, findings from studies of similar conditions could be combined to provide an adequate sample size for requisite analyses.

6.2 A central source should be identified where the results from many previous small investigations could be stored, organized, and managed. The studies preferably would be of the cohort, case-control or prevalence types; however, they may be merely observational studies from dentists' practices, as long as standardized recording formats are used. Depending on the disorders, clinical data in these studies could be comprised of results from oral examination, laboratory tests, magnetic imaging, radiographs, study casts, biopsies, DNA probes, or any of the myriad other types of new biotechnology techniques developed using molecular and cell biology.

6.3 The system should have an image display capability for this database, so that pictures, radiographs, and results from various newer imaging techniques are able to be transferred to videodisc, fully integrated into the database, and completely accessible to all users. There have been very few such systems developed for oral diseases and conditions.[39]

iv) Health Services Research

Recommendation # 7: Develop Databases for Health Services Research

7.1 National, regional and state data concerning the delivery and financing of dental care should be collected in the national automated information system of computer-based resources for oral health. These data can be provided by governmental agencies, purchasers of care in the private sector, insurance organizations, and group dental and medical-dental practices.[40] The existence of such a repository for data will enable access to on-line information by oral health services researchers for such topics as utilization rates, services mix, and costs for various combinations of providers, population groups, and payment sources.

7.2 Resources collected as part of the epidemiological and clinical care data banks discussed previously would be accessible to health services researchers using the national information system. The availability of larger databases will enable more experimental designs, rather than the traditional survey and descriptive methods, for research involving such areas as utilization of dental services, quality assurance and assessment, appropriateness of care, alternate delivery systems, needs of special population groups, satisfaction with care, standards of care for general and specialty practices, cost-effectiveness and cost benefit analyses.[41]

v) Biotechnology Information Resources

Molecular and cell biology have had major effects on oral health research. For example, recombinant DNA techniques have greatly contributed to our understanding of the structural regulatory genes related to the expression of dental tissues during craniofacial development. The methods and results from various studies employing these techniques soon will be used "for the synthetic production of dental biomaterials, for the augmentation or replacement therapy of dental diseases - enamel, dentin, and cementum replacement, facilitation of periodontal tissue attachment to tooth surfaces, and overt replacement of alveolar bone."[42]

Over the past few years, there has been a spurt of research in the area of biological markers for detecting oral conditions, with an emphasis on DNA probes for periodontal diseases,[43,44,45,46,47,48] and on microbiological or immunological markers for salivary pathology,[49,50] periodontal diseases,[51,52,53,54] dental cysts,[55] and dental caries.[56,57,58]

However, problems have arisen in biotechnology research as genetic and biochemical information has appeared much faster than it can be published in the scientific literature. Data production is expected to increase by at least a thousand times in the next five years alone.[59] To accomodate all this new knowledge in molecular and cell biology and assist in its dissemination, basic researchers have become increasingly dependent on automated tools to store and manipulate the massive bodies of data describing the structure and function of important substances. Many information resources recently have become available, including computer-assisted data banks for sequences of nucleic acids, proteins, and carbohydrates; molecular structure; human genetic maps; restriction enzymes, vectors, microbial strains, cell lines, and hybridomas. By 1989, there were over 50 such information resources in biotechnology.[60]

The National Library of Medicine has established several programs to coordinate these activities and provide retrieval of information from several different sources related to the same concept. These include the National Center for Biotechnology Information (NCBI), an intramural component that serves as both a repository and distribution center and as a laboratory for developing new information analysis and communication tools needed for advancement in the field. The NLM also has developed a Directory of Biotechnology Information Resources (DBIR) which, in 1989, contained over 1,400 separate descriptions of information resources describing a broad spectrum of biotechnology resources relating to medicine, molecular biology, microbiology, and other sciences. The directory is easily accessible by computer.

Recommendation # 8: Develop Data Resources for Molecular Biology Studies of Oral Disorders

8.1 To facilitate future oral health research, there should be a specific sub-section of the resource bases maintained by the NCBI and DBIR for basic science information related to oral conditions.

8.2 Specific molecular, cellular, and microbiological research results about the orofacial area or conditions should be forwarded by oral health scientists for inclusion in these databases.

8.3 Researchers and clinicians should be able to combine these biotechnology resources with the epidemiology and clinical care databases described previously by accessing the national automated information system of computer-based resources for oral health. Various types of expert systems could be used to facilitate the retrieval.

Since future practitioners will be educated in the molecular and cellular bases of oral health and disease, they will be able to use the combined information from this proposed resource base for clinical decision analyses in developing diagnoses and assessing risk among patients, thereby expanding further the research basis of clinical practice.

B) Applying Computer Technology to Generating Information in Oral Health Research and Delivery of Clinical Care

The second, and most frequent way so far, that informatics has been employed in dentistry involves computer-assisted approaches to generating information about various aspects of oral health research and dental practice. These include developing tools for and conducting research in such areas as (i) simulation modeling, (ii) diagnostic and therapeutic decision-making, (iii) interpretation and processing of radiographic and magnetic images, and (iv) design and manufacture of dental restorations and prostheses.

i) Computer Simulation for Research and Practice

One of the most frequent informatics technologies applied to oral health involves the use of computers to simulate various clinical conditions. In applied clinical research, computer simulation has been used recently for such purposes as predicting results of: orthodontic procedures,[61] surgery[62,63] occlusal adjustment,[64,65] and medication.[66]

In more basic investigations, computer simulations have been employed recently for developing and testing biological models of: tooth eruption,[67] structure of periodontal ligament fibers,[68] occurrence of periodontal breakdown,[69] caries development,[70] and clearance of fluoride from the oral cavity.[71]

ii) Computer-Assisted Decisions for Diagnosis and Treatment

Another common usage of computer technology in dental research and practice has been to develop diagnostic and treatment expert systems and decision models for particular oral conditions. These have included: general oral medicine,[72,73,74,75] orthodontic disorders,[76,77,78,79,80,81] periodontal diseases,[82,83] care of high-risk patients,[84] surgery,[85] jaw diseases,[86,87] craniomandibular disorders,[88] facial pain,[89,90] endodontics,[91] and salivary gland diseases.[92]

iii) Computer-Assisted Image Interpretation and Processing

Computer technology has been applied extensively to clinical dentistry and oral health research in the area of imaging methods — the use of computers to assist in the processing of radiographic, magnetic, and other types of images, and in their interpretation for developing diagnosis and monitoring treatment.

The most frequently applied techniques in dental research and practice include digital subtraction radiography, especially for studies in periodontology,[93,94,95,96,97,98] endodontics,[99,100] cariology,[101] and salivary gland diseases;[102] X-ray computed tomography for studies in temporomandibular disorders,[103,104] implantology,[105,106,107,108,109] oral-maxillofacial surgery,[110] and salivary gland diseases;[111,112] and magnetic resonance imaging for studies in facial pain and temporomandibular disorders,[113,114,115,116,117] and salivary gland pathology.[118]

Other examples of specific oral health research applications of computerized imaging techniques include: classification of periodontal diseases,[119] epidemiological investigations of periodontal diseases,[120] computer-based thermal imaging of human gingiva,[121] measurement of tooth root surfaces,[122,123] evaluation of bone resorption through radiographic changes by computer-assisted densitometric image analysis (CADIA),[124,125,126,127,128] determination of the level of alveolar bone height;[129,130] examination of dentinal lesions;[131] development of microcomputer systems for analysing dental radiographs,[132] evaluation of the RadioVisioGraphy system,[133] general digital image processing and transmission methods;[134,135,136] evaluation of surgical procedures,[137] estimation of outcomes for various types of surgical treatments for cosmetic dentistry procedures;[138] screening of the quality of dental restorations using new biomaterials;[139] computer analysis of radiographs regarding tooth positions and soft tissue profiles,[140] study of the usefulness of computer-aided photograph analysis (CAPA) for demonstrating intraoral tissue changes;[141] study of root canal morphology;[142] diagnosis of craniomandibular disorders;[143] and detection of malignancy among salivary gland tumors[144]

iv) Computer Technology in Restorative Dentistry

One of the more promising research frontiers with direct applicability to clinical practice lies in restorative dentistry. The most exciting advance, computer-aided design and computer-aided manufacturing (CAD/CAM), integrates engineering aspects of automation to create dental prostheses and restorations. A CAD/CAM system eliminates the need for impressions, temporary prostheses, dies, castings, and laboratory assistance, and completes the entire procedure in one appointment.[145,146,147] These systems have also been used for designing dental implants,[148] and have a potential for other types of prosthetic rehabilitation devices for soft and hard tissues.[149,150] All of these procedures may eventually be performed by "robotic" techniques and computer-assisted surgery.[151]

Recommendation # 9: Apply Computer Technology to Generating Information in Oral Health and Diseases

9.1 Basic and applied oral health research should be pursued for such areas as: computer simulation modeling; computer-assisted diagnostic and therapeutic decision-making; computer-assisted interpretation, processing and application of imaging techniques, such as digital subtraction radiography, X-ray computed tomography, and magnetic resonance imaging; and computer-assisted restorative dentistry.

9.2 Information about or generated by research in these areas should be incorporated in the proposed national automated information system of computer-based resources for oral health.

9.3 Where appropriate, every effort should be made to link and integrate materials and information developed in these areas with resources from the epidemiology, clinical care, health services, biotechnology, and DENTLINE information bases discussed in Recommendation # 2.

9.3.1 Expert systems should be developed to assist in the integration process.

9.3.2 Evaluation should be conducted to determine the effect of the database linkages on resulting research or clinical performance of users of the information system.

C) Creating a Cadre of Well-Trained Researchers in Dental Informatics

To pursue research in the areas delineated above, it is essential to have a well-trained group of available dental informaticians. These individuals also could serve on study sections and review groups of the major funding agencies that consider research proposals in dental informatics. However, there are few people at present who are able to articulate dentistry with computers and health care with information science. The National Library of Medicine does support several training programs, either through institutional or individual fellowship awards. In 1989, over fifty postdoctoral and predoctoral trainees were supported; only one was a dentist.

Based on the curriculum for medical informatics training programs[152] and the research topics discussed above, a core curriculum in dental informatics research training might consist of subjects such as the following: (1) clinical dentistry (meaning the dental or related degree); (2) oral epidemiology; (3) research methodology; (4) basic computer science (programming languages, symbolic systems, machine architecture, data structures, and artificial intelligence; (5) basic decision making (basic probability theory, Bayesian statistics, decision analysis, and experimental design techniques); (6) applied computer science in health care delivery (state of the art and future frontiers of medical and dental computing; computer applications in dentistry and medicine; computer-assisted medical decision making; dental and medical applications of Bayesian statistics, decision analysis and artificial intelligence); (7) a major programming project to develop an actual system using expert system shells, decision analysis software, and standard programming language; and (8) health policy and social issues (topics related to national health policy, health care financing, ethics, and pertinent legal topics).

II. Potential Sources of Funding in the United States for Dental Informatics Research

There are at least three possible Federal support sources for dental informatics research in the United States, depending on the particular activity. These are the National Institute of Dental Research, National Library of Medicine, and Agency for Health Care Policy and Research.

National Institute of Dental Research

The National Institute of Dental Research (NIDR) would be a potential funding source for investigations of oral health issues that seek to: 1) generate basic science, clinical, behavioral, and epidemiological information which could be included in the proposed national automated information system of computer-based resources for oral health and in DENTLINE; 2) utilize and analyze the data included in various knowledge resource bases to investigate oral health issues; 3) develop and/or apply to oral health research and practice computer-assisted approaches for such techniques as simulation modeling, decision analysis, image processing and interpretation, and clinical dentistry; and 4) disseminate contents of the national information system.

The recent NIDR portfolio includes several studies that apply informatics and computer technology to oral health research topics. Below are a sample of the informatics and computer-assisted research topics that have been supported by NIDR grants between 1988-1990.

a) Generating and compiling information for local data banks and centers in the following topics:

- genetic aspects of cleft lip and palate
- localized juvenile periodontitis
- skeletal muscle transplants
- dental composites
- unified computer coding system for microbial information
- clinical dental data combined with service utilization data for an elderly male population
- oral facial trauma

b) Computer Simulation Modeling

- constructing molecular structures generated by computer modeling to define the relationships between conformation of salivary molecules and their biological functions
- elucidating molecular structure-taste relationships among various peptide sweeteners through nuclear magnetic resonance imaging, computer simulation, biosysnthesis, spectroscopy, and other such techniques
- using computer-assisted molecular sequence analysis to develop a simulation model for the structure of the receptors for oral bacterial adhesins involved in periodontitis
- investigating the behavior of epithelial stem cells in   mice through computer simulation in conjunction with cell   labeling, autoradiography, tissue culture and other techniques
- developing a microsimulation model to forecast tooth loss, dental health conditions, and dental services use for a national population and sub-populations based on age, sex, socioeconomic status, and other such variables

- simulating natural tooth appearance properties in crown and bridge restorations
- investigating the applicability of computer solids modeling to restorative dentistry and orthodontics by developing a device to capture the three-dimensional geometry of the oral cavity in digital form
- testing the reliability and validity of constructing computer synthesized three-dimensional cephalometric landmark data, through steriophotogrammetry
- adapting three-dimensional CT scans and facial light scans for surgical simulation software and the analysis of surface form for the treatment of congenital craniofacial anomalies
- developing computer simulation models to predict both growth and form patterns in craniofacial structure and nasorespiratory function, using a longitudinal database created through NIDR support

c) Systems to store and integrate clinical data:

- storing and integrating data from physical measurement, graphics, three-dimensional techniques, photographs, radiographic images, cast models, and text for various treatments of dentofacial defects (such as malocclusions and osseous dysphasias)
- collecting longitudinal cephalometric data sets on normal, abnormal and altered growth and development in humans and other primates

d) Imaging techniques to assess oral diseases:

- performing automated assessment of adult periodontal diseases by computer digital imaging of bitewing radiographs, via sophisticated image processing hardware and software from NASA's LANDSAT satellite remote sensing instruments
- developing a computerized dental radiographic system to produce images which can be subtracted to show small changes in tissues occurring over long intervals of time
- using computer-assisted enhancement of bite-wing radiographs to improve consistency of diagnosis of alveolar bone loss
- reconstructing CAT scans of skeletal and soft tissue anatomy of patients with craniofacial anomalies to three-dimensional forms by a CEMAX-1 computer system, which will summate the 3-D slices from areas of interest and calculate volume
- elucidating the structure of salivary cycloneoglycopeptides using nuclear magnetic resonance spectroscopy (NMR), X-ray crystallography, and computer modeling
- developing the foundations of a standardized methodology to optimally acquire, process, and interpret magnetic resonance images of the temporomandibular joint, and subsequently implementing these image

processing techniques to further aid in localizing and characterizing certain anatomical structures in the joint

e) Computerized techniques for clinical dentistry:

- developing a system for computer-aided design and manufacture of dental restorations (CAD/CAM) that will be capable of automating the currently practiced restoration fabrication techniques from impression through final restoration (system will utilize robotics, three-dimensional vision systems, stereophotogrammetry, computer graphics, and computer integrated engineering)

- developing and testing the merit and feasibility of interactive videodiscs in preparing patients for orthognathic surgery, TMJ surgery, orthodontics in preparation for surgery, third molar extractions, osseointegrated implants, and full-mouth extraction followed by immediate dentures

Thus the NIDR has supported research that involves the application of informatics techniques and computer-assisted approaches to oral health topics, usually in combination with other types of technology.

National Library of Medicine

The National Library of Medicine (NLM) is the central Federal organization for the medical informatics field. In addition to its own extramural and intramural programs, the NLM works closely with the rest of the National Institutes of Health and other government agencies to complement their information dissemination and knowledge-management activities. The NLM encourages co-funding or research with other appropriate NIH Institutes for projects that would have a "major positive impact in both the field of primary study and the medical informatics field."[153] Priorities include clinical research studies using decision-support and expert system technologies. In the field of medical informatics, the NLM is interested especially in research that combines health specialty knowledge with the information and computer sciences, computational linguistics, and cognitive science to investigate fundamental questions about information in decision-making, innovative systems for maintaining and retrieving biotechnology information, the planning and operation of large-scale institution-wide integrated information networks, and the development of basic information access services at local and smaller health facilities. The NLM also supports research training in informatics. Regarding the issues about dental informatics discussed in this chapter, the NLM probably would be the primary source of support and technical expertise for constructing the system of computer-based resources for managing oral health research information, as well as any fundamental research in decision-making and expert systems.

Agency for Health Care Policy and Research

The Agency for Health Care Policy and Research (AHCPR, formerly the National Center for Health Services Research and Health Care Technology Assessment) in the U.S. Public Health Service supports studies on the outcomes of health care services and procedures used to prevent, diagnose, treat, and manage illness and disability. This includes the use of decision analysis, and the design and development of new data bases and enhancement of existing data bases that are useful for patient outcomes research and clinical decision-making. New data sets may be primarily clinical, epidemiological, economic, administrative, or a combination. They may consist of original data or a new combination of existing data. They may constitute prototypical research resources, or serve as registries for treatments that are new or have not been previously studied. Enhancements to existing data bases should make them more useful for patient outcomes research by the addition of pertinent new variables or cases, or by linkages with other data sets. An important aspect of data base development is the standardization of concepts and measures to facilitate aggregation and/or comparison of data from different sources and the standardization of methods to adjust or control for variables that change over time. The AHCPR also supports research intended to identify the relative effectiveness of various ways to disseminate research findings to diverse audiences and to evaluate the effect of alternative dissemination strategies. Regarding dental informatics, AHCPR would be the primary source of support for research in the area of health services, and probably for developing certain data bases, testing and evaluating information systems, and identifying innovative ways for disseminating knowledge resources to dental practitioners.

III. Considerations When Submitting Dental Informatics Research Proposals for Funding

A) Basic Elements for Any Research Proposal

There are certain basic elements of a successful grant application, regardless of the funding source. These have been discussed elsewhere[154,155,156] and will only be summarized here.

The most successful research is that which is hypothesis-generated and directed towards an important issue, problem, or mechanism of action. The hypothesis should be testable (able to be proved or disproved by the proposed experiments), and its rationale well defined. Each hypothesis should have a set of focused aims clearly and uniquely related to it. Similarly, the research methods should be specifically related to each aim. The scope of work proposed should be achievable in the proposed grant period. The next logical stage of research beyond the currently proposed project should always be identified. In general, observational research should be avoided, since that is usually just a data gathering exercise.

The experimental design of a research project includes the study and control groups, technical methodology, data collection procedures, and data management and analysis. These are the areas in which shortcomings are most often found in applications submitted to the NIH. Each experiment should be responsive to a specific aim and fit into a reasonable overall approach. Justification and rationale should be provided for the particular methods selected, and then compare this approach with related alternative methods. In any methodological approach, appropriate and available controls should be selected, avoiding methods with excessive, noncritical selection. It is most important to design the experiment to gather the data in a manner which will answer the questions needed to test the hypothesis.

A critical assessment of the proposed work must be shown. For example, there should be a clear exposition of the assumptions and limitations of the planned research; possible problems and the planned solutions should be identified; the precise criteria for evaluating when a specific test is a success or failure must be defined.

The statistical aspects of the application must be addressed correctly. For example, precision and accuracy of the proposed methods must be clearly defined. Statistical power calculations should be used, when appropriate, to determine the number and type of experiments.

The principal investigator and staff must demonstrate their qualifications and experience in the area of proposed research through previously published research, thorough familiarity with the literature, preliminary data, and appropriate collaborations at levels of commitment sufficient to assure success.

Finally, there should be reasonable availability at the investigator's institutional setting of resources (support staff, laboratory/clinical facilities, equipment, access to patient populations) necessary to the proposed research.

B) Specific Criteria for Research Proposals in Medical/Dental Informatics

Practically all medical informatics research grants in the United States are supported by the National Library of Medicine. Therefore the particular considerations by members of the NIH peer review group which assesses applications for the NLM in the area of informatics should be examined.[157] In addition to the general issues described above, there are several other points that are relevant for research in medical/dental informatics.

The first point concerns the selection of a topic. The ultimate goal of every informatics research project should be to open a new segment of biomedical knowledge or a new aspect of clinical practice to computer-based accessibility. The topic selected should be one where either an interesting new methodology can be applied convincingly and/or a biomedical dilemma exists. Further, the methodology should have implications beyond a single implementation of the proposed project. As recommended in its Long Range Plan, the NLM places maximum emphasis on basic issues and fundamental work in the research it supports. Awardees are expected to make contributions to science, and not just adapt an existing technique to a new problem or area[158] (they should not modify or apply an expert clinical decision analysis system developed for a particular medical problem to a dental situation, since this will likely produce no new insights). A strong justification must be provided for why the proposed work will represent a significant advancement over any similar previous projects. "The problem selected should be neither a simplistic program that is useful to a minimal area of biomedicine nor a sophisticated, complex computer science approach to a trivial health problem."[157]

The second step is to design the research project. It is essential to provide details about the following: (i) the intended field and scope of the informatics program's data/knowledge base; (ii) the size of the data/knowledge base in representative units (such as patients in sample, conditions covered, and decision rules); (iii) examples detailing the structure and function of data/knowledge base units, using nontrivial medical/dental examples taken from the intended project topic; (iv) realistic assessments of the amount of programming, programmer's time, and medical/dental experts' time required to design and/or construct the program's data/knowledge base; (v) examples of the proposed man-machine interface and the structure of an interactive session; (vi) a realistic appraisal of how the data/knowledge base will be maintained over time, how rapidly will the base's contents become obsolete, and how will errors of omission and commission be detected and corrected; (vii) description of a specific evaluation procedure for the project, especially testing the knowledge base with real patient data, and specifying in detail which aspects of the system are (and are not) to be evaluated and when, how, and where the evaluation will be done.

IV. Dental Informatics Research and the Practicing Dentist

One of the basic premises of this chapter is that research in dental informatics ultimately should be relevant to the specific information needs of dental practitioners. The future dentist will have to be able to access, assimilate, and utilize the multitude of findings from basic and clinical research. This must be attainable through a system that is relatively easy to employ and fulfills specific needs inherent in the delivery of care. Information dissemination to the clinician will be accomplished most often through automated data systems and electronic computer networks. These will help to make the practitioner aware of the most current knowledge, research findings, biomaterials, medications and techniques that are relevant for particular clinical conditions and oral health issues which will be found in future patient populations.

To develop the most useful and acceptable automated information system(s), the first tasks of dental informatics researchers will include: (a) identifying the perceived information needs of clinicians; (b) constructing processes and approaches to provide knowledge that will meet these needs in a way that will be willingly integrated into practice by most dentists; and (c) testing and evaluating the effectiveness and usefulness of the systems that are developed. These tasks will require a joint effort among dental practitioners and researchers from at least the behavioral and information sciences.

Initially, research will focus on the application of computers in dental practice, since information transmission in the clinical setting will occur primarily through such automated technology. In several recent surveys about computers in the dental office,[159,160] practitioners indicated that the most important uses of a computer were mainly administrative and business management functions, such as scheduling appointments, billing, maintaining patient records and accounts payable, preparing correspondence, and processing third-party insurance claims electronically. Very few respondents utilized computers for purposes such as providing access to relevant clinical information that could be used for diagnosis or treatment planning. (It should be noted that this is most likely due to the dearth of existing programs that perform these functions.) When asked about possible additional needs that could be met by computers, suggestions included computer-generated marketing reports to help build or increase a practice, such as referral sources and patient demographics, clinically-related software as for periodontal charting and cephalometric tracing, and business or clinical programs that worked via voice recognition. These surveys, as well as numerous other articles about computers in dentistry frequently found in the "popular" dental magazines and publications usually read by practitioners,[161] seem to indicate that the current major applications and interests are mostly for practice management activities.

However, more rigorous, methodologically-sound studies must be conducted by social scientists, with extensive assistance from clinicians, regarding the perceived uses for computers in practice and types of information felt to be needed by different segments of the dental community.

Since most dentists are not currently utilizing (and are most likely not even aware of the existence of) such information sources as MEDLINE, efforts should be made to introduce clinicians to the types of knowledge that could be obtained through these sources. This would have to be done through the development and testing of clinically relevant databases and user-friendly systems that are easily applied in the office by all members of the dental team. A cadre of practicing dentists should be recruited to assist at every step of the development process.

Several groups of interested clinicians throughout the country should be identified by researchers and encouraged to participate in activities such as the following:

A. Development of Information Systems

1. Become familiar with existing systems such as MEDLINE using GRATE-FUL MED. Practitioners could then indicate other types of information that they would find useful to receive through such an approach.

2. Develop practice-oriented and user-friendly knowledge bases. These should provide at least: (a) assistance about what to do in various situations, when to do it, and how to interpret clinical evidence; (b) access to large quantities of information that combine such clinically relevant information as image data, graphics, three-dimensional objects, and text. Such a system was discussed earlier in Recommendation Number 2, which proposed a clinical-biomedical database for dentists called DENTLINE. Practicing dentists should be involved in constructing such a system if it is to succeed.

3. Initiate prototype projects to integrate diverse information database systems, such as in clinical decision-support research for various oral conditions.

4. Establish electronic network communication systems so that information dissemination and specific collaborations can take place rapidly and conveniently.

B. *Participate in the Accumulation of Information Related to Risk Assessment*

1. Develop a standardized patient dental record that, in addition to oral, medical and personal background data, contains information about potential risk factors, including particular host factors, environmental measures, and behavioral variables.

2. Establish an electronic communication system whereby such data would be collected periodically from computerized dental records of a selected group of clinicians throughout the country who have been educated to maintain complete records. The information would be stored in a national database clearinghouse, and could be accessed by clinicians, researchers, private industry (such as insurance companies), and governmental agencies. The information could be incorporated into DENTLINE or other such systems.

As core groups of knowledgable dental clinicians are identified (or, perhaps initially, trained through various continuing education offerings), they will be able to develop and maintain a partnership with informaticians in academia and private industry to pursue together research activities such as those described earlier in this chapter. In this way, the dental profession, through informatics, will be better able to realize the potential that exists for the "new" dentistry in the coming decade.

V. A Proposed Strategic, Long-Range Plan for Dental Informatics Research

To close this chapter, a strategic, long-range research plan for dental informatics is proposed. The plan has been developed by abstracting and integrating parts of the nine overall recommendations offered earlier according to whether they can be pursued or started in the short-term (the next two to three years), intermediate-term (over the coming three to ten years), or long-term (within the next 10-20 years). Several long-range activities not discussed in the chapter also have been included.

Short-Term Objectives (to be started within the next two to three years)

1. Determine the various needs and uses of information among dental practitioners: who, when, for what purposes, what is the outcome, who benefits, and how satisfied are the users.

a) Identify additional types of information in which dentists would be interested.

b) Identify types of existing databases utilized by practicing physicians or faculty in dental and medical schools that might be relevant to practicing dentists.

2. Investigate the feasibility of developing prototypes for practice-oriented and user-friendly knowledge bases oriented primarily to the information needs of dental practitioners, based on the results from the previous objective. Initial efforts should focus on the utilization of MEDLARS and GRATEFUL MED.

a) Assess the adequacy of dental and oral health coverage in MEDLARS, especially MEDLINE, and the usefulness of the current organizational structure, especially the indexing terms employed for oral health topics using the current structure and content of Medical Subject Headings, or MeSH terms.

b) Improve, where necessary, the coverage and utility of the existing biomedical databases in MEDLARS.

3. Establish electronic network communications, using automated information systems, through oral health research and dental practitioner communities so that information dissemination and specific collaborations can take place rapidly and conveniently.

4. Initiate new approaches to collecting information about oral diseases

a) Develop descriptive databases that utilize records from such existing data sources as national statistical reports, disease registries, hospital records, third-party claims, and medical records.

b) Perform epidemiological surveys of purposive samples or special groups to collect an adequate amount of information about specific conditions encompassed by the broadened scope of dentistry, so that national knowledge bases could be developed at a later time for purposes of decision analysis.

5. Begin local or national training programs in dental informatics.

6. Apply computer technology to the prevention, diagnosis and treatment of oral conditions and diseases

a) Develop computer-assisted systems to investigate oral health topics. Areas of research can include:

- simulation modeling
- diagnostic and therapeutic decision-making
- interpretation, processing and application of imaging techniques, such as digital subtraction radiography, X-ray computed tomography, and magnetic resonance imaging
- robotics, for use in restorative dentistry
- speech recognition systems, for charting of clinical examination data

Intermediate-Term Objectives (to be initiated during the coming three to ten years)

1. Develop a knowledge base system that contains at least all references in MEDLARS related to oral health and diseases. This could be called DENTLINE, and made available through GRATEFUL MED or a similar mechanism.

DENTLINE would contain databases with information about such topics as: (a) new dental products; (b) drugs most relevant for practitioners; and (c) major new clinically-relevant research findings from journal articles, books, news conferences and releases reported in the popular press, and other sources. Information could be grouped according to clinical issues, such as: prevention, frequency, cause, assessment for risk, diagnosis of oral diseases; treatment, its outcome, and its cost-effectiveness. Alternately, data could be classified by specific conditions/diseases, or clinical specialty.

2. Develop new approaches to collecting data for risk assessment databases.

a) Collect data periodically from computerized dental records of a selected group of clinicians distributed throughout the country who are trained to maintain complete, standardized records and additional information regarding potential risk factors, including host factors, environmental measures, and behavioral variables.

b) Coordinate additional data collection with other ongoing studies in related fields where other variables associated with general health are being studied.

c) Develop central registries, similar to those for cancer, to monitor oral conditions.

d) Establish a national data clearinghouse to which state, federal, and individual investigators could submit oral health data for compilation and sharing, thereby facilitating the establishment of small, multisite longitudinal studies of potentially high-risk populations from many different geographic regions.

3. Develop national databases and systems for decision analysis.

a) Develop standardized clinical recording formats to be used in all studies involving particular conditions.

b) Combine findings from studies of similar conditions to provide an adequate sample size for requisite analyses. This will be necessary to provide the data which can be used by practitioners to determine the values and knowledge bases needed for constructing decision analytic models and expert systems, especially in cases of less common oral conditions.

c) Identify a central source where the results from many previous small investigations could be stored, organized and managed.

d) Include in the system an image display capability so that pictures, radiographs, and results from various newer imaging techniques are able to be transferred to videodisc, fully integrated into the database, and completely accessible to all users.

4. Develop databases for health services research.

a) Collect national, regional and state data concerning the delivery and financing of dental/oral health care, including quality assurance and analysis of cost-effectiveness. These data can be provided by governmental agencies, purchasers of care in the private sector, insurance organizations, and group dental and medical-dental practices.

5. Develop data storage resources for molecular biological studies of oral disorders and conditions.

a) Collect in one central repository specific molecular, cellular, and microbiological research results about the orofacial area or conditions that have been submitted by oral health scientists.

6. Prepare and maintain a directory of studies in all relevant areas that can be disseminated to researchers and clinicians so that multiple sources of information can be easily accessed, when needed, through automated systems.

Long-Term Objectives (to be started within the next 10-20 years)

1. Develop an integrated National Automated Information System of Computer-Based Resources for Oral Health that could be accessed by dentists and researchers via personal computer.

a) Integrate information from databases and resources developed during the intermediate phase of the plan, such as: bibliographic databases; national and local epidemiological surveys; practice-linked data banks; health services research databases; biomedical research data banks; and biomedical knowledge bases, consultation systems, and decision analysis systems. Various types of expert systems could be used to facilitate the retrieval.

b) Work closely with the National Library of Medicine (NLM) on activities that will lead to an integrated dental component in the Unified Medical Language System (UMLS), and other aspects of the NLM overall effort. This component would be accessible through the proposed national information system.

c) Develop a system to continually incorporate the most current information into the national automated information system.

d) Develop expert systems to assist in the integration process.

2. Develop and conduct an extensive, ongoing evaluation program to assess the effect of database linkages on resulting research and clinical performance of those who utilize the information system.

3. Improve the methods of information collection and dissemination in the dental office through such technologies as voice- or speech-generated systems for requesting and obtaining information from central repositories, and super computers for pooling and analysis of data and facilitating decision-making processes.

4. Enhance the use of computer-assisted clinical procedures for diagnostics (e.g., analysing molecular and cellular probes, and imaging intra- and extra-oral structures), and treatment (such as simulating aesthetic and anatomical outcomes, and employing robotic techniques for such areas as prosthetics, endodontics, orthodontics, and maxillofacial surgery).

VI. Summary and Conclusion

In the near future, dentistry will be responsible for the prevention, diagnosis, and management of a much broader scope of orofacial diseases and conditions than at present. The practitioner will employ routinely such approaches as molecular and cellular biology for diagnosis, and computer-assisted technology, lasers, and improved biomaterials for treatment. The field of informatics will be of great relevance to this "new" type of dental practice for several reasons. One is that the rapidly increasing knowledge base which will form the basis of clinical practice soon will become practically unmanageable by most of the current, nonautomated methods. Second, appropriate application of this burgeoning information to clinical practice will necessitate greater emphasis on the processes of informed decision-making and problem solving.[162] The major focus of this chapter was on nine research recommendations for dental informatics that would be helpful in achieving the typical automated dental practice of the future, as described elsewhere.[163] Based on these recommendations, a three-stage strategic plan for dental informatics research was proposed.

The first stage consisted of several short-term goals which established the groundwork for future activities. They concerned:

- identifying information needs perceived by practitioners, researchers, and informatics experts
- developing prototype methods to collect, store, and disseminate the needed information
- determining and constructing various computer technologies that might be applicable to future dental practice and research
- establishing programs to train and educate clinicians and researchers in the field of informatics

The second stage, or intermediate-term goals, concentrated on the development of methods for collecting, maintaining, and communicating an extensive set of specific knowledge bases and other information resources that would facilitate the following for the dental practitioner and scientist:

- obtaining the most current information about basic and clinical research
- assessing the risk of disease occurrence in private practice or community populations
- performing such procedures as decision analysis, quality assurance, and cost-effectiveness analysis

The third stage, or long-term objectives, involved the construction of a method that integrated the large variety of informatics products developed during the previous two phases. A National Automated Information System of Computer-Based Resources for Oral Health was proposed for this purpose. Other long-range goals were the establishment of a mechanism to evaluate the integration of informatics, clinical practice, and research; and preparation of several new types of computer-assisted technologies that could improve the delivery of care in the dental practice.

Realistically, it is not possible to predict accurately the future status of dental informatics or what the major themes will even be for a period beyond several years from now. The future of dental informatics will depend on such factors as the following:

1) Changes in the level and sophistication of computer technology and information science, such as what types of hardware and software will be available, and

how extensively developers and manufacturers will adapt the technoloqy to information needs of dentists;

2) Changes in medical informatics, from which many of the ideas and techniques for dental informatics will come;

3) Information and technology needs and interests of dentists, which will be shaped by such things as:

- the organization of dental practice in the future (primarily solo, partnership or large group structure)
- economic situation, involving the number of practicing dentists and their business; income levels; and most common types of payment mechanisms - fee-for-service, third-party reimbursement
- scope of diseases and conditions treated
- delivery of care - continued emphasis on primarily technical skills or shift to more diagnostic and medical orientation; mainly general practitioners, or increased number of clinical specialists and even appearance of new clinical specialties
- state of scientific and clinical knowledge

Other topics discussed in this chapter involved potential sources of funding in the United States for dental informatics research, considerations when submitting dental informatics research proposals to funding agencies, and ways that dental practitioners could become involved in informatics research.

In conclusion, pursuit of the dental informatics research activities recommended in this chapter should facilitate acceptance of informatics and computer technology throughout dental practice and research. With this foundation, the profession will be better prepared to assume the expanded scope of activities that should lead to the exciting "new" dentistry envisioned for the coming century.

References

1. Salley JJ, Zimmerman JL, Ball, MJ., eds. Dental informatics: strategic issues for the dental profession. Berlin: Springer Verlag, 1990.
2. This is adapted from the National Library of Medicine. Long Range Plan, Report of Panel 4: Medical Informatics. National Institutes of Health, 1986.
3. National Library of Medicine. GRATEFUL MED - User's Guide, Version 5.0. Bethesda, MD: U.S. Department of Health and Human Services, National Institutes of Health, 1990.
4. National Library of Medicine. Long Range Plan - Report of the Board of Regents. Bethesda: National Institutes of Health. 1987; p.25.
5. Humphreys BL and Lindberg DAB. Building the unified medical language system. In: Kingsland LC, ed. Proceedings - the thirteenth annual symposium on computer applications in medical care. Washington: IEEE Computer society Press, 1989: p. 475-480.
6. Barnett 0. Computers in medicine. J Amer Med Assoc. 1990; 263:2631-2633.

7. Lindberg DAB. Keynote address: informatics in dentistry. In: Salley JJ, Zimmerman JL, Ball, MJ, eds. Dental informatics: strategic issues for the dental profession. Berlin: SpringerVerlag, 1990; p. 9-16.

8. Burt BA, Albino JE, Carlos JP, et al. Advances in the epidemiological study of oral-facial diseases. AdV Dent Res. 1989; 3:30-41.

9. Bhat M, Li SH. Consumer product-related tooth injuries treated in hospital emergency rooms: United States, 1979-87. Community Dent Oral Epidemiol. 1990; 18:133-138.

10. Friedman RB, Cornwell KA, Lorton L. Dental characteristics of a large military population useful for identification. J Forensic Sci. 1989; 34:1357-1364.

11. Diehl MC. Design of an automated dental epidemiology system. Milit Med. 1984; 149:454-456.

12. Tala H. Information systems for oral health. Int Dent J. 1987; 37:215-217.

13. Pilot T, Barmes DE, Leclercq, et al. Periodontal conditions in adults, 35-44 years of age: an overview of CPITN data in the WHO Global Oral Data Bank. Community Dent Oral Epidemiol. 1986; 14:310-312.

14. Wilson MA. New information resource, the National Practitioner Data Bank. Public Health Rep. 1989; 104:311-312.

15. Burt BA, Albino JE, Carlos JP, et al. Advances in the epidemiological study of oral-facial diseases. Adv Dent Res. 1989; 3:30-41.

16. Eklund SA. Data bases for detecting and assessing caries risk factors. In: Bader JD, ed. Risk assessment in dentistry. Chapel Hill: University of North Carolina Dental Ecology, 1990 .

17. Weintraub JA. Reactor paper: data bases for detecting and assessing caries risk factors. In: Bader JD, ed. Risk assessment in dentistry. Chapel Hill: University of North Carolina Dental Ecology, 1990.

18. Weinstein MC, Fineberg HV, Elstein AS, et al. Clinical decision analysis. Philadelphia: W. B. Saunders Co., 1980.

19. Sox HC, Blatt M, Higgins MC, et al. Medical decision making. London: Butterworths, 1988.

20. Fletcher RH, Fletcher SW, Wagner EH. Clinical epidemiology. Baltimore: Williams & Wilkins, 1988.

21. Kramer MS. Clinical epidemiology and biostatistics. Berlin: Springer-Verlag, 1988.

22. Bauer JG, Cretin S, Schweitzer SO, et al. The reliability of diagnosing root caries using oral examinations. J Dent Educ. 1988; 52(11):622-629.

23. Tulloch JF, Antczak AA, Wilkes JW. The application of decision analysis to evaluate the need for extraction of asymptomatic third molars. J Oral Maxillofac Surg. 1987; 45:855-863.

24. Tulloch JF, Eng RCS, Antczak-Bouckoms AA. Decision analysis in the evaluationof clinical strategies for the management of mandibular third molars. J Dent Educ. 1987; 51:652-660.

25. Tzukert A. Pulpitis and root canal therapy: is a diagnostic radiograph of value? Oral Surg Oral Med, Oral Pathol. 1986; 61:284-288.

26. Thoden van Velzen SK, Duivenvoorden HJ, Schuurs AHB. Probabilities of success and failure in endodontic treatment: a Bayesian approach. Oral Surg, Oral Med, Oral Pathol. 1981; 52:85-90.

27. Maryniuk GA, Haywood VB. Placement of cast restorations over direct pulp capping procedures: a decision analytic approach. J Amer Dent Assoc. 1990; 120:183-187.

28. Tsevat J, Durand-Zaleski I, Pauker SG. Cost-effectiveness of antibiotic prophylaxis for dental procedures in patients with artificial joints. Am J Pub Health. 1989; 79:739-743.

29. Antczak-Bouckoms AA, Weinstein MC. Cost-effectiveness analysis of periodontal disease control. J Dent Res. 1987; 66:1630-1635.

30. Klausen B, Helbo M, Dabelsteen E. A differential diagnostic approach to the symptomatology of acute dental pain. Oral Surg, Oral Med, Oral Pathol. 1985; 59:297-301.

31. Douglass CW, McNeil BJ. Clinical decision analysis methods applied to diagnostic tests in dentistry. J Dent Educ. 1983; 47:708-712.

32. Kantor ML, Zeichner SJ, Valachovic RW et al. Efficacy of dental radiographic practices: options for image receptors, examination selection, and patient selection. J Amer Dent Assoc. 1989; 119:259-268.

33. Douglass CW, Valachovic RW, Berkey CS, et al. Clinical indicators of radiographically detectable dental diseases in the adult patient. Oral Surg Oral Med Oral Pathol. 1988; 65:474-482.

34. Tulloch JF, Antczak-Bouckoms AA, Berkey CS, et al. Selecting the optimal threshold for the radiographic diagnosis of interproximal caries. J Dent Educ. 1988; 52:630-636.

35. Zeichner SJ, Ruttimann UE, Webber RL. Dental radiography: efficacy in the assessment of intraosseous lesions of the face and jaws in asymptomatic patients. Radiology. 1987; 162:691695.

36. Douglass CW, Valachovic RW, Wijesinha A, et al. Clinical efficacy of dental radiography in the detection of dental caries and periodontal diseases. Oral Surg Oral Med Oral Pathol. 1986; 62:330-339.

37. Pliskin JS, Shwartz M, Grondahl HG, et al. Incoporating individual patient preferences in scheduling bitewing radiographs. Meth Inform Med. 1985; 24:213-217.

38. Priddy RW, Yip L. ORPAMS: a data-management system for oral pathology. Oral Surg Oral Med Oral Pathol. 1986; 61(6):590596.

39. Southard TE. Radiographic image storage via laser optical disk technology. A preliminary study. Oral Surg Oral Med Oral Pathol. 1985; 60:436-439.

40. Burt BA, Albino JE, Carlos JP, et al. Advances in the epidemiological study of oral-facial diseases. Adv Dent Res. 1989; 3:30-41.

41. Burt BA, Albino JE, Carlos JP et al. Advances in the epidemiological study of oral-facial diseases. Adv Dent Res. 1989; 3:30-41.

42. Slavkin HC Splice of life: toward understanding genetic determinants of oral diseases. AdV Dent Res. lg89; 3(1):42-57.

43. Abraham J, Stiles HM, Kammerman LA, et al. Assessing periodontal pathogens in children with varying levels of oral hygiene. ASDC J Dent Child. 1990; 57:189-193.

44. Yasui S. Development and clinical application of DNA probe specific for Peptostreptococcus micros. Bull Tokyo Med Dent Univ. 1989; 36:49-62.

45. Moncla BJ, Braham P, Dix K, et al. Use of synthetic oligonucleotide DNA probes for the identification of Bacteroides gingivalis. J Clin Microbiol. 1990; 28:324-327.

46. Larjava H, Sandberg M, Happonen RP, et al. Differential localization of type I and type III procollagen messenger ribonucleic acids in inflamed periodontal and periapical connective tissues by in situ hybridization. Lab Invest. 1990; 62:96-103.

47. Kisby LE, Savitt ED, French CK, et al. DNA probe detection of key periodontal pathogens in juveniles. J Pedod. 1989; 13:222-229.

48. Tanner A, Bouldin HD, Maiden MF. Newly delineated periodontal pathogens with special reference to selenomonas species. Infection. 1989; 17:182-187.

49. Janin A, Konttinen YT, Gronblad M, et al. Fibroblast markers in labial salivary gland biopsies in progressive systemic sclerosis. Clin Exp Rheumatol. 1990; 8:237-242.

50. Prause JU, Jensen OA, Paschides K, et al. Conjunctival cell glycoprotein pattern of healthy persons and of patients with primary Sjogren's syndrome. J Autoimmun. 1989; 2:495-500.

51. Masada MP, Persson R, Kenney JS, et al. Measurement of interleukin-1 alpha and -1 beta in gingival crevicular fluid: implications for the pathogenesis of periodontal disease. J Periodont Res. 1990; 25:156-163.

52. Curtis MA, Sterne JA, Price SJ, et al. The protein composition of gingival crevicular fluid sampled from male adolescents with no destructive periodontitis: baseline data of a longitudinal study. J Periodont Res. 1990; 25:6-16.

53. Bowers MR, Fisher LW, Termine JD, et al. Connective tissue-associated proteins in crevicular fluid: potential markers for periodontal diseases. J Periodontol. 1989; 60:448-451.

54. Wilton JM, Curtis MA, Gillett IR, et al. Detection of high-risk groups and individuals for periodontal diseases: laboratory markers from analysis of saliva. J Clin Periodontol. 1989; 16:475-483.

55. Smith AJ, Matthews JB, Mason GI, et al. Lactoferrin in aspirates of odontogenic cyst fluid. J Clin Pathol. 1988; 41:1117-1119.

56. Okahashi N, Sasakawa C, Yoshikawa M, et al. Molecular characterization of a surface protein antigen gene from serotype c streprococcus mutans, implicated in dental caries. Mol Microbiol. 1989; 3:673-678.

57. Gibbons RJ. Bacterial adhesion to oral tissues: a model for infectious diseases. J Dent Res. 1989; 68:750-760.

58. Kuramitsu HK. Recent advances in defining the cariogenicity of mutans streptococci: molecular genetic approaches. Eur J Epidemiol. 1987; 3:257-260.
59. National Library of Medicine. Report of the Board of Regents Long Range Plan. Bethesda, Md: U.S. Public Health Service, National Institutes of Health, 1987: p. 29.
60. Colwell RR, ed. Biomolecular data - a resource in transition. Oxford: Oxford University Press, 1989: p.351-358.
61. Takahashi I, Takahashi T, Hamada M, et al. Application of video surgery to orthodontic diagnosis. Int J Adult Orthodon Orthognath Surg. 1989; 4:219-222.
62. Kobayashi T, Ueda K, Honma K, et al. Three-dimensional analysis of facial morphology before and after orthognathic surgery. J Craniomaxillofac Surg. 1990; 18:68-73.
63. Lambrecht JT, Brix F. Planning orthognathic surgery with three-dimensional models. Int J Adult Orthodon Orthognath Surg. 1989; 4:141-144.
64. Mack PJ. A computer analysis of condylar movement as determined by cuspal guidances. J Prosthet Dent. 1989; 61:628-633.
65. Koolstra JH, van Eijden TM, Weijs WA, et al. A three-dimensional mathematical model of the human masticatory system predicting maximum possible bite forces. J Biomech. 1988; 21:563-576.
66. Jacobson JJ, Schweitzer S, DePorter DJ, et al. Chemoprophylaxis of dental patients with prosthetic joints: a simulation model. J Dent Educ. 1988; 52:599-604.
67. Katona TR, Boyle AM, Curcio FB, et al. Mechanisms of tooth eruption in a computer-generated analysis of functional jaw deformations in man. Arch Oral Biol. 1987; 32:367-369.
68. Katona TR, Tackney VM, Keates JK. A computer model of the periodontal ligament space in man. Arch Oral Biol. 1988; 33:839-844.
69. Manji F, Nagelkerke N. A stochastic model for periodontal breakdown. J Periodont Res. 1989; 24:279-281.
70. Dibdin GH. Plaque fluid and diffusion: a study of the cariogenic challenge by computer modeling. J Dent Res. 1990; 69:1324-1331.
71. Lagerlof F, Oliveby A. Computer simulation of oral fluoride clearance. Comput Methods Programs Biomed. 1990; 31:97-104.
72. Hubar JS, Manson-Hing LR, Heaven T. COMRADD: computerized radiographic differential diagnosis. Oral Surg Oral Med Oral Pathol. 1990; 69:263-265.
73. Abbey LM. An expert system for oral diagnosis. J Dent Educ. 1987; 51:475-480.
74. Ralls SA, Cohen ME, Southard TE. Computer-assisted dental diagnosis. Dent Clin North Am. 1986; 30:695-712.
75. Ralls SA, Southard TE, Cohen ME. A system for computer-assisted dental emergency diagnosis. Milit Med. 1986; 151:639-642.

76. Slavicek R. Clinical and instrumental functional analysis for diagnosis and treatment planning. Part 6. Computer-aided diagnosis and treatment planning system. J Clin Orthod. 1988; 22:718-729.

77. Slavicek R. Clinical and instrumental functional analysis for diagnosis and treatment planning. Part 7. Computer-aided axiography. J Clin Orthod. 1988; 22:776-787.

78. Sims-Williams JH, Brown ID, Matthewman A, et al. A computer- controlled system for orthodontic advice. Br Dent J. 1987; 163:161-166.

79. Guess MB, Solzer WV. Computer-generated treatment estimate. J Clin Orthod. 1987; 21:382-383.

80. Levy-Mandel AD, Venetsanopoulos An, Tsotsos JK. Knowledge-based landmarking of cephalograms. Comput Biomed Res. 1986; 19:282-309.

81. Wilkoff R. MacCeph: orthodontic computer database and diagnostic generator. Funct Orthod. 1989; 6:26-28.

82. Giovampaolo PP, Giancarlo A, Pierpaolo C, et al. Computer- assisted periodontal evaluation. Int J Periodontics Restorative Dent. 1988; 8:78-87.

83. Sild E, Bernardi F, Carnevale, G, Milano F. Computerized periodontal probe with adjustable pressure. Int J Periodontics Restorative Dent. 1987; 7:53-62.

84. Logan H, Baker K, Cowen H. Initial results of the use of a drug-interaction system. Spec Care Dentist. 1988; 8:252-255.

85. Hiranaka DK, Kelly JP. Stability of simultaneous orthognathic surgery on the maxilla and mandible: a computer-assisted cephalometric study. Int J Adult Orthodon Orthognath Surg. 1987; 2:193-213.

86. White SC. Computer-aided differential diagnosis of oral radiographic lesions. Dentomaxillofac Radiol. 1989; 18:53-59.

87. Wiener F, Laufer D, Ribak A. Computer-aided diagnosis of odontogenic lesions. Int J Oral Maxillofac Surg. 1986; 15:592-596.

88. Fricton JR, Nelson A, Monsein M. IMPATH: microcomputer assessment of behavioral and psychosocial factors in craniomandibular disorders. CRANIO. 1987; 5:372-381.

89. Matsumura Y. RHINOS: a consultative system for diagnosis of headache and facial pain. Comput Methods Programs Biomed. 1986; 23:65-71.

90. Matsumura Y, Matsunaga T, Hata R, et al. Consultation system for diagnosis of headache and facial pain: RHINOS. Med Inf. 1986;11:145-157.

91. Hyman JJ, Doblecki W. Computerized endodontic diagnosis. J Am Dent Assoc. 1983; 107:755-758.

92. De Rossi G, Focacci C. A computer-assisted method for semiquantitative assessment of salivary gland diseases. Eur J Nucl Med. 1980; 5:499-503.

93. Grondahl K. Computer-assisted subtraction radiography in periodontal diagnosis. Swed Dent J Suppl. 1987; 50:1-44.

94. Okano T, Mera T, Ohki M, et al. Digital subtraction of radiograph in evaluating alveolar bone changes after initial periodontal therapy. Oral Surg Oral Med Oral Pathol. 1990; 69:258-262.

95. Hausmann E, Dunford R, Christersson L, et al. Crestal alveolar bone change in patients with periodontitis as observed by subtraction radiography: an overview. AdV Dent Res. 1988; 2:378-381.

96. Schmidt EF, Webber RL, Ruttimann UE, etal. Effect of periodontal therapy on alveolar bone as measured by subtraction radiography. J Periodontol. 1988; 59:633-638.

97. Jeffcoat MK. Assessment of periodontal disease progression: application of new technology to conventional tools. Periodont Case Rep. 1989; 11:8-12.

98. Bragger U. Digital imaging in periodontal radiography. A review. J Clin Periodontol. 1988; 15:551-557.

99. Orstavik D, Farrants G, Wahl T, et al. Image analysis of endodontic radiographs: digital subtraction and quantitative densitometry. Endod Dent Traumatol. 1990; 6:6-11.

100. Kullendorff B, Grondahl K, Rohlin M, et al. Subtraction radiography for the diagnosis of periapical bone lesions. Endodont Dent Traumatol. 1988; 4:253-259.

101. Halse A, White SC, Espelid I, et al. Visualization of stannous fluoride treatment of carious lesions by subtraction radiography. Oral Surg Oral Med Oral Pathol. 1990; 69:378-381.

102. Rinast E, Gmelin E, Hollands-Thorn B. Digital subtraction sialography, conventional sialography, high-resolution ultrasonography and computed tomography in the diagnosis of salivary gland diseases. Eur J Radiol. 1989; 9:224-230.

103. Larheim TA, Johannessen 5, Tveito L. Abnormalities of the temporomandibular joint in adults with rheumatic disease. A comparison of panoramic, transcranial and transpharyngeal radiography with tomography. Dentomaxillofac Radiol. 1988; 17:109-113.

104. Schiffman E, Anderson G, Fricton J, et al. Diagnostic criteria for intraarticular T.M. disorders. Community Dent Oral Epidemiol. 1989; 17:252-257.

105. Berman CL. Osseointegration. Complications, prevention, recognition, treatment. Dent Clin North Am. 1989; 33:635-663.

106. Schwarz MS, Rothman SL, Chafetz N, et al. Computed tomography in dental implantation surgery. Dent Clin North Am. 1989; 33:555-597.

107. Wishan MS, Bahat 0, Krane M. Computed tomography as an adjunct in dental implant surgery. 1988; 8:30-47.

108. Truitt HP, James R, Altman A, et al. Use of computer tomography in subperiosteal implant therapy. J Prosthet Dent. 1988; 59:474-477.

109. Andersson JE, Svartz K. CT-scanning in the preoperative planning of osseointegrated implants in the maxilla. Int J Oral Maxillofac Surg. 1988; 17:33-35.

110. Donlon WC, Young P, Vassiliadis A. Three-dimensional computed tomography for maxillofacial surgery: report of cases. J Oral Maxillofac Surg. 1988; 46:142-147.

111. Cooper RA, Tempany CM, Farrell B. Conventional and computed tomographic sialography in evaluating disorders of the parotid gland. Entechnology. 1988; Sept. 20-35.

112. van den Akker HP. Diagnostic imaging in salivary gland disease. Oral Surg Oral Med Oral Pathol. 1988; 66:625-637.

113. Schellhas KP, Wilkes CH, el Deeb M, et al. Permanent Proplast temporomandibular joint implants: MR imaging of destructive complications. AJR Am J Roentgenol. 1988; 151:731-735.

114. Schellhas KP. Medical imaging in the evaluation of facial pain. Semin Neurol. 1988; 8:265-271.

115. Kerstens HC, Golding RP, Valk J, et al. Magnetic resonance imaging of partial temporomandibular joint disc displacement. J Oral Maxillofac Surg. 1989; 47:25-29.

116. Sanchez-Wodwoorth RE, Katzberg RW, Tallents RH, et al. Radiographic assessment of temporomandibular joint pain and dysfunction in the pediatric age group. ASDC J Dent Child. 1988; 55:278-281.

117. Helms CA, Kaplan P. Diagnostic imaging of the temporomandibular joint: recommendations for use of the various techniques. AJR Am J Roentgenol. 1990; 154:319-322.

118. Curtin HD. Assessment of salivary gland pathology. Otolaryngol Clin North Am. 1988; 21:547-573.

119. Hildebolt CF, Vannier MW. Automated classification of periodontal disease using bitewing radiographs. J Periodontol. 1988; 59:87-94.

120. Wouters FR, Lavstedt S, Frithiof L, et al. A computerized system to measure interproximal alveolar bone levels in epidemiologic, radiographic investigations. II. Intra- and inter-examiner variation study. Acta Odontol Scand. 1988; 46:33-39.

121. Barnett ML, Gilman RM, Charles CH, et al. Computer-based thermal imaging of human gingiva: preliminary investigation. J Periodontol. 1989; 60:628-633.

122. Verdonschot EH, Sabders AJ, Plasschaert AJ. A computer-aided image analysis system (IAS) for area measurement of tooth root surfaces. J Periodontol. 1990; 61:275-280.

123. Graves CN, Feagin FF. A method of semi-quantitative microradiographic analysis of root surface lesion remineralization. J Oral Pathol. 1988; 17:241-249.

124. Steffensen B, Pasquali LA, Yuan C, et al. Correction of density changes caused by methodological errors in CADIA. J Periodont Res. 1989; 24:402-408.

125. Braegger U, Pasquali L, Weber H, et al. Computer-assisted densitometric image analysis (CADIA) for the assessment of alveolar bone density changes in furcations. J Clin Periodontol. 1989; 16:46-52.

126. Bragger U, Pasquali L, Kornman KS. Remodelling of interdental alveolar bone after periodontal flap procedures assessed by means of computer-as-

sisted densitometric image analysis (CADIA). J Clin Periodontol. 1988; 15:558-564.

127. Bragger U, Pasquali L, Rylander H, et al. Computer-assisted densitometric image analysis in periodontal radiography. A methodological study. J Clin Periodontol. 1988; 15:27-37.

128. Braegger U, Litch J, Pasquali L, et al. Computer-assisted densitometric image analysis for the quantitation of radiographic alveolar bone changes. J Periodont Res. 1987; 22:227-229.

129. Hausmann E, Allen K, Dunford R, et al. A reliable computerized method to determine the level of the radiographic alveolar crest. J Periodont Res. 1989; 24:368-369.

130. Fredriksson M, Zimmerman M, Martinsson T. Precision of computerized measurement of marginal alveolar bone height from bite-wing radiographs. Swed Dent J. 1989; 13:163-167.

131. Heaven TJ, Firestone AR, Feagin FF. Quantitative radiographic measurement of dentinal lesions. J Dent Res. 1990; 69:51-54.

132. Verrier J, Waite I, Linney A, et al. A microcomputer system for the analysis of dental radiographs. Br Dent J. 1989; 167:135-139.

133. Mouyen F, Benz C, Sonnabend E, et al. Presentation and physical evaluation of RadioVisioGraphy. Oral Surg Oral Med Oral Pathol. 1989; 68:238-242.

134. Kassebaum DK, McDavid WD, Dove SB, et al. Spatial resolution requirements for digitizing dental radiographs. Oral Surg Oral Med Oral Pathol. 1989; 67:760-769.

135. Jager A, Doler W, Schormann T. Digital image processing in cephalometric analysis. Schweiz Monatsschr Zahnmed. 1989; 99:19-23.

136. Kolling JN, Price RB, Miller RL, et al. Evaluation of a digitizer and computer system designed to analyze articulatorgenerated occlusal tracings. J Prosthet Dent. 1988; 59:499503.

137. Hing NR. The accuracy of computer-generated prediction tracings. Int J Oral Maxillofac Surg. 1989; 18:148-151.

138. Guess MB, Solzer WV. Computer-generated diagnostic correction of anterior diastemas. J Prosthet Dent. 1988; 59:629-632.

139. Roulet JF, Reich T, Blunck U, et al. Quantitative margin analysis in the scanning electron microscope. Scanning Microsc. 1989; 3:147-158.

140. Watson RM, Bhatia SN. Tooth positions in the natural and complete artificial dentitions, with special reference to the incisor teeth: an interactive on-line computer analysis. J Oral Rehabil. 1989; 16:139-153.

141. Heyden G, Mattson U. Computer-aided photograph analyses in oral medicine - a pilot study. Swed Dent J. 1988; 12:93-99.

142. Gullickson DC, Montgomery S. The study of root canal morphology using a digital image processing technique. J Endod. 1987; 13:158-163.

143. Kircos LT, Ortendahl DA, Hattner RS, et al. Bayesian-deblurred Planar and SPECT nuclear bone imaging for the demonstration of facial anatomy

and craniomandibular disorders. Oral Surg Oral Med Oral Pathol. 1988; 66:102-110.

144. Layfield LJ, Hall TL, Fu YS. Discrimination of benign versus malignant mixed tumors of the salivary gland using digital image analysis. Cytometry. 1989; 10:217-221.

145. Mormann WH, Lutz F, Gotsch T. CAD-CAM ceramic inlays and onlays: a case report after 3 years in place. J Am Dent Assoc. 1990; 120:517-520.

146. Leinfelder KF, Isenberg BP, Essig ME. A new method for generating ceramic restorations: a CAD-CAM system. J Am Dent Assoc. 1989; 118:703-707.

147. Rekow D. Computer-aided design and manufacturing in dentistry: a review of the state of the art. J Prosthet Dent. 1987; 58:512-516.

148. Benjamin LS. Versatility of the subperiosteal implant utilizing CAD-CAM multiplanar diagnostic imaging. J Oral Implantol. 1983; 13: 282-296.

149. Radcliffe DF. Computer-aided rehabilitation engineering CARE. J Med Eng Technol. 1986; 10:1-6.

150. Marsh JL, Vannier MW, Stevens WG, et al. Computerized imaging for soft tissue and osseous reconstruction in the head and neck. Clin Plast Surg. 1985; 12:279-291.

151. Terranova VP, Jendresen M, Young F. Healing, regeneration, and repair: prospectus for new dental treatment. Adv Dent Res. 1989; 3:69-79.

152. Shortliffe EH, Fagan LM. Research training in medical informatics: the Stanford experience. Academic Medicine. 1989; 64:575-578.

153. National Library of Medicine. Long Range Plan, Report of Panel 4: Medical Informatics. National Institutes of Health. 1986; p. 71.

154. Gordon SL. Ingredients of a successful grant application to the National Institutes of Health. J Orthopaed Res. 1989; 7:138-141.

155. Cuca JM, McLoughlin WJ. Why clinical research grant applications fare poorly in review and how to recover. Cancer Investig. 1987; 5:55-58.

156. Cuca JM. NIH grant applications for clinical research: reasons for poor ratings or disapproval. Clin Res. 1983; 31:453-461.

157. Miller RA, Patil R, Mitchell JA, et al. Preparing a medical informatics research grant proposal: general principles. Comp Biomed Res. 1989; 222:92-101.

158. National Library of Medicine. Long Range Plan - Report 4: Medical Informatics. National Institutes of Health. 1986; p.69.

159. Jay AT. Using computers and actually liking it. Dental Management. October 1990:30-41.

160. Academy of General Dentistry. AGD looks at computers in the dental office. AGD Impact. 1989; 17:21.

161. For example, Dental Management, Dental Economics, Dental Products, Dentist, and Dentistry Today.

162. Blois MS, Shortliffe EH. The computer meets medicine: emergence of a discipline. In: Shortliffe EH, Perreault LE, eds. Medical informatics: com-

puter applications in health care. Massachusetts: Addison-Wesley Publ Comp, 1990: p. 20.

163. Stikeleather J, Hensel JS, Baumgarten SA. The computerized dental office of the future. Dental Clinics of North America. 1988; 32:173-190.

16
Informatics in Dental Education: The Administrative Perspective

William R. McCutcheon

The latter portion of the 20th Century finds dental education assuming a "catch-up" posture in yet another arena. The electronic storage, synthesis, and distribution of information has instituted a revolution in how the world functions, but schools of dentistry, not unlike other professional schools, have been slow to join this revolution and exploit its potential for enhancing the process of educating dental practitioners.

The nature of this situation poses some interesting dilemmas for the dental school administrator. On the one hand are the demands of substantial capital outlay for hardware, software and technical staffing along with requests for curriculum time to begin teaching the application of the new technology to dental practice. On the other hand are the promises of monetary savings through enhanced management systems and reduction in personal service budget items, as well as relief of curriculum crowding by altering both the form and substance of what is taught.

Someplace in the middle of these opposing forces reside the faculty and staff. Their motivation to be at the forefront of all that is new and relevant to their areas of responsibility is buffered by a natural resistance to change which is fortified by the inevitable institutional barriers to change.

The administrator in dental education, faced with the realities of an explosion in scientific information and increasing costs of education, confronts a climate that demands change. Pressures dictate that dental schools produce practitioners capable of meeting the oral health needs of a more complex patient living in an increasingly complex environment, and that this task be accomplished without an additional expenditure of time and its associated costs. Obviously this situation is, in large measure, a product of the technical advancement that has generated information handling capacities not dreamed of in the not-too-distant past. It is equally obvious that this same technology is the key to meeting the new challenges.

Informatics and Strategic Planning in Dental Education

Strategic planning seems to mean somewhat different things to different people and organizations. Perhaps one of the most comprehensive definitions is that put forth by Grant and King.[1] They define the strategic planning system as "a set of interrelated organizational task definitions and procedures for seeing that pertinent information is obtained, forecasts are made, and strategy choices are addressed in an integrated, internally consistent, and timely fashion." In other words an organization must assess its evolving environment and develop a plan that operationalizes its mission and goals as a function of this changing environment.

Translating this process to the dental school model requires that the institution first look carefully at both external and internal environmental factors that impact its mission. Typical external factors include such things as:

- Demographic and epidemiologic profiles of the population served by the typical graduate
- Demographic profile of the professional population into which the typical graduate enters
- Funding pattern projections for the dental educational program
- Operant environment external to the dental school per se (for example, the relationship to a larger university of which it is a part).

Typical internal environmental factors are:

- Overall curriculum status including adequacy, currency, degree of crowding, and flexibility
- Demographic profiles of faculty and staff including non-traditional areas of expertise
- Organizational behavior (how policies are formulated and how change actually occurs)
- Results of dental education program outcome assessments.

Given the state of rapidly changing demographics and its concomitant impact on epidemiologic patterns of oral disease, dramatic new approaches to the understanding and treatment of all disease processes, and a crowded, tradition-bound curriculum, it is inevitable that a dental school undergoing a strategic planning process must come to terms with the technology of information management.

Changing demographics will require the practitioner's focus to shift from routine preventive and restorative procedures to conditions and therapies associated with an aging, dentate population, such as chronic periodontal disease, craniomandibular dysfunction, and implantology. Furthermore, patients presenting with these concerns will more likely fit the medically compromised and/or polypharmacy categories. The implications for dental education are myriad. Prevailing curriculum design and teaching methodologies can not accommodate the amount of new information necessary to meet this challenge. Either the length of the curriculum must be increased or fairly drastic new ways of teaching must evolve.

Pragmatic concerns restrict dental education's freedom to lengthen the predoctoral curriculum. The cost of education continues to soar in both the absolute (tuition) and relative sense (society's burden in underwriting the cost of educating its health care providers). Therefore, ways must be found to meet the challenge within a similar time frame. The only reasonable solution, short of restructuring the practice of dentistry, is to evolve a curriculum that develops thinking skills (that is, problem-based) and emphasizes accessing information vis-a-vis committing it to memory. The role of information technology in such a venture is inescapable.

For informatics to play a significant role in resolving the problems presented by these evolving environmental factors, planning must first identify program target areas. Tira, et al[2] defined four such areas as (1) instruction-education, (2) administration-management, (3) research, and (4) professional and personal development. This author would suggest a slight modification of this classification arrived at by adding administration to the three traditional responsibilities of an academic institution (teaching, research, and service), thus providing a base on which a model of these target areas can be constructed. The model's appearance for a typical dental school is illustrated by the following diagram.

Dental School Program Target Areas for Informatics Planning

Administration

-Fiscal Management

-Personnel Management

-Faculty Evaluation

-Development Activities

-Alumni Tracking

-Inventory Management

-Electronic Mail

-Word Processing/Desktop Publishing

Research

-Bio-technical Support

-Epidemiology

-Educational Methods/Content

-Practice Management

Teaching

-Computer Assisted Instruction

-Artificial Intelligence

-Simulation

-Curriculum Tracking/Design

-Curriculum Evaluation

-Library Resources and Access

-Continuing Professional

-Education

Service (Patient/Clinic Management)

-Registration/Scheduling

-Billing

-Patient Records

-Quality Assurance

Development of the target area model brings into focus the final planning phase, addressing the impact on facilities and budget allocations. These issues must also be addressed on an evolving basis since it is impossible to predict comprehensive infrastructure needs at a point in time for a system undergoing constant change. This situation is not unmanageable even given the characteristic bureaucratic structure with which the dental school administrator must deal. However, it does require thoughtful and sometimes creative planning to build the necessary flexibility into an otherwise rigid structure.

Promoting Dental Informatics in the Educational Environment

At the outset it is important to appreciate that a major attitudinal barrier exists in the form of resistance to change. To be resistant to and/or threatened by change is a very human response. Informatics is a technology capable of pervading virtually every facet of an individual's working environment. Computer software can be designed to either take over, modify or augment every day-to-day task undertaken by a faculty or staff person. Therefore the administrator is attempting to promote something that constitutes a major assault on the status quo of the functional working environment of his/her institution. It is little wonder that resistance can be of considerable magnitude.

Useful clues to overcoming attitudinal barriers can be gleaned from some of the ideas of social psychology, especially those suggested by small group theory. The dental school administrator would be well-advised to take advantage of natural groupings afforded by his/her organization (the departmental structure) and deploy group process techniques such as collective goal setting, competition, and "public" commitment. The process of people working together in small groups where external commitments are made to the accomplishment of mutually developed goals is a highly effective way to overcome resistance to the change represented by those goals.

In a practical vein Arms[3] has pointed out that for major changes to occur at an institution, three factors are necessary - leadership, excitement, and the ability to move the process of change rapidly. These factors are especially cogent when one addresses faculty and staff issues in promoting informatics for the dental educational environment.

Using the Arms[3] paradigm it is important to identify faculty/staff leadership early on in the process. There are always one or more individuals present in these ranks who respond to challenges. These people must be nurtured so that their amenability to and interest in change serve as a catalyst for those around them. The administration must facilitate their actually acquiring the resources, using the innovation, and sharing both process and outcomes with their peers. Programs for general faculty meetings and retreats provide an ideal forum for accomplishing such objectives.

There are many dimensions to generating and maintaining excitement, but perhaps the two most important are involvement and rewards. Every effort should be made to involve people using new technology in the decision-making processes. As Arms[3] points out this task can often be accomplished by including discretionary funds in the budget and allowing these people to decide how they should best be spent. Of conceivably greater significance is the attention that must be paid to the reward system. Specific references to efforts in informatics must be factored into promotion and tenure guidelines for faculty as well as job descriptions and classifications for staff. Such things as software development can be fitted neatly into the research category of promotion and tenure guidelines whereas specific applications characteristically fall under instructional methodology portions of the teaching category. Staff job descriptions can contain merit pay provisions tied to informatics development and application.

The third factor (the ability to move the process of change rapidly) offers the greatest challenge to the dental school administrator. The process of change is usually driven by budget, and the institutional budget does not lend itself readily to any process involving rapid change. For one thing there are the long budget cycles which make anticipation of all needs extremely difficult. This difficulty is bolstered by traditional academic conservatism and the characteristic employment of committee structure for decision making.[3] However, as with so many other matters of process, to be forewarned is to be forearmed; planning with all of these constraints in the model can minimize their impact on the outcomes. One useful ploy available to most dental school administrations is to move as much as possible of the essentially fixed and/or predictable organizational costs into the budget section over which the least control can be exercised. Then less predictable costs such as informatics development can be funded from more discretionary portions of the budget (such as clinic income revenues).

Since this chapter addresses the informatics issues from the administrator's perspective, it can be assumed that the factors of leadership, excitement, and rapid change are in place at the administrative level. What remains in the promotional sense is to clarify the central issue of resource commitment vs. return. The Carnegie Commission noted in 1972[4] that the new electronic technology is tending to add to rather than replace older approaches. It is incumbent upon the dental school administrator to make certain that this finding is without foundation at his/her institution or the entire initiative will likely fail. The administration must be convinced that the resource commitment will result in a streamlining and increased efficiency of the existing system, not simply another addition.

If an innovation can be configured to generate a need for its existence, it will not be construed as excess baggage. Fortunately the generation of need with informatics technology is not difficult, particularly at the administrative level. The first and most obvious way to meet this objective is by facilitating routine operations. Such things as the budget process, personnel management, electronic mail, wordprocessing, and inventory are all readily addressed by available software and, hence, available to provide early returns on resource commitment.

Having established a working presence with these base level operations, the informatics initiative can address more sophisticated functions such as analyses related to the accreditation process, development activity, alumni tracking, and continuing education. These applications are laden with many returns to please administrators.

Like other institutions of higher learning, dental schools are periodically stirred into some degree of disruptive activity by the prospect of putting together a comprehensive report for an accreditation site-visit team. The task is disruptive because it typically requires existing responsibilities (mainly administrative) to be refocused into achievement of a short-term goal (the accreditation self-study). Informatics applications provide a ready means of lightening this task by maintaining ongoing records of multiple institutional processes; records that give quick access to information concerning school operational data, student performance data, and curriculum content and analysis.

With institutional development assuming an ever-increasing role in dental education, the application of information management technology to alumni tracking and capital fund raising is important. This entire activity can be greatly enhanced through alumni tracking, profiling, and geographical clustering, not to mention basic activities such as creation and distribution of mailings.

Since virtually all dental schools include continuing education as part of their mission statement, it too should be considered in an informatics initiative. Aside from the obvious applications to the mechanics of distribution and mailing, planning for future sophisticated linkages between the private practitioners and the school should occur from the outset. Not only will the private practitioner be able to access the school's learning resources center for in-office continuing education and updates, but he/she may also link up for various practice monitoring services offered by the school. The latter could include things such as time studies for practice management and epidemiologic profiles of patient populations.

With all the upper level activity that an initiative as broadly based as informatics can generate in a school, it is easy to overlook the basic responsibility of education. Although students characteristically occupy a somewhat passive role in regard to what the faculty and administration feel to be in their best interest, they must accept the new technology and ultimately benefit from it. The key to accomplishing this goal is twofold: (1) the innovations must be helpful and relevant from the student perspective and (2) none of the innovations should be viewed as gimmickry.

These axioms are somewhat interrelated. There is the ever-present temptation for educators to push for wholesale adoption of promising innovations without a sufficient record of outcomes. Dental education saw this situation occur in the 1960s and 70s when early forms of computer-assisted instruction were viewed as the answer to many of the ills poised by crowded curricula and classrooms. Unfortunately, students did not share this view in that once the novelty of new technology had worn off, the branched programs were so lacking in stimulus and human interaction that little learning took place.

For informatics to realize its full potential as an educational tool, some fundamental pedagogical changes already alluded to are in order for dental education. The informatics perspective is one where technology provides the virtually unlimited storage capacity for facts and education can no longer be concerned with teaching facts but rather with teaching how to properly access them. Complete adoption of this stance obviously is not realistic for dental education. The health sciences continue to rely on a doctor-patient relationship that requires a basic store of factual knowledge, since one can ill afford to consult the computer in a clinical emergency. However, reorientation of the dental curriculum to provide a problem-oriented approach employing critical thinking skills is central to meeting the challenge of using information technology to overcome the growing problem of curriculum crowding and the compression of specialized knowledge. With this approach the dental graduate will be able to apply the most up-to-date knowledge to any clinical situation by virtue of having learned to access data banks appropriate to that situation as determined by the specialized knowledge gained from his/her professional education.

To make such fundamental changes in pedagogy is an enormous challenge for the dental school administration. However, it is not an insurmountable obstacle. The key is evolution - not revolution. One begins by challenging individual departments and/or course directors to design and implement one course using a problem-oriented approach. This effort will usually require input from an educational consultant and can be accomplished in the most economic fashion by collective exposure through faculty development programs. As with so many innovations, once the process is begun as a challenge from the administration, the subsequent spread of its application will be much easier.

Finally, the realization of the informatics initiative in a dental school brings with it a new set of concerns that impact all levels — students, faculty, staff and administration. New sets of technical decisions must now be made concerning such issues as hardware compatibility, maintenance, and information security. Ethical dilemmas concerning copyrights and distribution will present themselves. However, when one reviews the experiences of institutions that have begun participating in the informatics revolution (Graham et al),[5] the benefits that seem to rapidly accrue place all of these concerns into a manageable perspective.

Conclusions

The Report of the Steering Committee[6] for the Symposium on Medical Informatics summarized the growing concerns of dental education when they noted that humans have a finite limit on the number of information items they can manage cognitively at one time. To address even moderately complex clinical situations can be compromised by this limitation.

In the same set of proceedings, Tosteson[7] suggested that computers will change the role of physicians in the direction of having the doctor do more of what humans do better than machines — personal interactions requiring breadth of perception and a range of awareness. He then concludes that if physicians will be doing different things, then medical education must change.

These two conceptualizations translate easily to the dental profession and, consequently, to dental education. All of the administrative issues noted in this chapter are but small parts of this larger picture and as each one is addressed, dental education moves closer to more adequately preparing practitioners for the 21st Century.

References

1. Grant, J.H., and King, W.R. The Logic of Strategic Planning. Little, Brown and Co. 1982, Boston/Toronto.
2. Tira, D.E., Tharp, L.B., and Lipson, L.F. Computers in dental education, in Dental Clinics of North America, 30:4, pp. 681-84, Oct. 1986.

3. Arms, W.Y. Institutional decision-making and commitment to computers in education. In Medical Education in the Information Age: Proceedings of the Symposium on Medical Informatics. Association of American Medical Colleges, 1986, pp. 101-07.

4. Carnegie Commission on Higher Education. The Fourth Revolution: Instructional Technology in Higher Education. Hightstown, N.J., McGraw-Hill, 1972.

5. Graham, W.L., Biddington, W.R., Richmond, W.A., and Sizemore, R.M. ODONTICS: Omnibus dental online treatment and information control system. Cause/Effect, July 1982, pp. 4-8.

6. Report of the steering committee on the evaluation of medical information science in medical education. Medical Education in the Information Age: Proceedings of the Symposium on Medical Informatics. Association of American Medical Colleges, 1986, p. 11.

7. Tosteson, D. Medical education in the computer age. In Medical Education in the Information Age: Proceedings of the Symposium on Medical Informatics. Association of American Medical Colleges, 1986, pp. 71-78.

Section 3
Planning for the Future

17
Integrating Information Technology in Healthcare

Marion J. Ball and Judith V. Douglas

Today computing and communications technologies are a force for integration, especially in areas such as healthcare which are information dependent. Healthcare professionals are working as individuals and as members of professional associations to realize the benefits that technology offers.

The technology of the 1990s will build upon open architecture system design, which enables computers to talk to one another and to share data, even if the computers are made by different manufacturers and the applications run on different software.[1,2] On a technical level, integration involves the development of seamless interfaces between systems and menu-driven access for users. The concept of integration goes far beyond technical linkages and interoperable computers, however.

Technically, microcomputers are bringing their capabilities to the desktop. Increasingly, practitioners use personal computers for a host of applications, including practice management. As networking becomes more common, practitioners are accessing electronic conferences of professional interest. A small investigation is now being funded by the National Library of Medicine to determine whether GRATEFUL MED, the Library's microbased search tool for its massive holdings, might be of help to practicing dentists.[3] Development of databases in many areas is being discussed, such as one on dental materials.

These activities and countless others promise new capabilities, just as surely as the networked desktop computer offers a powerful tool. The technology is already here and it can be dazzling, but integration, not technology, is critical.

Moving Toward Integration

In the 1970s, computer applications became standard in biomedical research, clinical laboratories, and hospital accounting offices. Automated library systems and information databases were coming into their own. Leaders, among them Lindberg and Matheson, advocated using information technology to address the explosion in biomedical knowledge.[4] In 1986, the Association of American Medical Colleges (AAMC) set forth plans for reforming medical education to incorporate information handling skills.[5]

The National Library of Medicine

In its long range plan published in 1986,[6] the National Library of Medicine (NLM) detailed sixteen goals in five domains, including professional education and medical informatics. In the words of Donald A.B. Lindberg, Director of the NLM.

The top discretionary efforts must be to prepare the Library and the Nation's health professionals for the optimal utilization of the burgeoning electronic technology for knowledge management.

For the Library, this means using its resources to provide advanced information handling services and to develop integrating and coordinating systems, as the Library is doing with databases in molecular biology and biotechnology.[7]

The integration concept is also at the heart of the Integrated Academic Information Management Systems (IAIMS) initiative, launched by the National Library of Medicine (NLM) in the early 1980s to encourage academic health centers across the country to create new information environments.[8,9,10]

In its call for proposals, the NLM articulated a three-phase process, beginning with strategic planning, moving through model development or pilot implementation, and concluding with full scale implementation. Since 1983, sixteen institutions have been awarded IAIMS funds. Four campuses were named phase one strategic planning sites in 1984; by 1990, four institutions had been designated phase three implementation sites.

In 1990, at the second invitational IAIMS symposium, participants meeting at Georgetown University reviewed accomplishments and sketched out visions of the future. Outlining challenges of the 1990s, the Director of the NLM, Dr. Donald Lindberg, reported on exponentially more powerful computers now being developed within the scientific community and of the need of biomedicine to prepare to take advantage of them. IAIMS representatives broke into four working groups to address education, workstations, funding, and networking. All four reports to the plenary body generated interest; networking, or linkages, elicited consensus and action points. What was patently clear, however, was that integration remained elusive, despite the technology available and the systems.

Hospitals and Health Level 7 (HL7)

Efforts in the healthcare delivery system mirror those in academic medicine. In the report of the outreach panel chaired by Dr. Michael DeBakey,[11] the NLM targeted community hospitals and practitioners through their Regional Medical Library network. The American College of Obstetrics and Gynecology (ACOG) became an IAIMS site and worked to link all its members through a national network.

In the hospital sector, the promise of software linkages under Health Level 7 (HL7) was perhaps the hottest topic at the Healthcare Information and Management Systems Society (HIMSS) convention in 1990.[12] Hospitals are now calling upon technology to help them obtain a competitive advantage in the marketplace, address regulatory concerns, and ensure professional accountability and quality of care.

Today hospitals are looking beyond financially-oriented hospital information systems (HIS).[13,14] Today hospitals need information systems which support patient care as well as generate bills. Such systems must link the many technology applications now up and running, making information available to the healthcare professional through a single access point. This is no easy task, with the volumes of information created in clinical and other specialized laboratories, in imaging centers, on the nursing floor, and elsewhere throughout the healthcare system.

Where Caring and Technology Meet

The profession of nursing has highlighted the need for integrated information systems. As caregivers, nurses have long been responsible for coordinating information from multiple sources, from doctors to dieticians and many more. It was inevitable, therefore, that implementation of HIS required nurses to input data. Nurses became the professionals upon whose involvement and commitment the success of HIS depended.

Accordingly, nurses began to ask that HIS serve their needs as well as those of the accounts office. Nurses took on new roles as individuals and within their professional groups, both regional and national. In 1983, nursing was accorded Working Group status by the International Medical Informatics Association (IMIA). In 1991, the Working Group hosted its fourth triennial international symposium on computers in nursing in Australia.

Nursing education also recognized these changing roles. A master's degree in nursing informatics was established at the University of Maryland in 1989, the first program of its kind.[15] In 1990, Maryland moved to extend nursing informatics to the doctoral level. In addition, a second master's degree program has been launched at the University of Utah in Salt Lake City.[16]

Technology in Care

In general, however, curricula change slowly, compared to actual practice.[17] Point of care terminals, at the bedside or handheld, are transforming the way patient care is delivered.[18,19] Nurses can be free of the need to return to the nursing station to enter or to confirm orders. They can enter vital signs at the moment they are taken; they can even ask for graphic displays of a particular sign over time. Such changes reduce the time spent in data entry and retrieval and decrease the probability of error. They also integrate the technology into nursing care, making the handheld terminal as basic as the stethoscope or the digital thermometer.

An innovation which promises to change patient care dramatically is the use of existing barcode scanning technology for positive patient identification.[20] Integrating the ubiquitous barcode into patient care would support quality assurance functions and professional accountability. Specimens could be tracked, drug administration monitored, and all actions by any care provider verified through searching automatically generated records. The yield here is not so much from the technology itself, but from the integration of that technology into the actual delivery of healthcare.

The same is true for dentistry. Technology exists today which can significantly alter the way dentists practice. In a profession which relies heavily upon visual information for diagnosis and treatment, videodisks can be invaluable for education, research, and clinical care, giving ready access to images of conditions rarely encountered in practice.

In delivering care, dentists are extraordinarily dependent upon their tools in ways in which few other health professionals are. Integrating information technology with those tools can revolutionize dentistry. For example, periodontal probes could both measure and record, performing a vital function without deviation. Graphic capabilities known as CAD/CAM could (and do) provide simulations for reconstructive work.

Still another innovation, this one from medicine, holds promise for dentistry. Dr. Louis Abbey has built upon the work of Dr. Lawrence Weed and developed computer based programs which link the dentist's knowledge of specific problems to biomedical knowledge.[21] These couplers can offer real support to the dentist, documenting the processes involved in diagnosis and treatment. With inputs clearly stated, the evaluation of outcomes will become possible.

In dentistry, as in nursing and medicine, the practitioners themselves must be the ones to define integration and to determine how information technology can serve the profession. It is this role which the evolving field of healthcare informatics addresses. However healthcare informatics is defined, it invariably involves integration of technology with healthcare, of information science with computing, of profession with profession.

References

1. Sharrott LH. Centralized and distributed information systems: two architectural approaches for the 90s. In: Ball MJ, Douglas JV, O'Desky RI, et al, eds. Healthcare information management systems: a practical guide. New York: Springer-Verlag, 1991: p. 306-315.
2. Gabler JM. Information systems: a competitive advantage for managing healthcare. In: Ball MJ, Douglas JV, O'Desky RI, et al, eds. Healthcare information management systems: a practical guide. New York: Springer-Verlag, 1991: p. 199-208.
3. Zimmerman JL. National Institute of Health/National Library of Medicine. A study of clinical dentistry information needs using GRATEFUL MED, Contract 467-MZ-001213, 1990.
4. Matheson NW, Lindberg DAB. Subgroup report on medical information science skills. Journal of Medical Education. 1984;59:155-159.
5. Association of American Medical Colleges. Medical education in the information age: proceedings of the symposium on medical informatics. Washington, DC: Association of American Medical Colleges, 1986.

6. National Library of Medicine. Long range plan: report of panels 1-5. Bethesda: National Institutes of Health, 1986.
7. National Library of Medicine (U.S.) Board of Regents. Long range plan. Bethesda: National Institutes of Health, 1987.
8. Ball MJ, Douglas JV. Tying it all together: the integrated academic information management system being implemented at Maryland. CRC Critical Reviews. 1988;1:311-322.
9. Symposium on Integrated Academic Information Management Systems (lst: 1984:National Library of Medicine). Planning for Integrated Academic Information Management Systems. Bethesda: National Institutes of Health, 1984.
10. Symposium on Integrated Academic Information Management Systems (2nd: 1986:National Library of Medicine). IAIMS and Health Sciences Education. Bethesda: National Institutes of Health, 1986.
11. National Library of Medicine (U.S.) Board of Regents. Improving health professionals' access to information: report of the board of regents. Bethesda, MD: National Institutes of Health, 1989.
12. American Hospital Association. Proceedings of the 1990 Annual Health Care Information Management Systems Conference. Chicago: American Hospital Association, 1989.
13. Ball MJ, Douglas JV, O'Desky RI, et al, eds. Healthcare information management systems: a practical guide. New York: Springer-Verlag, 1991.
14. Ball MJ, Hannah KJ, Gerdin Jelger U, et al, eds. Nursing informatics: where caring and technology meet. New York: Springer-Verlag, 1988.
15. Heller BR, Romano CA, Damrosch SP, et al. The need for an educational program in nursing informatics. In: Ball MJ, Hannah KJ, Gerdin Jelger U, et al, eds. Nursing informatics: where caring and technology meet. New York: Springer-Verlag, 1988.
16. Ball MJ, Douglas JV. Informatics programs in the United States and abroad. M.D. Computing. 1990;7: 172-175.
17. Ball MJ, Douglas JV, Zimmerman JL, et al. Informatics education and the professions. Journal of the American Society for Information Science. 1989;40:368-377.
18. Tranbarger RE. Nurses and computers: at the point of care. In: Ball MJ, Douglas JV, O'Desky RI, et al, eds. Healthcare information management systems: a practical guide. New York: Springer-Verlag, 1991: p. 95-102.
19. Hughes S. Bedside information systems: state of the art. In: Ball MJ, Hannah KJ, Gerdin Jelger U, et al, eds. Nursing informatics: where caring and technology meet. New York: Springer-Verlag, 1988: p. 138-145.
20. Rappoport AE. Positive patient and specimen identification. In: Ball MJ, Douglas JV, O'Desky RI, et al, eds. Healthcare information management systems: a practical guide. New York: Springer-Verlag, 1991: p. 32-41.
21. Weed LL. New premises and new tools for medical care and medical education. New York: Springer-Verlag, in press.

18
Strategic Planning for Informatics in Dentistry

Judith V. Douglas and John J. Salley

Concepts and Corollaries

Strategic planning for information technology is critical in dentistry as well as in other fields. Critics label the term a buzzword and allege that there is no such concept as strategic planning. In their judgment, strategic planning is merely a new name for the established practice known as long-term planning.

The literature of change suggests otherwise. In The Planning of Change behavioral scientists set forth theories, primarily social, and suggested processes and methodologies for planned change.[1] In the 1980s, futurists Toffler and Naisbitt described the new information age. The concept of change as a driving force is now widely accepted, especially in the area of information technology.

Unlike long range planning, which plans for tomorrow by extrapolating the trends of today, strategic planning recognizes the unpredictable nature of change. Although models for strategic planning differ, the basic principles remain constant. Strategic planning is an ongoing process, practiced to maximize the opportunities and to minimize the negative impacts of unexpected events.

Strategic planning has received special attention in the information technology area. The rapid development of both computing and communications technologies has made long range planning difficult, perhaps impossible. Applications and capabilities are quickly outdated, and linear planning becomes ineffectual. An iterative process with multiple options becomes imperative, although some important decisions remain that are not strategic in nature.

Strategic planning is closely linked to other trends evident in the 1980s, notably the information resources management (IRM) approach and the chief information officer (CIO) position.[2] Originating in the business sector, these trends stress the importance of information as a valuable resource in an increasingly competitive and unpredictable environment. They also emphasize the need to assign information policy level importance.

All three trends can be observed in both profit and non-profit enterprises. The financial services and airline industries have been transformed by computing and communications technologies. Other sectors, including healthcare and higher education, invested heavily in information technology in the 1980s and now expect (even demand) a return on their investment.

Models and Methods

Given differences in organizational cultures and leadership styles, would-be planners should choose from available models and adapt the process selected to fit their institution. The very first step, however, is to analyze why the institution is entering upon a formal planning process and to evaluate its history, focusing on organizational style and decision making patterns. It is prudent to evaluate past planning efforts, identifying biases against planning as well as supporters and detractors. Most important, "The resulting insights should be reflected in the charge to plan *and the model itself* [italics added for emphasis]."[3]

Strategic planning is not an easy process, as its practitioners acknowledge. According to Penrod, its success is dependent upon a number of factors. Organizationally, there must be top-level support from the board and the chief executive officer and a strong sense of participatory ownership among those involved in the planning process. There must be a formalized process which has identifiable outcomes and is characterized by comprehensiveness and accountability. Finally, there must be incorporation of the resulting plan into policies, procedures, and operating decisions, including budgetary and resource allocations.[4]

Drawing upon Shirley's work in higher education and Bryson's with public nonprofit organizations, Penrod developed a planning model for healthcare and applied it in an academic health center.[5] The steps of the model are listed below. For more detail consult James I. Penrod, "Methods and Models for Planning Strategically," in Healthcare Information Management Systems: A Practical Guide, eds. Ball, Douglas, O'Desky, and Albright, New York: Springer-Verlag 1991.

The Penrod Model for Strategic Planning

Step 1: Establish planning parameters
- Purpose, steps, reports, roles/teams, resources, requirements

Step 2: Assess the environment
- External: forces presenting opportunities, threats, and constraints
- Internal: organizational strengths and weaknesses

Step 3: Determine values
- Primary stakeholders or constituencies

Step 4: Specify areas for strategic decisions
- Organizational mission and purpose
- Clientele to be served

- Goals and outcomes
- Service mix
- Geographic service area
- Comparative advantage

Step 5: Form functional strategies
- Pose questions
- Group strategic issues by area
- Formulate strategies
- Establish timelines and operational pararneters
- Link to broad based, multi-year budget

Step 6: Develop action plans
- Relate to functional parameters (such as finances and facilities)
- Purpose, steps, reports, roles/teams, resources, requirements.

The first four steps lay the groundwork for the plan; the input they provide is essential to the successful formulation of functional strategies and action plans. The last two steps build the bridge between strategic planning and implementation. Measurable elements identified within those steps thus provide a basis for evaluating the planning process and documenting accountability. In health care and in higher education, a host of issues make accountability critically important. Fiscal constraints, malpractice considerations, and outcome studies all require measures of input and output and the ability to study the relationships between/among them.

Planning for Change in Healthcare

Within healthcare, the National Library of Medicine (NLM) has advanced the strategic planning concept through its own work as an agent of change. To this end, the NLM established the Integrated Academic Information Management System (IAIMS) program, with grant funding to support institutions initiating, piloting, and implementing strategic plans for information technology. In 1986, the NLM developed its own plan for the Twenty-First Century, and more recently, in 1989, convened a national outreach panel. Plan and panel alike advocate using technology to make information available to healthcare professionals where, when, and how they need it.

The Association of American Medical Colleges (AAMC) supported these NLM initiatives, conducting key studies assessing the changing information environment. In the 1980s, in the report on the general professional education of the physician (GPEP), the AAMC acknowledged the importance of independent learning skills in dealing with the knowledge explosion. A subsequent group sponsored by the AAMC concluded that "medical informatics is basic to the understanding and practice of modern medicine," and recommended actions by academic health centers, the National Library of Medicine, and professional societies and scientific journals. Medical informatics programs of varying degrees of formality can be found, from basic literacy requirements to MD/PhD degree granting programs. The NLM continues to support medical informatics training sites at a number of schools.

If, as theorists suggest, strategic planning is most effective in areas experiencing some (not excessive) stress, informatics technology in healthcare is primed for such an approach. Certainly, all of healthcare faces hard decisions as to how to deliver quality care and contain costs. As cost-justifying information technology increases in rigor, strategic planning will be critical in assessing environmental factors in healthcare and in proposing technological alternatives.

Stress clearly exists within the healthcare professions as well. Nursing, for example, faces personnel shortages and declining enrollments. Issues of career ladders and professional practice in nursing thus assume a vital importance to healthcare. Nursing informatics is evolving to address these issues and to offer new roles for nursing. Since 1988, the University of Maryland has offered a master's degree program in nursing informatics; the University of Utah was the second to do so. This new field has received support of a small group of dedicated nurses, who have worked within their professional organizations on behalf of informatics. Nursing has for some time enjoyed working group status within the International Medical Informatics Association (IMIA); in 1991,the working group sponsored its fourth international conference in 12 years.

In 1990, the American Association of Colleges of Pharmacy invited Dr. Marion J. Ball, now President Elect of the International Medical Informatics Association, to speak on informatics development. The widespread use of drug databases and of automated pharmacy systems may well prepare this profession for more formalized informatics program development. Should they wish for a model for futher efforts, they might well look to dentistry and its efforts these past two years, launched at the Aspen conference.

Strategic Planning in Dentistry

Among the health professions dentistry is neither in the vanguard nor the rearguard in the field of informatics and application of information technologies. In point of fact there have been important advances in this field by individual dentists and selected organizations in dentistry. Like the other health professions, however, dentistry has been slow to develop a broad and coordinated strategic plan for the profession as a whole to take full advantage of information science and technology.

Individual members of the profession, primarily in dental education, have used computer aided instruction (CAI) for many years. More recently they have developed methods for applying computer-aided design and manufacturing (CAD/CAM) to clinical restorative dentistry. Case simulations for dental student instruction are now in use in several schools, and clinical decision support systems utilizing artificial intelligence, expert systems and neural network technologies are under development. A large number of dental practitioners use computers for practice management. In the dental practice sector, the American Dental Association has estimated that by the year 2000 better than three quarters of U.S. dentists will have personal computers in their offices.

Among national dental organizations, the American Association of Dental Schools is the only one which has formulated a strategic plan for dental informatics utilization in the nation's schools of dentistry. In August 1989, representatives of the major dental organizations in the U.S. and the Federal dental services attended a conference at the Aspen Conference Center at Wye Island, Maryland, designed to explore the current status of dental informatics in the practice, education and research sectors of the profession.[6] An important outcome of this conference (which was supported by the Westinghouse Corporation and the University of Maryland at Baltimore) was the identification of significant strategic issues surrounding dental informatics as an emerging discipline. Another of its significant outcomes was a call for the organizations and agencies represented to come together to develop a strategic plan for the entire profession of dentistry.

In recognition of the early momentum of dental informatics in Europe and Asia as well as the United States, the International Medical Informatics Association (IMIA) approved the formation of a dental working group. Likewise, the American Medical Informatics Association (AMIA) recognized the activity of dental informaticians in the United States through the establishment of a Professional Specialty Group. Perhaps this latter group will take the lead and accept the challenge developed at the Aspen Conference to convene a consortium of national dental organizations for strategic planning.

As has been pointed out elsewhere in this book, at this early stage of evolution and development of dental informatics, work in the field is strong and relevant but it is fragmented and lacks coordination and integration of effort. Dentistry simply has not developed a broad vision for dental informatics; at the same time, the opportunity for the profession to become the leader among health providers in this endeavor is present. Dentistry has circumscribed limits, both biologically and professionally, that make it less encumbered than some other health areas with broader perspectives and more extensive patient care responsibilities. This advantage for dentistry does not necessarily simplify the problem, but it can make the process of planning more manageable.

The ultimate goal of informatics can and should be improving the quality of dental health care. Early work and experiences in the field confirm the feasibility of this premise; it now remains for the leadership in dental practice, education and research to forge a program designed to achieve this goal.

References

1. Bennis WG, Benne KD, Chin R. The planning of change (second edition). New York: Holt, Rinehart and Winston, Inc., 1961,1969.
2. Penrod JI, Dolence MG, Douglas JV. The chief information officer in higher education. In: CAUSE, Professional Paper Series #4. USA: CAUSE, 1990: p. 1-41.

3. Penrod JI. Methods and models for planning strategically. In: Ball MJ, Douglas JV, O'Desky RI, et al, eds. Healthcare information management systems: a practical guide. New York: Springer-Verlag, 1991: p. 180.
4. Ibid. p. 181.
5. Ibid. p. 181-185.
6. Salley JJ, Zimmerman JL, Ball MJ, eds. Lecture notes in medical informatics. Heidelberg: Springer-Verlag, 1990.

19
Informatics, Professional Societies, and Interpersonal Networking

John L. Zimmerman, Marion J. Ball, and Judith V. Douglas

There is a great deal to learn about informatics from other health care professionals as well as computer and information specialists. Often more can be learned from a few minutes casually conversing with peers and colleagues than from several hours of reading journals and books. Professional societies offer both structured meetings and presentations and informal discussions. Often these societies provide opportunities to learn about exciting new techniques and research from other disciplines that have not been applied to dentistry. To gain knowledge of information technology and informatics, dental professionals should seek membership in three types of organizations.

- Affiliation with multidisciplinary associations whose focus is health care computing. Membership in this type of organization allows dentists to maintain and expand their expertise in the use of information technology

- Continuing affiliations with dental professional organizations for the dual purpose of providing leadership and sharing ideas and information within the dental community. Some of the established dental organizations hold great promise as developers of informatics-based activities, but need to mature and develop leaders in this field

- Membership in vendor-sponsored user groups.[1]

Included in this chapter are descriptions and addresses for professional organizations that play either a major or supporting role in the field of informatics. Some of these organizations are specific to dentistry while others, with a significant influence on the field, may not be exclusively targeted to a dental audience. Dentists stand to gain a great deal from attending meetings with other health care professionals. The cross-fertilization of ideas can be very exciting and give insight across disciplinary boundaries. Professionals can learn from one another's experiences and by evaluating their similarities and differences. Synergism would be lost in the field of informatics if each profession chooses to establish its own professional organizations and not to interact with other health care fields.

Multidisciplinary Informatics Professional Associations

The largest and most widely known health informatics organization in the United States is the American Medical Informatics Association (AMIA). In existence since 1990, AMIA was incorporated in the District of Columbia in 1988 to bring together two other professional associations solely devoted to medical informatics. These were the American Association for Medical Systems and Informatics (AAMSI) and the American College of Medical Informatics (ACMI). The College continues to function within AMIA, with an annual election of leading informaticians to membership. Today AMIA is a multidisciplinary membership organization with representation from the various health professions as well as the information sciences, computer sciences, informatics, health administration, government, and industry. It is now responsible for the major annual meeting in the field, the Symposium on Computer Applications in Medical Care (SCAMC). The AMIA bylaws state its organizational purposes are to advance the public interest through charitable, scientific, literary, and educational activities, as well as to promote the development and application of medical informatics in the support of patient care, teaching, research, and health care administration. The activities of AMIA include:

- Serving as an authoritative body in the field of medical informatics, and providing representation with respect to such matters in international forums
- Fostering liaisons between disciplines involved in health care, computers, information, communications, systems sciences, engineering and technology
- Promoting training and development of professional and allied health manpower necessary to support medical informatics
- Planning and conducting scientific, technical, and educational meetings and programs
- Publishing and distributing educational materials through various media
- Coordinating medical informatics activities with other national and international organizations to better advance the public interest
- Carrying on such other activities necessary, suitable, and proper for the fulfillment of AMIA's charitable, scientific, literary, and educational purposes.

AMIA also sponsors a spring congress. In the spring of 1990 the dental members of AMIA formed a Professional Specialty Group (PSG) within AMIA. PSG 4 Dental Informatics provides a forum for AMIA members to increase their professional knowledge and to interact with others in the field of dental informatics. The emphasis is on the use of dental information systems, computer technology, and telecommunications to improve patient care, research, and education.

Membership in AMIA provides a means of staying abreast of the rapid changes in health systems and informatics, and is open to anyone with an interest in the field. Student membership is available at a reduced cost in accordance with

AMIA's commitment to support and encourage those planning to enter the discipline.

American Medical Informatics Association
Suite 700
1101 Connecticut Ave, NW
Washington, DC 20036

AMIA is the designated organization for the United States and joins with other health informatics organizations from other nations to make up the membership of the International Medical Informatics Association (IMIA). The IMIA information brochure (1982/83) defines itself as

> an international and world representative federation of national societies of health informatics and affiliated organizations. It does not have individual members. Although there may be several delegates from each country as observers, each country has only one designated representative with one vote.

IMIA states its primary function as education and dissemination of health information processing, that is, informatics. One method of achieving this goal is the sponsorship of a World Congress on Medical Informatics, known as MEDINFO, every three years at different locations around the world. MEDINFO 92 will be held in Geneva, Switzerland; the location of the 1995 Congress will be announced at that time. The MEDINFO Congresses promote all aspects of medical and health care computing from all countries of the world. They encourage the participation of health information scientists, medical computing specialists, public health and hospital administrators, dentists, physicians, nurses, and other allied health professionals, as well as consultants from various health fields. Topics for these meetings include imaging, general practice and ambulatory care systems, drug information systems, administrative and financial systems, impact of new technologies, modelling and simulation, education and training, privacy, confidentiality, and security, epidemiology and statistics, clinical decision support systems, and many other topics too numerous to include here.

In addition to these large and broadly scoped triennial congresses, IMIA sponsors working groups on special topics such as informatics education, dentistry, nursing, and confidentiality, security and privacy. These working groups hold conferences, approximately 20 in the past ten years, on such wide ranging topics as hospital information systems, data security, and nursing. In April 1989, IMIA extended formal approval of Working Group 11, Dental Informatics, in response to a petition from several individual dentists and dental educators located in the United States. The objectives of Working Group 11 are to:

- Identify and define the elements which constitute the field of dental informatics and how they can impact on dental practice, education, and research
- Identify individuals who are leaders in research, development and application of dental informatics in all sectors of dentistry
- Promote the utilization of information technologies in all sectors of the dental profession

- Identify areas in dental informatics where joint ventures can develop between individuals, other health professionals, organizations, institutions, and nations to expand the field
- Identify specific areas of research and development to expand the knowledge base of dental informatics
- Promote training programs to increase the number of dental informaticians
- Plan and sponsor meetings, conferences, and symposia to focus on research, development, and applications of dental informatics
- Maintain liaison with appropriate national organizations with an interest in medical informatics generally and dental informatics specifically.

The Working Group consists of 20 to 25 members with a wide geographical representation. IMIA's goal is to promote needed cross communication, information sharing, and collaboration among dental informaticians with a long range outcome of improved oral health care.

Dental Professional Associations and Their Interaction with Informatics

American Association of Dental Schools (AADS)

In March 1988 at the AADS Annual Meeting in Montreal, Canada, several individuals met to discuss the feasibility of an international organization with dental informatics as its focus. The AADS Board later created a Committee on Information Technology. The AADS and the University of Maryland at Baltimore, with funding support from Westinghouse Electronic Corporation, sponsored a 1989 leadership conference on dental informatics. The proceedings, Dental Informatics: Strategic Issues for the Dental Profession, describe the recommendations for development and application of informatics in dental education, research, and practice, which were endorsed by the conference participants. AADS is also actively involved with the American Medical Informatics Association; as a leader in dental informatics, AADS has been instrumental in bringing together other dental organizations to discuss the role of informatics in the dental profession.

The feasibility of establishing several informatics-related consortia is being explored by the AADS Committee on Information Technology. The consortium possibilities include patient simulations on dental diagnosis and treatment, interactive videodiscs on dental anatomy for dental and dental hygiene students, curriculum consortium on sharing curricular data on scheduling, course outlines, and key content areas, clinical database development, and decision support systems. Further information can be obtained by contacting:

Assistant Executive Director for Educational Affairs
American Association of Dental Schools
1625 Massachusetts Avenue, NW
Washington, DC 20036

American Dental Association

The American Dental Association has historically maintained a cautious and remote interest in the informatics project, but recently that has changed. Several of the Councils have ongoing projects in informatics topics, such as computerized office systems, information retrieval, electronic claims submission, and data base standards. They established a Department of Information Science in 1990 to oversee and coordinate informatics initiatives within the association as well as for the membership. For further information on ADA activities contact:

Dr. Anthony Kiser
Director, Information Science American Dental Association
611 East Chicago Ave.
Chicago, IL 60611.

Vendor-Sponsored User Groups

DECUS - Digital Equipment Corporation Users Society

DECUS is an independent professional computer society operated by approximately 600 volunteers. The mission of DECUS is to promote the exchange of information processing-related information among users of Digital Equipment Corporation's computing products. The exchange of information takes the form of user-to-user, user-to-Digital, and Digital-to-user. The members of this organization come from industry, government, research laboratories, and universities. Membership is free, and a variety of services includes conferences, software library, newsletters, and electronic conferencing.

Digital Equipment Computer Society
219 Boston Post Road (BP02)
Marlboro, MA 01752-4605

SHARE

SHARE is a nonprofit organization similar to DECUS, but its membership is comprised of users of larger IBM systems. SHARE has over 1,200 members and is the oldest organized user group in this field. The mission of SHARE is to foster support and communication among its members as well as between users and IBM. SHARE sponsors two major meetings each year and smaller interim meetings and seminars throughout the year.

Traditionally SHARE has focused on large, complex (mainframe) IBM systems, but due to the changing computing environment and the importance of distributed computing to the workplace, SHARE has started to address broader issues. SHARE's strategic plan now includes:

- maintaining its status as the IBM user group that provides in-depth, high quality technical information about large scale IBM computing environments

- expanding its scope to include the use of technologies beyond those that qualify an establishment for membership in SHARE
- providing a forum to address the interconnection of IBM equipment in a multivendor computing environment

being the most effective user group in these areas.

SHARE, Inc.
One Illinois Center
111 E. Wacker Drive
Chicago, IL 60601 312/822-0932

SAS Users Group International - SUGI

The SUGI Executive Board encourages and authorizes the formation of Regional SAS Users Groups. A regional group may be composed of several local, inhouse, or special interest groups whose primary interest is SAS Institute software and services. A very active and representative regional SAS users group is the Northeast SAS Users Group (NESUG). NESUG covers the geographical area of New England, New York, New Jersey, Pennsylvania, Maryland, and Washington, DC. The organization represents the local users and coordinates local activities, liaisons with the SUGI/SAS Institute, and is the centralized information resource for the region. The information maintained by the group includes trainers, consultants, vendors, meeting calendars and sites, speaker directories, and prospective employers/employees. NESUG also organizes regional conferences, provides shareware libraries of statistical programs and utilities, and maintains electronic bulletin boards containing information such as homegrown SAS applications, tips, and tools.

SUGI SAS Institute, Inc.
SAS Campus Drive
Cary, NC 27513

Informatics: An Evolving Field

Increasingly, health care professionals are coming to recognize the promise of informatics. In medicine, informatics training programs supported by the National Library of Medicine continue to attract pre- and post-doctoral students. In nursing, concerted professional networking of the sort advocated here and in *Using Computers in Nursing*[1] has resulted in wide ranging activities. Among its successes are the establishment of two master's degree programs in nursing informatics and the promise of a doctoral program at the University of Maryland.

In dentistry, after holding a ground-breaking conference on dental informatics, a core group has obtained working group status in IMIA. Hopefully, dentistry will build upon these accomplishments and, like nursing, support an ever-growing body of informatics activities through its own professional organizations. Hopefully, like nursing, dentistry will continue to grow in influence and importance within the wider arena of health care informatics. Without a doubt, dental informatics today stands poised to change the profession of dentistry. Its successes there will enrich and empower informatics throughout health care.

References

1. Ball MJ, Hannah K. Using Computers in Nursing. Reston, Virginia: Reston Publishing Company, Inc., 1984: p. 238-248.

Author Index

Subject Index

Contributors

LOUIS M. ABBEY, D.M.D., M.S.
Professor of Oral Pathology, School of Dentistry, Virginia Commonwealth University, Richmond, VA 23298, USA

HOWARD L. BAILIT, D.M.D., PH.D.
Tufts University, University of Michigan, Harvard University, Vice President of Medical Policy and Programs EBD Aetna Life and Casualty, Hartford, CT 06156, USA

MARION J. BALL, ED.D.
Associate Vice Chairman, Information Resources, University of Maryland at Baltimore, Baltimore, MD 21201, USA

JAMES F. CRAIG, ED.D.
Professor, Chairman, Department of Educational and Instructional Resources, and Director, Division of Dental Informatics, Baltimore College of Dental Surgery, Dental School, University of Maryland at Baltimore, Baltimore, MD 21201, USA

JAMES J. CRALL, D.D.S., M.S., S.M.
University of Connecticut Health Center, Pediatric Dentistry, Behavioral Sciences and Community Health, Farmington, CT 06030, USA

MARK DIEHL, B.S., D.D.S., M.A.
Commander, Dental Corps, United States Navy, Corporate Information Management, Medical Function Group, Falls Church, VA 22041, USA

JUDITH V. DOUGLAS
Information Resources, University of Maryland at Baltimore, Baltimore, MD 21201, USA

JOHN E. EISNER, D.D.S., PH.D.
Head, Section on Informatics, Office of Educational Planning, State University of New York at Buffalo, School of Dental Medicine, Buffalo, NY 14214, USA

LYNN A. JOHNSON, M.A.
Project Coordinator, Department of Oral Pathology and Diagnosis, The University of Iowa, College of Dentistry, Iowa City, IA 52242, USA

LESLIE A. JONES
Former Senior Vice President, Dentsply International Inc., York, PA 17404, USA

ANTHONY L. KISER, D.D.S., M.P.H.
Director, Council on Dental Practice, American Dental Association, Chicago, IL 60611, USA

JAMES A. LIPTON, D.D.S., PH.D.
Chief, Office of Planning, Evaluation, and Data Systems, National Institute of Dental Research, NIH, Bethesda, MD 20892, USA

WILLIAM R. MCCUTCHEON, D.D.S., M.P.H.
Associate Dean, Academic and Student Affairs, West Virginia University, School of Dentistry, Morgantown, WV 26506, USA

BRIAN D. MONTEITH, M.CH.D.
Professor and Chairman, Department of Prosthodontics, Medical University of Southern Africa, Medunsa 0204, Republic of South Africa

ERNEST F. MORELAND, ED.D.
Associate Dean Academic and Student Affairs, and Professor, Department of Educational and Instructional Resources, Baltimore College of Dental Surgery, Dental School, University of Maryland at Baltimore, Baltimore, MD 21201, USA

JOHN J. SALLEY, D.D.S., PH.D.
Dean Emeritus, Dental School, University of Maryland, Urbanna, VA 23175, USA

WERNER SCHNEIDER, PH.D, MDHC
Center for Human-Computer Studies, Uppsala University Datacenter, Uppsala S-750-02, Sweden

JANE TERPSTRA, ED.S.
Instructional Designer, Training and Education Programs, Division of Substance Abuse Medicine, Medical College of Virginia, Richmond, VA 23298, USA

INA-VERONIKA WAGNER, DR. MED. DENT.HABIL.
Center for Human-Computer Studies, Uppsala University Datacenter, Uppsala S-750-02, Sweden, and Medical Academy, Dresden, Germany.

JOHN L. ZIMMERMAN, D.D.S.
Director, Academic Computing and Health Informatics, University of Maryland at Baltimore, Baltimore, MD 21201, USA

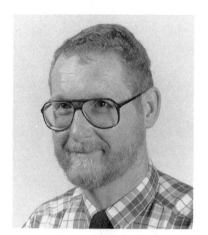

Louis M. Abbey

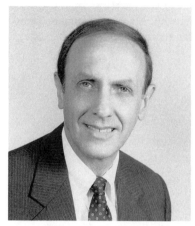

Howard L. Bailit

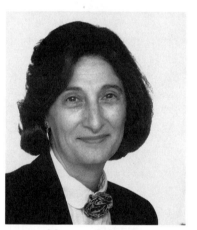

Marion J. Ball

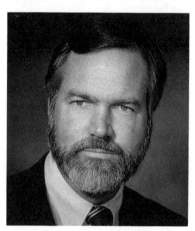

James F. Craig

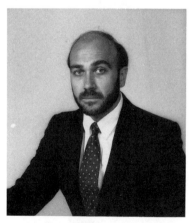

James J. Crall

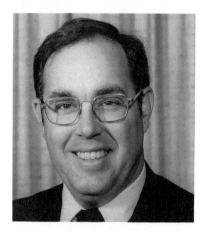

Mark Diehl

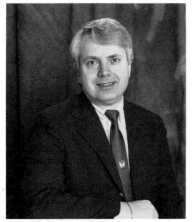

JOHN E. EISNER

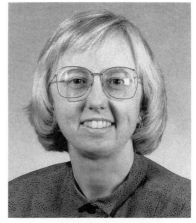

LYNN JOHNSON

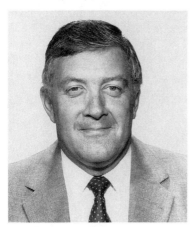

LESLIE A. JONES

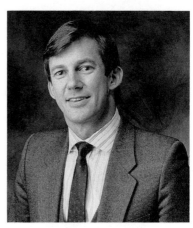

ANTHONY L. KISER

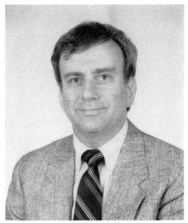

JAMES A. LIPTON

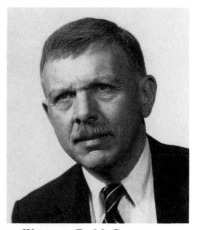

WILLIAM R. McCUTCHEON

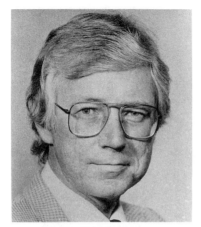

BRIAN D. MONTEITH

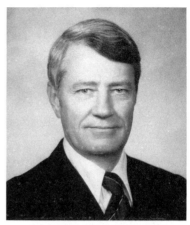

JOHN J. SALLEY

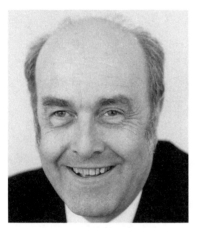

WERNER SCHNEIDER

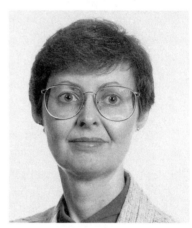

JANE TERPSTRA

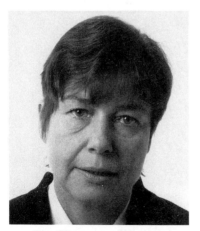

INA-VERONIKA WAGNER

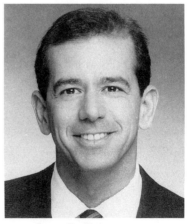

JOHN L. ZIMMERMAN